ACTA UNIVERSITATIS UPSALIENSIS

Studia Latina Upsaliensia

28

Four Eighteenth-century Medical Dissertations under the Presidency of Nils Rosén

Edited and translated, with an introduction and commentary

by

URBAN ÖRNEHOLM

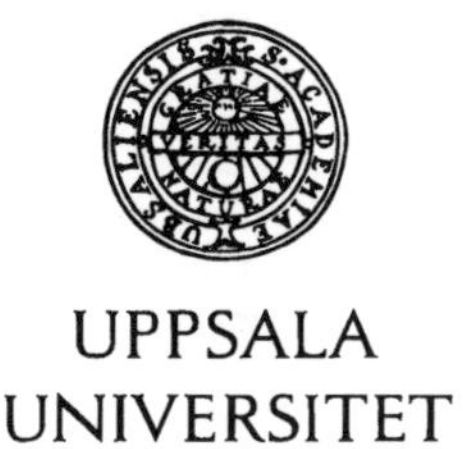

UPPSALA
UNIVERSITET

Thesis for the Degree of Doctor of Philosophy in Latin, Uppsala University, 2003

ABSTRACT

Örneholm, U, 2003: Four Eighteenth-century Medical Dissertations under the Presidency of Nils Rosén. Edited and translated, with an introduction and commentary by Urban Örneholm.
Acta Univ. Ups, *Studia Latina Upsaliensia* 28. 284 pp. Uppsala. ISBN 91-554-5789-4.

Nils Rosén (von Rosenstein) (1706–73), Professor of medicine at Uppsala University, is less known than his colleague Linnaeus, but has, mainly through his textbook *Underrättelser om Barn-Sjukdomar* (1st monograph ed. 1764), had an enormous influence on the care of children throughout Europe.

In this thesis, four Latin dissertations, put forth under the presidency of Nils Rosén, are edited, with translation, commentary, and introduction. These dissertations quite clearly represent the latest medical knowledge of the mid 18th century, and recent theories are propounded, discussed, and examined against practical and empirical knowledge; the texts are thus representative examples of the kind of academic dissertations that communicated and discussed relevant factual matter as opposed to those that just constituted an amount of text, suitable for elaborating on during the disputational ceremony.

In my introduction, I mainly concentrate on medical and pharmacological technical terminology, but more general aspects on scholarly and scientific Neo-Latin are also dealt with. The dissertations edited are *De variolis praecavendis* (1751), *De variolis curandis* (1754), both treating smallpox; *De epilepsia infantili* (1754), on children's epilepsy, and *De morbis infantum* (1752), dealing with the health care of children *in genere*, and interesting as an early Latin version of parts of *Underrättelser*.

Key-words: Neo-Latin, dissertations, terminology, nomenclature, Nils Rosén, history of medicine, smallpox, paediatrics.

Urban Örneholm, Department of Classical Philology, Uppsala University, Box 527, SE-751 20 Uppsala, Sweden.

ISSN 0562-2859
ISBN 91-554-5789-4

Printed in Sweden by Elanders Gotab 2003

Distributor: Uppsala University Library, Box 510, SE-751 20 Uppsala, Sweden

Acknowledgements

To begin with, there are of course a lot of people who indirectly have contributed to this thesis ultimately being written, such as my grandparents, who did nothing to prevent my taking an interest in anything "old" (which meant everything in their attic), and my parents, who on an early stage introduced me to the public library (in Knutby, 43 kilometers east of Uppsala, for those who wonder). As a result of this, the smell of old library-bound books still makes me just as happy as the smell of coffee.

Next in line are all those school teachers who managed to make their various subjects interesting; in my early teens, thus, I developed a certain taste for chemistry and biology, which eventually has come out handy.

As for languages, however, I did not realise that such stuff could be fun until high school, and even then, being thoroughbred working-class, I never got the idea that university studies could be a decent occupation.

Consequently, I started working, first as a mental warden and later as a nurse; these professions have of course contributed to the choice of subject for this thesis, but have also improved my self-discipline.

During my seventeen-year career at the hospital, the need for some kind of a hobby ultimately made me settle for Latin, which turned out to be even more fun than I had imagined.

As we are now closing in on those who have been more directly important, I wish to thank the following persons: Jörgen Secher, Ph.Lic, who was my first teacher of Latin, and who also first suggested that I give the A-level Latin course a try; Professor Monica Hedlund, who took care of most of the A- and B-level teaching, (as well as, at times, of most things being done at all in the department); Professor Sten Eklund, who is guilty of having admitted me in the first place, and who has always been willing – and able – to answer even stupid questions, and to discuss not only Latin matters but almost anything.

Among other members of the Latin seminar in Uppsala – to which, in its entirety, I am grateful for valuable suggestions on several matters – I want to mention in particular Krister Östlund, Ph.D, Georg Stenborg, Ph.Lic, and Peter Sjökvist, Ph.Lic. candidate.

My tutor, Professor Hans Helander, deserves a paragraph for himself; his encouragement and enthusiasm have of course been essential, as has his profound erudition, which he has always willingly communicated; one easily gets the impression that the man has read every existing book of any importance.

I also wish to thank Professor Lars Thorén and Stig Ekström, Dr. Pharm, of the Museum of Medical History, Uppsala, as well as Docent Irène Sjögren, for their interest and their valuable suggestions; my own language (except for this very page) has been corrected by Donald MacQueen, B.A, of the Department of English.

Last but not least: essential for my entire existence are my wife Ingela Ekrelius and my sons Frans and Filip Örneholm.

Uppsala, October 2003

Urban Örneholm

Contents

Introduction

Medical theory

The iatromechanistic or iatrophysical[1] school of medicine, with which Nils Rosén generally is associated, is one of three main systems prevalent in 18th-century medicine, the other two being the iatrochemical and the vitalistic system.

The idea of the human body as a machine, which constitutes the basis for iatromechanistic medicine, is generally seen as having its origin in René Descartes' posthumously published *De Homine* (1662), considered by some the world's first work on physiology. Descartes regards the body as a machine, dependent on directions by the soul, which he locates in the pineal gland;[2] the most extreme mechanistic position, however, was probably that of Julien Offray de la Mettrie (1709–51), who had studied under Herman Boerhaave, and who in 1748 published *L'Homme Machine*, which eventually got him exiled to Frederick the Great of Prussia.

One of the representatives of the iatromechanical school that were most admired by Rosén was Friedrich Hoffmann (1660–1742), probably the most prominent and influential proponent of the iatromechanistical theories, who himself described his theories as derived *ex solidis physico-mechanicis et anatomicis principiis*.[3] Hoffmann emphasized the need for a theoretical background, as opposed to pure empiricism, even if he, as is pointed out by I.W. Müller,[4] regarded medical practice from a rather eclectic point of view; he thus considered Hippocrates a valuable predecessor, in spite of the empirical methods used by the latter; partly, Hippocrates could be excused, since no theories could have existed at the beginning of medicine. To some extent, Hippocrates had in fact tried to form a system: inasmuch as he had carefully observed the symptoms in his patients, he had formulated general rules from his observations, and he had stressed the importance of studies in anatomy and "natural history", all of which, according to Hoffmann's view, would ultimately lead to a system, much like his own; in fact, Hippocrates could be called the first iatromechanic.[5]

As for Hoffmann's view upon more contemporary theories, he despises the iatrochemical school and its founder Paracelsus (1493–1541), basically, as it seems, on the ground that Hoffmann regards Paracelsus as too quickly dubbing a remedy "specific" to a certain illness, without a sufficient number of case studies, which puts paracelsism too close to pure empiricism; on the other hand, chemistry as a natural science – regarded as a branch of physics – would provide explanations of certain processes in the human body, such as digestion.[6]

According to Hoffmann, however, the foremost of the modern sciences was anatomy; not only did the findings as regards the joints of the skeleton, the respiratory apparatus, etc, seem to support the mechanistic view, but the early microscopical

---

[1] These two terms are often used synonymously in the literature; as is pointed out by I.W. Müller, *Iatromechanische Theorie und ärztliche Praxis*, 1991, p 21, note 22, Hoffmann did not himself use the concept of 'physics' in a consistent way, and as mechanics furthermore is a part of physics, I will not try to make any distinction in this context.

[2] It should be noted, however, that related ideas about the bodily functions had been put forth already by Erasistratos (fl. c. 250 BC), who regarded such things as digestion and breathing as automatic processes; cf. *Der Neue Pauly* 4, 41sq, s.v. *Erasistratos*.

[3] From the full title of Hoffmann's *Medicina rationalis systematica*, 2nd ed, 1729.

[4] Müller, p 18sq.

[5] Ibid, p 25sq.

[6] Ibid, pp 21-24.

explorations had also shown fibres and blood vessels, rendering mechanical actions possible, to be present throughout the human body.[7]

Nevertheless, as mentioned above, in his medical practice Hoffmann took a more eclectic position; he disapproved of Galen, but regarded the idea of the *res non naturales*[8] as commendable; certain remedies recommended by Paracelsus were useful; gymnastics and riding, as recommended by Mercurialis[9] and Sydenham[10] respectively, were also regarded as healthful, etc.

Of even greater importance to the work of Nils Rosén, however, was Herman Boerhaave (1668–1738), professor of medicine, chemistry and botany at Leiden, and probably the most famous of all 18th-century physicians.

Boerhaave, like Rosén, incidentally, was the son of a clergyman, and started his studies with theology, mathematics and philosophy, then became interested in medicine, in which field he studied the authors from classical to modern time; he recieved his doctorate in Harderwijk in 1693 and was to spend ca. thirty years teaching medicine in Leiden.

The major feature of Boerhaave's system is probably his managing to form a synthesis of several prevailing medical theories of his time; his interest and skill in mathematics did put him close to iatromechanics, however, inasmuch as he believed that every problem of the human machine could be solved by physical and mathematical methods; even if he was fully aware of science's incomplete knowledge of nature, he rejected speculation; the physician should base his actions only on facts known from science.[11]

As regards the reasons for bad health, Boerhaave believed small particles to constitute the bodily fibres and fluids; when fluids became corrupt, "sharp" or "bitter" particles, *acria*, of different kinds could cause different states of disease: so knife-sharp particles would cause boils, for instance, while agglomerating particles would cause swellings.[12]

The bodily fluids would not, however, become corrupt by themselves, but from an external cause, such as an improper diet; this standpoint also underlines the usefulness of chemistry to the physician.

Another major feature of Boerhaave's system was the necessity of taking into consideration each individual patient's constitution and life situation; in principle he believed – as opposed to the representants of the vitalistic school, most notably Georg Ernst Stahl (1660–1734), professor of medicin in Halle – that a physician should not deal with the human soul at all. But despite his fundamentally mechanistic standpoint, he also carefully observed the mental state of his patients.

As regards Nils Rosén, even before his European journey he had studied the works of the iatromechanics, as will be seen from the dissertation *De usu methodi*

---

[7] Ibid, pp 24sq.

[8] These – air, food/drink, motion/rest, sleep/wake, excretions/retentions and emotions – are things essential to man, which do not depend on the nature of the human being – hence *non naturales* – but which can contribute to health or sickness according to how they are handled; cf. Martin 19.1; cf. also Zedler: *Universal-Lexicon*, s.v. *Ding*.

[9] Geronimo Mercuriale (1530–1606), Italian physician, most known for edd. of Hippocrates and Galen.

[10] Thomas Sydenham (1624–89), English physician, who above all stressed the need for the observation of symptoms, which e.g. led to the definition of scarlet fever.

[11] Anna-Lena Pehrsson, *Nils Rosén von Rosenstein and iatromechanics*, in *Nils Rosén von Rosenstein and his Textbook on Paediatrics*, 1964, p 77.

[12] Ibid.

mechanicae in medicina, 1728; as is pointed out by Anna-Lena Pehrsson,[13] even the title is almost identical to that of an address given by Boerhaave at Leiden in 1703: *De usu ratiocinii mechanici in medicina*.

When Rosén in 1730 put forth his doctoral dissertation at the University of Harderwijk, the subject was however of an apparently more Sydenhamian or Hippocratic kind:[14] *De historiis morborum rite consignandis*, but since even Sydenham would fit in into Boerhaave's theories, this does not at all contradict the labelling of Rosén as a iatromechanic.

Upon examining the four dissertations treated in this thesis, one does also find several instances where the reasoning is clearly influenced by iatromechanical theories, e.g. in Martin 13–14, where the Boerhaavian theories of the corruption of bodily fluids is the obvious theoretical background: *patet ... insignem [antimonii] esse ... utilitatem ... in vitiis lymphae emendandis* (13.2); likewise, the discussion of *mercurius dulcis* in 14.2 clearly hints at the conception of a purely mechanical effect in remedies: *tantum mercurii vivi additur, ut ejus globuli cum spiculis mercurii sublimati ... uniti, illa obtundant, quo mitius evadit mercuriale medicamentum*. In Martin 18.1, the arguments are also of a iatromechanical nature, inasmuch as the remedies discussed are thought to mechanically cleanse the blood vessels.

In Bergius, we might regard the views propounded in e.g. 5.29 as based on iatromechanical theory; the passage *Si tumorem faciei retrocedentem manuum & pedum non sequatur, nec copiosus compenset ptyalismus, pessimum jure censetur* seems to imply a direct communication between all fluids of the body, necessitating a decrease in one place to be compensated for by an increase elsewhere; other examples of iatromechanical influence in Bergius are the notes on diet in 7.6, where meat and eggs are ruled out as making the bodily fluids acrid, and the discussion of phlebotomy in 8.5, where the point is the reduction of the mechanical impact on the body by the red blood corpuscules.

In Sundius, corruption of bodily fluids is also mentioned; in 1.1 the acrid residue of meconium is said to bring about epileptic fits; in 2.1, one reason accounted for is *lactis vitium*; Schröder does not contain any theoretical discussion at all, which probably is due to that particular text's not being a dissertation *pro gradu*.

---

[13] Ibid, p 81sqq.
[14] Ibid, pp 87-89.

Biographical notes

Nils Rosén

The available biographical facts about Nils Rosén are rather incomplete.[15] Unlike his colleague Linnaeus, Rosén, as far as we know, never made any autobiographical notes, and what we have is the meagre and somewhat uncertain information that can be obtained from memorial speeches, letters etc.

Nils Rosén was born in 1706 and grew up in Sexdrega, not far from Gothenburg, where his father, Erik Rosenius, was a parson from 1709. Out of his eight brothers and sisters one brother, Eberhard, born 1714, from 1770 Rosenblad, was also later to become a professor of medicine; one, Sven,[16] a pietistic preacher, and two, Gabriel and Johan, doctors of theology. Even less is known about Roséns childhood than about his private life as an adult. Franzén mentions Rosén's interest, as a child, in playing with his own home-made toy pharmacy,[17] but also gives an account of how Rosén at the age of four contracted the plague and, after having been apparently dead for a day, woke up during the shrouding; an experience, which Franzén assumes was essential in directing Rosén's interest towards the medical profession. In 1723 Rosén began his studies at the University of Lund, under the assumption that he was to become a clergyman. As a member of *Natio Gothoburgensis* Rosén was advised by Andreas Rydelius, the famous professor of philosophy, who was also *inspector Nationis Gothoburgensis*, to concentrate on medicine, since it was obvious that this was more in line with his own wish. Rosén thus studied medicine under Kilian Stobaeus, who was acting professor of medicine in 1722–24 during the sick leave of professor von Döbeln; as far as we know, he also studied philosophy, mathematics, French, and German,[18] and seems to have improved his skill in the classical languages.[19] In 1725 he moved to Stockholm, where he made a living as a private tutor, and as a translator of German and French literature, while continuing his medical studies on his own, associating with, among others, Casten Rönnow, later physician-in-ordinary to the king of Poland. In 1727 Rosén, according to Lindroth,[20] studied mathematics under Anders Celsius in Uppsala, where the *adjunctus* of Medicine Petrus Martin had just died.

---

[15] For general surveys, see e.g S. Lindroth, *Svensk Lärdomshistoria; Frihetstiden*, 1975, esp. pp 472–480; T. Frängsmyr, *Svensk idéhistoria*, I, p 276sqq. All available information has been collected in *Svenskt Biografiskt Lexikon*, 30, pp 425–433, in an article by Eva Nyström.

[16] Sven Rosén is the subject of a doctoral thesis by Emanuel Linderholm: *Sven Rosén och hans insats i frihetstidens radikala pietism*, Upsala 1911.

[17] F. M. Franzén, *Minne af Archiatern och Medicinae Professoren i Upsala Nils Rosén von Rosenstein* in *Svenska Akademins handlingar*, 1814.

[18] David von Schulzenheim, *Åminnelse-Tal öfver Kongl. VetenskapsAcademiens framledne ledamot, Välborne Herren, Herr Nils Rosén von Rosenstein*, 1773.

[19] J. Floderus, *Parentalia Viro, dum in vivis erat, Generoso ac Nobilissimo Domino Nicolao Rosén à Rosenstein S.R.M:tis Archiatro et Eqviti de Stella Polari membr. reg. acad. scient. Stockh. et reg. societ. sc. Ups. oratione funebri facta*, 1775, p 14sq.

[20] Annerstedt, who also mentions these mathematical studies, quotes a letter from A. Celsius to E. Benzelius, where Celsius states that Rosén *förstår arithmetiquen och geometrien så grundeligen som någon mathematicus* ("understands arithmetic and geometry as thoroughly as any mathematician") while all other sources have it that Rosén was searched out in Stockholm after Rudbeck's having failed to locate any appropriate candidates in Uppsala.

Martin had been fulfilling the duties properly resting upon professor Olof Rudbeck, the Younger, and as Rudbeck was searching for a new *adjunctus*, he was recommended by Rönnow to ask Rosén, who was appointed on the condition that he put forth a dissertation,[21] and subsequently set out on a European journey to complete his education with a doctor's degree.[22] Rosén, travelling as the private tutor of a young nobleman, Mauritz Posse, spent two and a half years abroad, visiting Germany, France, Switzerland, Italy, Belgium and Holland. He stayed a couple of months in Halle, where he studied philosophy, almost one year in Geneva, where he took up a lasting correspondence – and friendship – with Albrecht von Haller;[23] he also studied for Friedrich Hoffmann at Halle, and probably got in touch with the prominent anatomist Jakob B. Winslow in Paris as well as with Herman Boerhaave at Leiden, where he otherwise seems to have been concentrating mainly on physics. During this time, he also put forth the dissertation *De historiis morborum rite consignandis*, whereby he achieved the degree of MD at the University of Harderwijk in 1730.[24]

Having returned to Uppsala, Rosén, still as a substitute for professor Rudbeck, had to take care of almost all medical education[25] at the university while being at the same time, according to Lindroth, almost the only practising physician in Uppsala. In

---

[21] *De usu methodi mechanicae in medicina*, 1728, put forth under Rudbeck's colleague, Lars Roberg.

[22] The degree of MD had, according to T. Neveus, *En akademisk festsed och dess utveckling*, pp 24, 27, been granted only once in Sweden before 1738, namely in 1681, when the degree was conferred upon one J. Rothman.

At least one more medical dissertation *pro gradu* from the 17th century does exist, viz. *De passione hypochondriaca*, defended by M. Detterberg under Rudbeck the Younger in 1697, but, according to Annerstedt, 2:2, p 151, the doctoral degree was apparently never conferred upon Detterberg.

During the following forty years, Swedish physicians generally took the degree abroad, even if there was nothing but tradition – and, perhaps, a lack of competent or interested teachers of medicine – to prevent a Swedish conferment.

[23] Albrecht von Haller (1708–77), Swiss anatomist, physiologist and botanist, who had studied and graduated under Boerhaave at Leiden, and subsequently perfected his education in London, Paris and Basel. At this time, Haller had just returned to Switzerland, where he was to stay until 1736, when he accepted a professorship in Göttingen, which he was to hold for seventeen years, during which time he upheld a vast correspondence with several colleagues all over Europe and published important medical works, such as *Primae lineae physiologiae* (1747), which was to be used by Rosén as a basis for his lectures.

From the still extant part of the correspondence, in French and Latin, between Rosén and Haller – thirty letters from Rosén and four from Haller were published by Fredrik Berg in *Nils Rosén von Rosenstein and his Textbook on Paediatrics (supplement 156 of Acta Paediatrica)*, 1964 – it is obvious that Rosén's interests went beyond medical questions: there are frequent comments also upon such things as O. von Dalin's historical works, the political situation, and Triewald's experiments in physics.

[24] At Harderwijk, the entire process from immatriculation to graduation could be completed in very short time (in Rosén's case, he spent two days at the university); the University of Harderwijk thus was a popular place for the perfection of a medical education, and not only Rosén, but several other Swedish physicians, e.g. Linnaeus (1735; he, on the other hand, needed almost three weeks), obtained their degrees at this place.

[25] Among other things, Rosén was also responsible for the lecturing and teaching in botany, which led to a conflict with Linnaeus, who, until the arrival of Rosén, had been in charge of the subject. When Rosén had replaced Rudbeck in 1740, and Linnaeus had been appointed successor to Roberg in the following year, the two professors, however, rearranged their subject, leaving Rosén responsible for anatomy and Linnaeus for botany, which also seems to have settled their conflict.

1732, without having submitted an application, Rosén was nominated for the professorship in physics at the University of Lund, but declined, after having been granted a higher income at Uppsala.

As for Rosén's achievements as *adjunctus*, it is obvious that medical education in Uppsala during this period prospered in comparison with the situation during the later years of the professorships of Roberg and Rudbeck the Younger, but even without such comparison, Rosén's activities are quite impressive; he lectured not only on medicine in a strict sense, but also on physiology, anatomy, pharmacology and botany, while, as is mentioned above, he was virtually the only available practising physician in town; irrespective of the fact that all this would have left him without any measurable amount of spare time, one might regard this combination of clinical and scientific activities as being quite in line with Rosén's general views on the task of the physician.

As regards the more practical side of medical education, Rosén had the old university hospital, *nosocomium academicum*, originally established by Roberg in 1708–09, restored and enlarged; there were still only the original eight beds, but an outpatient department, with opening hours twice a week, was added, where the poor could be examined and treated by the professor and students of medicine and, if they were suffering from any particularly interesting disease, hospitalized. He also restored the tradition of anatomical dissections[26] in the Gustavianum and by 1736 had edited his *Compendium anatomicum* (2nd enlarged ed. in 1738),[27] which was the first really useful anatomy book in Sweden, even if Roberg had put forth his *Lijkrevningstaflor* ('Tables of Anatomy') in 1718.

As is pointed out by Lindroth,[28] Rosén was an excellent teacher, who also, much through the aforementioned correspondance with Haller, kept in touch with the scientific achievements of his time; the number of medical students in Upsala soon began to increase, and since a more regular conferment of the doctoral degree in medicine at the University of Uppsala was established in 1738 – when the degree was conferred upon one P. Hamnerin by Professor Roberg – the prospects of achieving the degree without a trip to Harderwijk also attracted more students; in the mid 18th century, they numbered about fifty, and during his entire career, Rosén was to preside over forty-six disputations.[29]

In 1734 Rosén had married Anna Christina Hermansson – daughter of the *professor Skytteanus* Johan Hermansson – by whom he had three children, of which one daughter, Anna Margareta, would later marry Samuel Aurivillius, who was not only to become Rosén's son-in-law, but also his successor as a professor of medicine.[30] Of his other children one daughter died at the age of four in 1756 from smallpox, which she had contracted from variolation,[31] while her twin brother Nils would later become

---

[26] While corpses for the dissections had originally been available only through the executions of criminals, Rosén subsequently was granted access also to bodies from the hospital, the prison and the asylum, according to a royal letter from 1757.

[27] The *Compendium anatomicum* was written in Swedish, and explicitly intended to be read not only by physicians, but also by barber-surgeons and the general public (2nd ed, p 9sq).

[28] Lindroth, p 476.

[29] Even if the typical dissertation of this period seems to be regarded, by some, as little more than stage prop for the disputation, it was definitely also used to communicate scientific results etc, as will be seen below, in footnote 34.

[30] In 1756, apparently for health reasons, Rosén was allowed to trade positions with Aurivillius, thus becoming university librarian for one year before leaving the university altogether.

[31] According to some sources, among which is a passage in Linnaeus' *Nemesis Divina*, Rosén also lost a foster-daughter in this way; the girl is said by Linnaeus to have been the daughter of the

known as, among other things, secretary to the Swedish Academy and spokesman for the ideas of the Enlightenment.[32]

After leaving his professorship, Rosén devoted his time to his private practice in Stockholm, and, to quite a large extent, to his duties as physician-in-ordinary to the court. In 1762 Rosén, much because of his services to the court, was made a nobleman under the name of *Rosén von Rosenstein*.[33] In 1767 Samuel Aurivillius died, and after the death also of Rosén's daughter Anna Margareta in 1772, Rosén adopted his eight grandchildren, of which one of the boys, Carl, was to become Arch-bishop.

It seems evident that Rosén was always more inclined towards the practical side of medical science than towards any other aspect of the subject: all his major works, the *Compendium anatomicum*, *Underrättelser om Barn-Sjukdomar och deras Bote-Medel* ('Information on the Diseases of Children and their Remedies'), 1764,[34] and *Hus- och Rese-Apotheque* ('House and Travel Pharmacy'), 1765, were written in the vernacular, while he never put forth any traditional scientific work of weight equal to those published by e.g. Linnaeus or von Haller; his impact on popular health could nevertheless hardly be exaggerated.

Nils Rosén von Rosenstein died in 1773. None of his sons ever had any children, and thus the family name only lasted for one more generation; among his students, several were to be prominent men, such as Abraham Bäck, Johan Gottschalk Wallerius and David (Schultz) von Schulzenheim; among those who later became famous are also the *respondentes* of two of the dissertations treated in this thesis, namely Roland Martin and Petrus Jonas Bergius.

Roland Martin[35]

Roland Martin was born in Uppsala in 1726, the son of Rosén's predecessor, Petrus Martin, who died in 1727. After the death also of his mother in 1730, Roland Martin was brought up in the family of Pehr Ström, parson in Nora, in the province of Ångermanland. During the years 1736–40, he attended school in Härnösand, and in 1741–42, he went through the *gymnasium* of the same town.

---

former university librarian Andreas Norrelius. Rosén did nevertheless persist in his firm conviction, that variolation would contribute to a great extent to decrease the death rate among children.

[32] Nils von Rosenstein, as the son would call himself, is the subject of a biography by Torgny Segerstedt, *Nils von Rosenstein – samhällets människa*, Stockholm 1981.

[33] In fact, Rosén tells von Haller about this, and about the conferment of the order of *Stella Borealis* (sic!; instead of *Polaris*) upon him, in a letter dated as early as February, 20th, 1758; the heraldic bearings, a stone or obelisk flanked by two roses, were not issued until 1762, however.

[34] The origin of *Underrättelser* was a series of articles on health care, published in the calendars of the Royal Academy of Sciences from 1753 on, as a means to deal with the high rates of mortality among infants; the Academy subsequently wished to edit these articles as a book, which eventually was to appear in several European languages; the last Swedish edition was published in 1851.

As is indicated in the commentaries to Sundius and Schröder, much of the matter published in *Underrättelser* can also be found in the dissertations treated here; while Sundius might be dependent on the calendar texts – to which references are made in the dissertation – Schröder was published two years before the first calendar article, and this text might thus be regarded as a preliminary work to corresponding parts of *Underrättelser*.

[35] The contents of the notes on all four respondents are to a large extent derived from Sacklén, *Sveriges Läkare-historia ... I-II*, Nyköping, 1822–24.

In 1743(?), Roland Martin took up studies at the University of Uppsala, where he studied medicine under Rosén and Linnaeus.

In 1744, he published a complimentary poem in a dissertation by Nils Gissler; the same year he went back to Härnösand, maybe to practise the medical profession with Gissler as a tutor. During his stay in Härnösand, he acted as *respondens* for at least one dissertation in the *gymnasium* under the presidency of Gissler, who, in addition to his medical profession, lectured on physics.

In 1745, Martin was back in Uppsala, where he put forth, under the direction of Linnaeus, a botanical dissertation, *Plantae Martino-Burserianae explicatae*, whereby he continued a work, originally undertaken by his father, the aim of which was the cataloguing of a plant collection. Shortly afterwards, for economic reasons, he moved to Falun, in the province of Dalarna, where he took up a position, probably as a private tutor. From 1749 he, upon the recommendation of Rosén, became the private tutor of Nils Posse, a young nobleman and student at the university of Upsala, who was a boarder with Rosén, which gave Martin full access to his teacher and the teacher's library.

He then continued his medical education, and in 1751, following the defence of his dissertation *De variolis praecavendis*, the degree of MD was conferred upon him; later in the same year, he was elected a member of the *Collegium Medicum*.

In 1752, Martin married Eleonora Charlotta von Berco, and was appointed district medical officer in the province of Halland, where he was the only physician. Upon the death of his wife in 1753, Martin returned to Stockholm, and decided to leave Sweden to study abroad. After having been promised a professorship in anatomy and surgery upon his return, he left for Paris, where he studied and practised both subjects, and also bought necessary surgical instruments; according to Lindroth, Martin was probably the best educated Swedish physician of his time, as far as anatomy and surgery are concerned. In 1756 Martin took up his lecturing as a professor, which lead to certain conflicts,[36] and in 1759 he was elected a member of the Royal Academy of Sciences, where he published several observations on surgery and anatomy; his most important work, however, was a speech *Om nervers allmänna egenskaper* ('On the general properties of nerves'), which was delivered in 1763; an enlarged Latin edition was published in 1781.

In 1779, Roland Martin asked permission to resign his professorship, and he died on September 10, 1788.

Petrus Jonas Bergius

Bergius was born in 1730 in Eriksstad, in the province of Småland. Six weeks after his birth, he lost his father, and after his mother had also died seven years later, he spent one year together with his brothers and sisters under the supervision of his oldest brother before being sent away to be educated, first by a vicar, then at the school and, subsequently, *gymnasium* of Visingsö.

In 1746 Bergius, advised by his brother Bengt, went to the university of Lund, where he took up his medical studies.[37] After two years of studying languages and philosophy, but also medicine, under the brother of Nils Rosén, professor Eberhard Rosén, Bergius went to Uppsala to continue his education in anatomy and natural history. Having, as it seems, made quite an impression on Linnaeus, he defended a

---

[36] Cf. my commentary to **Martin 19.1**.

[37] Sacklén has it (I, p 725) that Bengt Bergius and the university secretary chose this education on behalf of Bergius, since his stammering made him less suited to practise theology or law.

minor dissertation, *Semina Muscorum detecta*, in 1750, and was sent in 1752 to the province of Gotland to collect plant specimens. In 1754 the degree of MD was conferred upon him after he defended his dissertation *De variolis curandis* under Nils Rosén.

Following his education, Bergius took up a medical practice in Stockholm, where he was elected a member of the Royal Academy of Sciences in 1758; in 1761 he received a professorship in natural history and pharmacy, and during the following years he was elected to several learned societies.[38]

Among the works published by Bergius, one of the most important was *Descriptiones plantarum ex Capite Bonae Spei*, 1767; he also published *Materia medica e regno vegetabili* I-II, 1778, which does not deal strictly with medical herbs, but also treats other useful plants.

Bergius never married, but lived together with his brother Bengt for twenty-eight years. After the death of Bengt Bergius in 1784, and of Petrus Jonas Bergius in 1790, their estate on what was then the northern outskirts of Stockholm was bequeathed to the Royal Academy of Sciences, to be turned into an important school of gardening and an institution for botanical experiments; due to the increasing need for housing areas in Stockholm, the Bergius Botanical Garden was moved in 1885, to the Frescati area, where it is still located, in the immediate vicinity of the University of Stockholm.

Petrus Sundius

Sundius was born in Stockholm, where his father was a chaplain, in 1725. The family later moved to the province of Ångermanland, and Sundius received his elementary education partly through a private tutor, partly in the *gymnasium* of Härnösand. In 1740, he was matriculated at the University of Uppsala, where he studied natural history and medicine, and in 1754, after practising medicine in Stockholm and defending his dissertation *De epilepsia infantili* under Rosén, he had the degree of MD conferred upon him.

In 1755, Sundius went to Norway, to become City Physician of Christiania (i.e. Oslo), and is reported to have died there in 1786.

Johannes Schröder

Very little is known about Schröder; he was born in Gothenburg in 1727, and arrived at the University of Uppsala in 1748, where he defended the dissertation *De morbis infantum* in 1752 under Rosén, and subsequently, after having put forth another dissertation, *Genera morborum*, under Linnaeus, in 1759, graduated as an MD, whereupon he was appointed 2nd City Physician of Gothenburg later this year, only to die in 1764.

---

[38] Sacklén (I, p 726) mentions societies in Montpellier and Vlissingen (1769), Philadelphia (1770), Rotterdam, Switzerland, and Zell (1771), Harlem (1773), Berlin (1775), St. Petersburg and Lund (1776), Uppsala (1777), London, Trondheim, and Göttingen (1778).

Language

Even if Neo-Latin is based upon ancient Latin, judging material of the kind at hand by the grammatical standards for classical Latin as known today would be rather unfair; not only was the notion of "classical Latin" wider than it is today, but rules for certain grammatical features were not to be formulated until the mid 19th century; as has been pointed out by e.g. Benner & Tengström (p 80sqq), and Östlund (pp 38, 41), such phaenomena as e.g. mood in subordinate clauses were little, or not at all, treated in the 17th and 18th century grammatical literature, while the main point seems to have been syntax of cases; other syntactical rules were, by and large, learnt by extensive reading (behold the virtues of long reading lists!) of Latin texts, not only in school, but throughout life; one has to remember that the universities in the 18th century were still basically Latin-speaking: during the period of immediate interest for this thesis, namely 1750–59, no less than ninety-seven percent of all dissertations at the University of Uppsala were written in Latin,[39] as was the major part of all reference literature used.

The author of any Latin dissertation, such as those treated here, would thus use a language, influenced partly by what he had learnt in school, partly by what he had studied at the university (and, indeed, in his spare time); a writer on medicine would be heavily influenced by other medical writers, both earlier and contemporary, and these influences would not be restricted to the use of technical terms, but would also comprise such features as e.g. the current words and expressions for discussing one's subject in a proper way; in a case where no unambiguous information as regards e.g. the correct choice of mood could be gathered from the experience of reading, the texts in question would necessarily have been regarded more as guidelines to how one *could* write than to how one *had to* write. At any rate, the focus of attention was on the advancement of medical science, and hence in such uncertain cases the choice of the correct term would probably be of more importance than the choice of construction.

The usage of language in this period is also rather eclectic as regards general vocabulary; as will be seen in the present material, several words from pre- and post-classical Latin are found, while the aberrations from classical Latin syntax are few; those uncovered do not prove to be of much relevance to the purpose of this thesis, and I will not provide any systematic treatment of syntactical "errors" in the texts; such divergences are mentioned in the running commentary, at most.

With that exception, there still are a few things to be said in this chapter; since my texts are of a kind similar to, and almost contemporary with, the Swedish dissertations edited by Krister Östlund (*Johan Ihre on the Origins and History of the Runes*, 2000), I will discuss these matters mainly in accordance with his corresponding chapter.

One quite fundamental difference between the present texts and those treated by Östlund, however, is that the dissertations discussed by him are dissertations on language, albeit not Latin, and on history, while those presented here deal with medical questions; one might perhaps suspect that a scholar – in the case of Johan Ihre a *professor eloquentiae et politices*[40] – writing on linguistic matters would consider his own usage of language more carefully than one who writes on medicine.

---

[39] Krister Östlund and Urban Örneholm, *Avhandlingsspråk vid Uppsala universitet 1600–1855*, in *Lychnos*, 2000, pp 180–183.

[40] The title pertains to a professorship, which had been created in 1622 by means of a donation from Johan Skytte (1577–1645), upon his being appointed chancellor of the University of

If, thus, the actual language for the medical writer was more of a vehicle for the factual matter which he wanted to discuss or propagate, this, as we shall see, by no means excluded the use of certain rhetorical ornament etc., which will be treated under "Style" below, as will the features that I regard as the most interesting ones of these texts, viz. what one might call *ways of discussing the matter*.[41]

Orthography

These texts quite naturally evince the same typical Neo-Latin ortographic features as does any other text from this period, and since those features have been treated on several occasions and by numerous authors,[42] I will not dwell upon them further here.

Morphology

Latin forms

In this field also, the phaenomena found are mostly those, typical of Neo-Latin;[43] the suffigated forms of *hic, haec, hoc*, viz. *hicce, haecce, hocce*, etc, are e.g. present; in the case of *hisce*, this form is in two of the texts (Schröder and Bergius) even more frequent than *his*.

The usage of *necesse/necessum* differs between the texts, inasmuch as Schröder has only *necessum* while the other three have only *necesse*; since the texts are short, and the occurrences are few altogether, it is quite possible that this is mere coincidence, as the two forms otherwise were considered equally correct,[44] even when used alternately in the same text.

Greek words

As might be expected, there are numerous words of Greek origin to be found in these texts, as there would be in any medical text. A large majority of these are of course medical technical terms, which will be treated separately below; of the very few non-medical Greek words printed in Latin type, only four are declined according to their Greek paradigm, namely *autoptae* (nom. pl.) (Bergius 7.8), *hebdomadas* (acc. pl.)

Uppsala; as is pointed out by Sven Lundström in *Faculty of Arts at Uppsala University*, p 50, this professorship was still a *de facto* professorship of Latin in the 18th century.

The holder of the chair was to be elected by the donor and his heirs, which principle was upheld until 1908 – even if the focus during the years gradually drifted from eloquence towards political science – in which year the terms were brought into line with those of other professorships; the heirs are, however, still to be consulted before the creation of a new *professor Skytteanus*, cf. Barbro Lewin: *Johan Skytte och de skytteanska professorerna* (1985).

[41] As for vocabulary, ancient Latin would also be more suited to a humanist subject than to the natural sciences, which, to be properly dealt with in the 18th century, would need a considerably larger number of neologisms, as will also be seen from "The medical word-stock" below.

[42] This matter is discussed by, among others, Berggren, pp 43–46, Östlund, pp 31–34.

[43] Cf. e.g. Östlund, pp 35–38.

[44] Even if *necessum* is basically an archaic form, known from e.g. Plautus, *Asinaria* 895 and Terence, *Phormio* 296, the notion of "the Classical period" was at the time sufficiently wide to include also these authors (by the way, there is also one occurrence in Celsus 8.2).

(Schröder 17),[45] *hypothesios* (gen. sg.) (Bergius 10.15), and *praxin* (acc. sg.) (Bergius 5.1, Martin 19.1), of which the dat. sg. form *praxi* is also found (Bergius 10).[46]

There are also three words of this category that are found declined only according to Latin paradigms; these are *diaphanus*[47] (Bergius 1.7); *hodegus*[48] (Schröder 4) and *nycthemerum* (Bergius 10.54). Finally, there are two terms originally pertaining to philosophy, in Greek type and of course declined according to their Greek paradigm, namely προκαταρτικοίς (sic!) and προηγουμένοις (both dat. pl.) in Martin 4.1.[49]

Choice of words

One noteworthy feature, even of the most scientifically oriented and least literary texts of this period – such as the average university dissertation – is the ambition to use the most elegant expression available whenever there is a choice.

On examining these particular texts, one will thus find a number of quotations from ancient Latin poetry, as well as other "choice expressions", which are further treated in the commentaries below, e.g:

illustris Werlhof, cui suum etiam calculum addit *summus Angliae Medicus Illustris Mead* (Martin 3.2)

Quod reliquum est, … Hahnii scriptum rotunde dilucideque *exponet* (Martin 3.5)

Operae pretium non ducimus allata variorum judicia convellere (Martin 4.7)

Quartum variolae emetiuntur *stadium … hisce indiciis* (Martin 6.8)

vana victoriae spe adducti Magno Boerhavio dicam scribere *sunt ausi* (Martin 8.2)

cum certum sit, quoad valeant humeri, *diligentissime hoc argumentum pertractare, fieri non potest, quin eum aliquando tramitem insistam* (Martin 12.4)

frigus cane angueque pejus *vitetur* (Bergius 9.6)

Dicas mihi ad quam, positis his, sacram confugiendum anchoram, & magnus mihi eris Apollo! (Bergius 10.34)

subito remitti debet febris … at in confluentibus non semper ita agitur; casu posito posteriore, pro certo signo haberi potest … pus e pustulis debito modo non evacuari, verum in sanguinem resorberi, novumque adeo addi calcar *febri* currenti. (Bergius 10.31)

---

[45] Also as Latin abl. sg. *hebdomade* in Sundius 9.

[46] One could perhaps regard *praxis* as a technical term in this context, even if the original Greek πρᾶξις has a more general meaning of 'action' etc.

[47] *Diaphanus*, Gr. διαφανής, seems in Neo-Latin to be an exclusively scientific term, found e.g. in Hoffwenius' *Synopsis physica*, cf. also OED, s.v. 'diaphanous' (and synonyms 'diaphanal' and 'diaphane') where the 17th and 18th century occurrences provided generally are found in a technical or scientific context.

[48] *Hodegus*, Gr. ὁδηγός, 'guide'; this word, on the other hand, is known from non-technical authors, such as historians Polybios, Dionysius of Halicarnassus, and Plutarch.

[49] Both terms, προκαταρκτικός and προηγούμενος meaning 'initial', and 'going first', respectively, refer to initial conditions; both are found e.g. in Chrysippos, but – more important in this context – also in Greek medical authors, such as Galen (cf. e.g. his περὶ τῶν προκαταρκτικῶν αἰτίων) and Dioscorides.

Variation

As in any other context, where one particular phaenomenon has to be frequently mentioned, the authors of these texts of course try to achieve variaton as regards choice of words and phrases; an illustrative example of a field where these ambitions are particularly prominent is that of the bowels and their function, where we find:

On the function of the bowels in general:

facultas excrementa exprimendi (Sundius 1.2)
alvi facilitas (Sundius 3.3)

On defecation and the results thereof:

excreta per alvum (Bergius 5.20)
alvi exoneratio (Bergius 8.17)
alvum deponere (Bergius 10.42)
excreta excernere (Bergius 10.48)
evacuationes (Bergius 10.51)
excreta alvi (Bergius 10.56)
depositiones alvi (Bergius 10.56)
sedes (Bergius 10.57)
excrementa dejicere (Sundius 2.2)
excretio per alvum (Schröder 13)
per alvum ejicere (Schröder 35)

On costiveness/constipation:

alvus stricta (Martin 6.1)
obstipatio alvi (Bergius 8.17)
adstrictior alvus (Sundius 0.3)
alvus adstricta (Sundius 1.1)
occlusa alvus (Sundius 1.2)
durior alvus (Sundius 1.2)
alvi durities (Sundius 4)
alvus contracta (Schröder 13)
alvus obstipata (Schröder 32)
claussa alvus (Schröder 35)

On the treatment of constipation:

alvum solvere (Sundius 7.5)

On looseness/diarrhoea:

laxa alvus (Sundius 9.5)
laxata alvus (Sundius 9.6)

Apart from these cases of directly mentioning the bodily functions in question, there are also examples of more elaborate circumlocutions:

> [*alvus*] *offici statim memor reddi debet* (Schröder 13)

> *Bis intra horas 24* [*alvi*] *beneficio gaudere debent* [*infantes*] (Schröder 33)

As a second example of variation, here follows a selection of phrases used to express 'indication' etc, e.g. of a disease reaching a new stage in its course:

> *haec exstant indicia* (Martin 6.1)

> [*stadium*] *internoscitur signis* (Martin 6.3)

> [*periodus*] *hisce notatur phoenomenis* (Martin 6.6)

> *indicium est* (Martin 6.6)

> [*stadium emetiuntur*] *hisce indiciis* (Martin 6.8)

> *indicio sunt* (Martin 7.2)

> [*Insultus epileptici*] *significant* (Bergius 5.5)

> [*Pulsus*] *signum ... dat* (Bergius 5.13)

> [*Variolae*] *... docent* (Bergius 5.15)

> [*maculae*] *... prodentes* (Bergius 5.19)

> [*Vomitus & Dolores*] *indicant* (Bergius 5.21)

> *Si ..., indicatur* (Bergius 5.22)

> *Si ..., malum indicans est* (Bergius 5.24)

> *Si ... , significatur* (Bergius 5.27)

> *indicia adsunt* (Sundius 0.3)

> *praebet indicium* (Sundius 9.6)

> *arguit* (Sundius 9.6)

A third example, in this case illustrating how variation can be used to avoid monotony in an otherwise catalogue-like passage, can be obtained from **Bergius 3**, where the suggestions of different authors as regards the causes of smallpox are referred to:

Sanguinis menstrui reliquias … caussam … statuebant olim Arabes (3.3)

Morbum haereditarium esse … crediderunt GENTILIS de FULGINEO … &c. (3.4)

Acidum ex reliquis lactis … exortum accusavit SYLVIUS (3.5)

A venenata bestiola variolas esse putavit M. LISTER (3.7)

Sideribus aliquam inesse vim … variolasque provocandi arrisit N CHESNEAU (3.8)

Nuperrime in liquore renum succenturiatorum caussam quaesivit Ph. VIOLANTE (3.9)

The medical word-stock

General principles

One feature of the "Latin" medical language that perhaps has not always been sufficiently stressed, is that there has been, from the beginning of Latin medical writing, a fundamental difference between the anatomical word stock, which, generally speaking, tends to be pure Latin, while pathological terms are of Greek origin;[50] one could e.g. compare the anatomical Latin term *ren*, 'kidney', to the pathological, originally Greek, term *nephritis* (from νεφρός, 'kidney'), meaning an inflammation of the same organ; likewise the anatomical term *ventriculus*, 'stomach', is Latin, while the pathological term *gastritis* is of Greek origin (from γαστήρ, 'belly').

This state of affairs is of course a result of the Roman habit of relying heavily on Greek physicians and their writings when in need of more subtle medical actions, while, even before forming any notion whatsoever of such a profession as that of the physician, they certainly had been in possession of vernacular names for such elementary things as the various readily observable parts of the body (and, indeed, for those pathological phaenomena which might be noted by laymen; see below). This is a point of importance when discussing the question of whether or not a certain word is to be regarded as a technical term.

Many Latin words for medically coloured phaenomena are used, even in their oldest extant instances by laymen, and thus difficult to regard with any certainty as technical terms, even if the matter of course would be treated in different ways by different authors; an example of rather strict criteria are those suggested by D. R. Langslow:

> a word is counted as a technical term if:
> 1) it is not generally understood in the linguistic community as a whole;
> 2) it is proper to a given specialist or technical discipline;
> 3) it is normalized or standardized in its usage in the discipline.[51]

These criteria, if strictly applied, would probably exclude quite a large part of the Latin anatomical terms on the ground that the word in question has been in use before the appearance of the medical profession, thus not fulfilling Langslow's second criterion above.

Taking into the account also, that medicine in the Roman society originally was no more an approved occupation for a native Roman of any importance than any other profession, and thus better left with Greek slaves, the Latin terms were probably never regarded as quite as technical as the Greek ones; even among laymen, *tumor* has denoted a morbid swelling of some part of the body from the beginning of Latin literature.

Yet another complication considering the application of such criteria as Langslow's to the present material is that they were never intended for categorization of 18th-century material: how would, e.g, the "linguistic community" of the first criterion above be defined, when dealing with a language which hardly anybody outside of the learned and scientific field uses?

---

[50] There are important exceptions to this general principle, as will be seen below, under "Words of Greek origin: General remarks".

[51] D. R. Langslow: *Medical Latin in the Roman Empire*, p 13.

ACTA UNIVERSITATIS UPSALIENSIS
Studia Latina Upsaliensia 28
Distributor: Uppsala University Library, Box 510, SE-751 20 Uppsala, Sweden

Four Eighteenth-century Medical Dissertations
under the Presidency of Nils Rosén.

Edited and translated, with an introduction and commentary

by

URBAN ÖRNEHOLM

Akademisk avhandling som för avläggande av filosofie doktorsexamen i latin vid Uppsala universitet kommer att offentligen försvaras i Ihresalen, SVC, fredagen den 12 december 2003 kl. 14.

ABSTRACT

Örneholm, U, 2003: Four Eighteenth-century Medical Dissertations under the Presidency of Nils Rosén. Edited and translated, with an introduction and commentary by Urban Örneholm.
Acta Univ. Ups, *Studia Latina Upsaliensia* 28. 284 pp. Uppsala. ISBN 91-554-5789-4.

Nils Rosén (von Rosenstein) (1706–73), Professor of medicine at Uppsala University, is less known than his colleague Linnaeus, but has, mainly through his textbook *Underrättelser om Barn-Sjukdomar* (1st monograph ed. 1764), had an enormous influence on the care of children throughout Europe.

In this thesis, four Latin dissertations, put forth under the presidency of Nils Rosén, are edited, with translation, commentary, and introduction. These dissertations quite clearly represent the latest medical knowledge of the mid 18th century, and recent theories are propounded, discussed, and examined against practical and empirical knowledge; the texts are thus representative examples of the kind of academic dissertations that communicated and discussed relevant factual matter as opposed to those that just constituted an amount of text, suitable for elaborating on during the disputational ceremony.

In my introduction, I mainly concentrate on medical and pharmacological technical terminology, but more general aspects on scholarly and scientific Neo-Latin are also dealt with. The dissertations edited are *De variolis praecavendis* (1751), *De variolis curandis* (1754), both treating smallpox; *De epilepsia infantili* (1754), on children's epilepsy, and *De morbis infantum* (1752), dealing with the health care of children *in genere*, and interesting as an early Latin version of parts of *Underrättelser*.

Key-words: Neo-Latin, dissertations, terminology, nomenclature, Nils Rosén, history of medicine, smallpox, paediatrics.

Urban Örneholm, Department of Classical Philology, Uppsala University, Box 527, SE-751 20 Uppsala, Sweden.

In short, it is quite clear that the present material must be treated in a different way; one possible approach, as far as original Latin terms are concerned, would perhaps be to regard those Latin words, which might have been learned at school (i.e. words found in an author likely to have been studied before the student's specializing in any particular field), as non-technical.

When applied to the works of ancient authors, this would lead to the inclusion of medical words found in Celsus – however "untechnical" they might have been to a contemporary reader[52] – with the exception of those also used by authors like Cicero or Livy.

The pure Latin terms found in Celsus might thus well have been regarded as non-technical terms by a contemporary reader, but since, in many cases, they would not mean exactly the same to the 18th century physician as to the contemporary layman, even if they both were skilled latinists, it would be appropriate to regard them as technical terms in this context.

Thus, we would do well to make the distinction, mentioned above, between different categories of authors. We should also add to the technical category those of the ancient, originally non-technical, Latin words that have since undergone any significant change of meaning,[53] or which do appear in fixed compound terms[54] giving them a more specific denotation, thereby making them more technical. The conclusion would be, I believe, that I shall have to treat such Latin words, and all Greek terms in my material, more thoroughly, while Latin terms, known from ancient Latin layman usage, and where the meaning has remained unchanged, will be briefly mentioned, at the most.

On word studies

Another field, where the direct application on Neo-Latin material of methods devised for the traditional classical philology would be quite inconvenient, is that of word studies.

Traditionally, the search for earlier occurrences of a word, when studying a text, has far too often started with, and stopped at, the oldest proof of earlier usage, whereupon the writer has been able to rest assured of having fulfilled his duties, according to the rules of philology.

---

[52] From Langslow's work (pp 118–121) it is quite clear that Celsus uses relatively few Greek words without mentioning their Greek origin; he also quite often provides the reader with a Latin translation or explanation. Keeping in mind that Celsus himself was neither a physician, nor writing for physicians, this seems quite a clear indication that the Greek terms in question should be regarded as technical terms, while their Latin counterparts should not, as regards Celsus' own time.

[53] As an example of such a word we might consider *humerus/umerus*, which to any Latin student outside of the medical field would only be associated with, roughly, the shoulder and upper arm of man, while in Celsus, apart from in this sense, it is also used as specifically denoting the bone of the upper arm (e.g. in 8.1.18), which still is the medical denotation.

[54] This is a particularly important category in anatomy; as we know, the anatomical science had made several new discoveries from Andreas Vesalius (1514–64) on, which had also lead to the need for new terms; such terms as *tuba Eustachii* (i.e. the auditory tube, a channel between the middle ear and the nasopharynx, named after the Italian anatomist Bartolommeo Eustachio (1520–74)) or *tuba Fallopii* (i.e. the uterine tube, after Gabriele Falloppio (1523–62)) might serve as examples; while *tuba* (a trumpet or tube) certainly in itself is no technical term from a medical point of view, the compounds in question definitely are.

Of course, there could be no doubt about the fact that ascertaining the first occurrence of a word in a language is of great value in itself; the problem, when dealing, as in my case, with texts from the last (or latest) period of a language's practical usage, is that an occurrence of e.g. a Greek medical term in an ancient, late, or mediaeval Latin manuscript would be of immediate interest from the Neo-Latinist's point of view only if it could be established with any certainty that the author of the Neo-Latin text dealt with has had any knowledge of the earlier work in question.

In many cases, however, to make such an assumption would mean to take for granted quite an extraordinary state of book learning among average writers; thus, when we have established e.g. that the first Latin occurrence of the word *cardia*, Gr. καρδία (i.e. the upper orifice of the stomach), is to be found in *Alphita*,[55] probably from the 13th century, we will have to consider the problem that if we wish to settle for this as a fully satisfactory explanation of the finding of *cardia* in a mid 18th century dissertation, then we must needs assume that *Alphita* has been read by our author, which certainly might be possible, but in most cases would seem rather far-fetched. Otherwise, a reference to *Alphita* would mean only that *cardia* is a word which has been used in Latin by someone, somewhere, at some point in history.

In order to avoid these kinds of methodological mistakes one should preferably start, not from the earliest, but rather from the latest proof of the word in question; thus, what are my author's immediate sources? what books are otherwise the most likely to have been read by, in this case, an 18th century physician? and so on. (It should be observed, that "Well, Alphita, of course!" is not likely to be the correct answer to any of these questions.)

After treating the matter according to these principles, one will probably have found quite a few occurrences of the words in question; in the sources of one's text, in important earlier works on the subject in point (e.g. Galen, when dealing with the field of medicine; see below), but also in various dictionaries, grammar books, etc. *from the appropriate period.*

The next step then would be the identification, if possible, of the sources of the sources, as it were, and so on, as far back in time as possible. However, when a word is found in any of the standard reference books of the time dealt with, this would of course often explain the usage both in the text being treated and in its primary sources; in the case of *cardia*, then, one will find this word in the Latin translation (about 1500 AD) of Galen, thus in a work, which is likely to have been studied by every medical writer well towards the end of the 18th century. An occurrence of a term in the Latin Galen therefore provides a somewhat stronger piece of evidence when trying to explain the 18th-century usage, than just a reference to *Alphita* would.

Since the study of Neo-Latin is a rather recent branch of philology, the tools ready at hand for the Neo-Latinist are quite limited in number; there is no explicitly Neo-Latin dictionary of equal weight with e.g. TLL or OLD for ancient Latin, or the standard mediaeval Latin dictionaries. Certainly, the collected stock of words of the Neo-Latin literature is to a certain extent identical to that of the ancient Latin literature, however not to such a degree that a Neo-Latin dictionary justly could be dubbed an unnecessary addition; especially during the 17th and 18th centuries, new terms, necessary to record the development of modern sciences, were continuously added. Moreover, as every Neo-Latinist knows, far from all identical words have also an identical meaning.

---

[55] ed de Renzi, p282.28

26

While waiting for this dictionary we will have to manage by trying to establish, at least for the various kinds of scientific texts, which constitute a very large part of the Neo-Latin literature,[56] some kind of standard starting-points for the search (that is, apart from the primary sources of our subject, if there are any).

In the present case then, dealing with medical texts, appropriate starting-points would naturally be the Renaissance Latin translations of the great Greek medical writers: even if particular Greek terms had of course already been incorporated into the Latin language by medical writers of the Roman empire[57] and of mediaeval Europe,[58] it was not until late 15th century that the complete works of e.g. Hippocrates and Galen were published in western Europe, both in Greek and in Latin translations.[59]

In the following three word lists, the medical terms of my texts have been distributed into the categories Greek terms, Latin terms, and names of pharmacological preparations, respectively.

Otherwise, we could distinguish three main categories of medical terms with regard to medical fields:

1) The words of anatomy, referring to various parts of the body.

2) The words of pathology and physiology, referring to illnesses and processes in the body.

3) The words of pharmacology, referring to drugs and preparations, consisting of ingredients from the botanical, animal and mineral realms.

In group (1) we find almost exclusively words of Latin and Greek origin, with a predominance for Latin terms, as remarked above. Group (2) likewise contains mainly Latin and Greek words, however with a predominance of the Greek, whereas group (3) consists of Latinized terms (very often compounds) of varied ethymological background, often Greek and Latin, certainly, but also words from Arabic and Persian among other languages, in addition to which there are also several eponymical terms to be found in this group.

Because of these special linguistic features, and because of these terms' specific denotata, often bordering upon the fields of chemistry and botany, I find it reasonable to give the pharmacological terms a special treatment; the particular words of a compound term might often be readily understood, while the exact meaning of a

---

[56] In the case of university dissertations, a majority of these were written in Latin as late as 1850 at the University of Uppsala (K. Östlund, U. Örneholm: *Avhandlingsspråk vid Uppsala universitet 1600–1855*, in *Lychnos*, 2000, pp 180–183).

[57] For a more thorough discussion on the incorporation of Greek medical terms into the Latin language of the Roman empire, see Langslow.

[58] As is pointed out by e.g. Richard J. Durling, *Galenus Latinus*, I, p VIIsq, texts of Galen had been translated directly from Greek manuscripts by the Italian judge Burgundio of Pisa (c. 1110–1193), even if the translation in most common use was that made from Arab manuscripts by Gerard of Cremona.

[59] Several editions of the great Greek medical authors appeared during the 16th and 17th century; Hippocrates was edited in Greek by Aldus in Venice 1526 and by Cornarius in Basel 1538, followed by Greek-Latin parallel editions by Mercurialis (Venice) in 1588; by v. Foës (Frankfurt) in 1595; by v. d. Linden (Leiden) in 1665, and by Chartier (Paris) in 1639–79. The first printed edition of Galen was that by Aldus in 1525, which was followed by the Basel edition by Linacre et al. in 1541.

specific compound at a specific time and place can be considerably more difficult to ascertain.[60] Another problem is the fact that every specific preparation was still made on request in the pharmacy and according to established local traditions, not necessarily according to the official pharmacopoeia.

As for the distribution between languages in different medical fields of the first two groups mentioned above, the present material could be divided into the following categories:

Table 1: distribution of terms from different medical areas between languages.

	Greek	Latin	Other
Anatomy	4	16	1
Pathology/Physiology	54	37	1
Therapy	6	1	-
Equipment	1	-	-

Here, even if the material is rather small, we note that the Latin terms clearly are in majority among the anatomical terms, while the Greek domination in the pathological field is not quite as obvious; one reason for the rather small difference between the languages in this field might be that among the pathological terms are seven Latin names of specific diseases, which had not been defined by the ancient authors, and thus had recieved their names at a time, when Greek was no longer the natural language for the physician.

Words of Greek origin

General remarks

It should first of all be observed that a majority of the Greek or latinized Greek words of the present material are to be referred to the field of pathology/physiology; of the remaining Greek terms, six belong to the field of therapy, and one significates a piece of medical equipment, which is also quite understandable from what we know about the dominance of Greek in ancient Roman medicine.

The remaining terms, finally, are anatomical, and might in two cases (*larynx* and *oesophagus*) have been preferred to their corresponding Latin terms (*faux* and *stomachus*) as being more univocal.[61] The adoption of *cardia* might be explained by that particular

---

[60] As an example might serve the preparation *aqua floris Acaciae* below, which in direct translation obviously is 'water with flowers of acacia', but which actually was made with flowers of sloe, at least in 18th-century Sweden.

[61] It should be observed that the sing. *faux* is not regarded as classical, and that the plur. *fauces* normally is used figuratively in classical Latin, denoting any kind of precipice, but also narrow doorways, river mouths, etc; the sing. is, however, to be found in Burgundio of Pisa's translation of Galen's *De interioribus*, where it is used to explain the meaning of *larinx*. As for *stomachus*, this is indeed also originally a Greek word that was already used in ancient Latin,

28

part of the gastrointestinal system being unknown to the Romans prior to the appearance of the medical profession; as for *lympha*, finally, even if this particular word, meaning water, had been quite common in Latin poetry from Lucretius on, it would not be used to denote ordinary water in a medical prose context,[62] and might thus have seemed a suitable adoption for describing a more water-like bodily fluid.

Earlier occurrences

When applying the method indicated above ("On word studies") to the Greek word list, the result is that out of the sixty-five terms of Greek origin to be found in my material, thirty-six are also found in the index volume (1542) to the 1541 Basel edition of the Latin translation of Galen (**GL**), and no less than fifty-three in the 1748 edition of Stephanus Blancardus' *Lexicon Medicum* (**B**).

In Table 2 below, the words of my list are checked against, in addition to Galen and Blancardus, Johannes Gorraeus' *Definitionum medicarum libri xxiiii*, 1564 (**G**), and to Bartholdus Castelli's *Lexicon Medicum*, 1713 (**C**).

All occurrences of a certain word is marked by an "x" in the table, while any occurrence of the word stem in any other form (e.g. when *chylus* is found, but not *chylosus*), is marked by an "o"; any instances of the exact word appearing, but in another sense than in my texts, is indicated by the sign "(x)". It should furthermore be observed, that all entries in Gorraeus are printed in Greek type and, of course, with Greek spelling, which is not indicated in the table.

We might also note that of the eight words which are not found in their exact form or sense in any of the sources accounted for in Table 2, two (*catarrhalis* and *chylosus*) are latinized adjectives, to which the corresponding noun is found in at least three of the sources; the formation of new adjectives by analogy is of course close at hand to a writer, who has the necessary knowledge of a certain noun; this kind of word formation would lead to such Latin forms out of Greek stems as those found here; cf. also the pure Latin adjectives on *-orius* (*excretorius* etc, the Latin word list).

Several original Greek adjectives have, on the other hand, been substantivized by losing a headword, such as νόσος, 'disease/illness', or φάρμακον, 'drug', while in other cases a neologism, or at least an apparent neologism, parallel to an already existent ancient Greek form, is found, e.g. when *spasmodicus* is used by Latin writers instead of the Hippocratic term σπασμώδης, which is found in Gorraeus, while no such word as *σπασμοδικός seems ever to have existed in the Greek language; a phaenomenon which might perhaps be regarded as a case of neologism brought about as a result of an original Greek term's lack of "Latin compatibility"; it might of course on the other hand be taken as an indication of Hippocrates being less frequently read than e.g. Galen.[63]

---

however, to denote both the stomach and the gullet. It would thus seem quite reasonable to adopt more specific terms for professional use.

[62] It is indeed to be found, probably in the general sense of 'water', in the medical *poetry* of Serenus Sammoniacus, see below s.v. *lympha*.

[63] It turns out, in fact, that very few words of the present list are found in Cornarius' Latin edition of Hippocrates (Basel 1554); so few, actually, that Hippocrates is excluded altogether from the table, as is, for the same reason, the 1523 Latin edition of Dioscorides.

Table 2: earlier Neo-Latin occurrences of Greek terms.

term \ work	GalenusL 1541	Gorraeus 1564	Castelli 1713	Blancardus 1748
achor				
agrypnia			x	x
amphemerina	x	x	x	x
anthraces	x	x	x	x
borborygmus	x	x	x	x
bubones	x	x	x	x
cardia	x	x	x	x
catarrhalis	o	o	o	o
catharsis		x	x	(x)
catheter	x	x	x	x
cephalalgia	x	x	x	x
chirurgus	x	o	x	x
chylosus	o	o	o	o
colicus	x	x	x	x
coma	x	x	x	x
corium		x	x	
coryza	x	x	x	x
crisis	x	x	x	x
diaeta	x	x	x	x
diaphoresis	o	x	x	x
diapnoë		x	x	x
diarrhoea	x	x	x	x
eclampsia			o	
epilepsia	x	x	x	x
ἐπινυκτίδες		x	x	x
erysipelas	x	x	x	x
ἐξανθηματικός		o	o	o
gangraena	x	x	x	x
haemoptoë	o			o
haemoptysis			x	x
haemorrhagia	x	x	x	x
hydroa				x
ichor	x	x	x	x
icterus	x	x	x	x
larynx	x	x	x	x
lethargus	x	x	x	x
lympha			x	x
meconium		(x)	x	x
melancholia	x	x	x	x
metastasis			x	x
miasma				x
nausea	x	x	x	x
nephriticus	(x)	o	(x)	x
oesophagus	x	x	x	x
paroxysmus	x	x	x	x

peripneumonia	x	x	x	x
phlebotomia	x		x	x
phlogosis		x	x	x
phrenesis			x	x
phrenitis	x	x	x	x
plethoricus	o		o	x
pleuriticus	(x)		x	
pleuritis	x	x	x	x
podagra	x	x	x	x
prognosis	o		x	x
prophylaxis	o	o	o	o
ptyalismus		o	x	x
scybala			x	x
spasmodicus		o	x	(x)
spasmus	x	x	x	x
sphacelus	x	x	x	x
stasis			x	
strabismus	x	x	x	x
symtoma	x	x	x	x
syncope	x	x	x	x

Greek word list

ACHOR, Sundius 5.2; scurf
Gr. ἄχωρ, 'scurf', 'dandruff'; in Latin found as *achora* (fem) in Theodorus Priscianus 13 (c. 4ᵗʰ–5ᵗʰ cent. AD): *achoras papillas dicimus quae per cavernas brevissimas umorem pinguissimum mittunt.*

In all probability, the word *achor* in itself does not actually denote 'the scabies', even if what is intended here is the skin manifestations of that particular disease, but rather any discharging or suppurating rash of the head; cf. Castelli (1607 ed.) s.v. *Achores* (*sic*).

AGRYPNIA, Bergius 10.58, Schröder 31; sleeplessness
Gr. ἀγρυπνία, Hippocrates *Aph.* 2.3 (5ᵗʰ cent. BC); in Latin Martianus Capella 2.112 (ca. 5ᵗʰ cent.?)(TLL). Found in C (Castelli 1713) and B (Blancardus).

AMPHIMERINA (noun, for *amphemerina*), Bergius 10.26; daily, not intermittent, fever
Gr. ἀμφημερινός, Hippocrates *Epid.* 1.6; in Latin Pliny (23–79) *NH* 28.66. Since this word is found in Pliny, it should perhaps not be regarded as a strictly medical term, according to the principles suggested above, but I doubt that Pliny was read *in extenso* in 18ᵗʰ century schools. The word is otherwise found in GalenusL(GL), where it is spelled *amphi-*, as in Bergius' text; in Gorraeus(G), and in both C and B (where it is an adjective).

ANTHRACES, Bergius 1.2, and **ΑΝΤΡΑΚΑΣ**, (acc pl, misprint for ἀνθράκας), Martin 3.2; a disease with pustules or carbuncles.
In Greek, ἄνθραξ originally means 'charcoal', but also a dark-red stone, whence the medical sense 'carbuncle' or 'malignant pustule'. The latter sense in Hippocrates *Epid.* 3.7; known in Latin in the medical sense from Aem. Macer (?–14 BC) *de Herb*. Martin

uses the Greek version quoting Richard Mead: *De variolis et morbillis liber*, where it however is spelled correctly (cf. ἐπινυκτίδες below). The word is found, in sg, in GL, G, C, and B. Today, the term denotes only infections caused by the *Bacillus Anthracis*.

BORBORYGMUS, Sundius 1.2; a rumbling sound from the bowels
Gr. βορβορυγμός (or κορκορυγμός), Hippocrates *Prog.* 11; not known from classical Latin; acc to *Mittellateinisches Wörterbuch* (MLW), the word *borborygmon* in *Gloss. med.* (c. 700) means 'troubled sleep'. In the ancient sense, it is found in GL, where the word is said to be *Graece dictus*, G, C, and B.

BUBONES (plur.), Bergius 1.2; boils
Gr. βουβών, 'groin'; the pl used for 'swollen glands' in Hippocrates *Epid.* 2.2.24. lat *Dub Nom gramm.* V.575.16 (7th cent? AD) (TLL); here 'boils', in which sense it is found in GL, G, C, and B.

CARDIA, Bergius 5.11; the upper orifice of the stomach
Gr. καρδία, 'heart' or 'stomach'; in the sense of 'orifice of the stomach' in Thucydides 2.49; Latin in this sense: *Alphita I* p 282.28 (c. 13th cent.)(MLW). Found in GL, in Greek letters, in G, C, and B.

CATARRHALIS (adj.), Martin 16.2; with symptoms, or in a state, of catarrh
fr. Gr. κατάρροος, (adj.) 'down-flowing', medically (noun) 'running from the head', 'catarrh', Hippocrates *Aph.* 3.12, Lat *catarrhus*, Isidorus *Orig.* 4.7.11 (?–636) (TLL). This adj. not found in ancient Latin, nor in GL, G, C, or B, whereas these four all have *catarrhus*. There is a Greek adj. καταρροώδης (Hippocrates *Vict.* 1.32), which however denotes a person, susceptible to catarrh. The creation of an adjective of this kind, where there is an extant noun from the same word stem, would of course be quite natural to a medical Latin writer. Stotz (II, § 75.1) points out the frequent formation of words by the suffix *-alis*, both in mediaeval and renaissance Latin, also (§75:4)from Greek word stems; cf. also the long list provided by Hoven (pp 403–405).

CATHARSIS, Bergius 8.16; cleansing or purging
Gr. κάθαρσις, in the medical sense: Hippocrates *Aph.* 5.36; in earlier Latin, *catharsis* seems not to have been used in this more general sense; it is used about the menstruation in Oribasius Lat 347.17; 348.1 (6th cent.) (Souter), which however is a direct translation from the Greek. This term is not found in GL, but in G and C in this sense; in B it is used as =*catharticum*.

CATHETER, Sundius 9.1; catheter
Gr. καθετήρ, in its medical sense: Galen 1.125 (2nd cent.); in Latin Caelius Aurelianus *Tard* 2.1.13 (5th cent?) (L&S). Found in GL, G, C, and B.

CEPHALALGIA, Bergius 8.3; headache
Gr. κεφαλαλγία, Hippocrates *Aph.* 3.13; in Latin (spelled *cephalargia*) *Gloss Med.* p 17.11(c. 700). In GL, G, C, and B.

CHIRURGUS, Martin 19.1; barber-surgeon
Gr. χειρουργός (noun), in this sense: Plutarch 2.486 (1st/2nd cent.); in Latin Celsus 7. *praef.* (the reign of Tiberius). Found in GL, C, and B, while G has χειρουργίη(*sic.* Hippocratic ionism). It should be observed that surgery still was not

regarded as a part of medical science in mid 18th century, and that the only occurrence
in the present material is of a rather pejorative nature.

CHYLOSUS (adj.), Martin 4.6, Schröder 14; mixed with intestinal fluid
from Gr. χυλός, 'juice', especially the result of the digestion: Galen *UP* 4; in ancient
Latin, the normal meaning of *chylus* seems to be that of the juice from a plant, while
the Greek medical sense is known in mediaeval Latin from Albertus Magnus *De
animalibus* 3.100. *Chylosus* is apparently known from Constantinus Afer (c. 1020–1087)
theor. 6.27, then in the general sense of (adj.) 'liquid'. The meaning here, however, is
not found in MLW or Bartal. In GL, G, C, and B, only the noun *chylus* is found.

COLICUS (adj.), Martin 6.1; pertaining to colic
from Gr. κωλικός 'suffering from colic', Dioscorides 2.54, Galen 8.40 (cf. κῶλον,
incorrect for κόλον (Isidorus *Etym.* 4.7.38)); known in mediaeval Latin from *Tract. de
aegr. cur* p 258.11 (12th cent.) (MLW). Found in GL, G, C, and B. Cf also
NEPHRITICUS and **PLEURITICUS** below.

COMA, Martin 6.4; unconsciousness
Gr. κῶμα, 'deep sleep', *Od.* 18.201; in Latin Paulus of Aegina *Cur.* 40 p 18.20 (7th
cent.)(MLW), which is a translation from a Greek original. Found in GL, G, and C. In
B. only in compounds, e.g. *coma somnolentium.*

CORIUM, Bergius 8.20; coating
Gr. χόριον, originally the membrane covering the foetus, Hippocrates *Nat. Puer.* 16; in
ancient Latin the skin or hide of an animal, Cato RR 135.3 (?–149 BC): In the sense
indicated here, of an 'inflammatory coating' on the blood, not known from ancient or
medieval usage. Found in G and in C, but only in the original sense.

CORYZA, Schröder 10; running of the nose
Gr. κόρυζα, Ruf. *Onom.* 33 (2nd cent.), in Latin Caelius Aurelianus *Acut.* 2.17.101
(L&S). Found in GL, G, C, and B.

CRISIS, Martin 8.2, Bergius 5.9
Gr. κρίσις, 'a separating', 'a judgement', etc; in a medical context 'the turning point'
of, or 'sudden chance' in, a disease. Known in Greek, in its medical sense, from
Hippocrates' περὶ ἀρχαίης ἰατρικῆς 19: διὸ καὶ κρίσιες καὶ ἀριθμοὶ τῶν χρόνων ἐν
τοῖσι τοιούτοισι μέγα δύνανται, and from Galen 9.550.

For the period dealt with here, we might suspect some uncertainty as to what,
exactly, was to be understood by a *crisis*, as C puts it (s.v. *crisis*):

> *Interdum enim crisis dicitur subita morbi in melius pejusve ad vitam, aut mortem mutatio;
> interdum ea, quae antecedit judicium, humorum agitatio; interdum integra totius morbi
> solutio; interdum illa tantum morbi solutio, quae ad bonum sit, nomine criseos venit.*

B, who does not discuss the exact meaning of the term, does however establish that
crisin a lunae & siderum motu, & influentiis dependere ... verum non est.

DIAETA, Bergius 7.6; diet
Gr. δίαιτα, 'way of life', in the medical sense of 'prescriptions regarding life-style'
Hippocrates *Vict.* 1.1; known in Latin from Vindicianus medicus 40 (fl. late 4th cent.
AD) (TLL). Found in GL, G, C, and B; cf. also Linnaeus' *Diaeta naturalis* and *Dietetik.*

DIAPHORESIS, Bergius 10.29; perspiration

Gr. διαφόρησις (from διαφορέω) originally meaning 'spreading or carrying around things', *Od.* 19.333; found, still as a Greek term, in Cicero *Fam.* 16.18.1: *Tibi* διαφόρησιν *gaudeo profuisse*, where the sense seems to be that of a cure. In Latin, meaning 'sweating', Theodorus Priscianus *De diaeta* 14 (L&S). Found in G, C, and B, while GL has noun *diaphoretica* (npl).

DIAPNOË, Martin 13.2; here transpiration

Gr. διαπνοή, Hippocrates *Alim.* 28. The word seems not to be known from ancient Latin, but is found in Burgundio of Pisa's (12th century) *De interioribus*, a Latin translation of Galen, with the explanation *idest transpiratio*. Found in G, C, and B.

DIARRHOEA, Martin 6.1, Bergius 5.20

Gr. διάρροια, Hippocrates *Aph.* 3.21. (pl); in Latin Caelius Aurelianus *Acut.* 3.19 (L&S). Found in GL, G, C, and B.

ECLAMPSIA, Bergius 5.5; a fit of epilepsy

From Gr. ἔκλαμψις, a 'shining forth' or 'beaming', also 'a sudden development', Hippocrates *Epid.* 6.1.4, of the rapid development in the puberty; the term seems today, at least in the medical language of Sweden, to be used about a general spastic state which does *not* originate from an epileptic disease or brain damage (Lindskog/Zetterberg). In Dorland, the term is used for the *eclampsia gravidarum* or *eclampsia parturientium*.

Not found in TLL or in any Mediaeval Latin sources, nor in GL, G, or B; C has *eclampsis*.

EPILEPSIA, Martin 6.2, Bergius 5.5, Sundius passim; epilepsy

Gr. ἐπιληψία, (ἐπί + λῆψις, from λαμβάνω, 'to take'); in its present, medical, sense, Hippocrates *Aph.* 3.22; in ancient Latin the equivalent would be *morbus comitialis* or, in Caelius Aurelianus, *passio sacra: Epilepsia ... appellatur etiam puerilis passio ... et sacra* (*Tard.* 1.4), whereas *morbus sacer* by OLD is said to be any of several skin diseases, e.g. erysipelas or herpes; the word *epilepsia* is known from e.g. ps. Soranos *Quaest. med.* 207 (TLL) which however is a translation from Greek. Found in GL, G, C, and B.

ΕΠΙΝΥΚΤΙΔΕΣ (in the text ἐτινυκτίδας (ack.pl.)), Martin 3.2; a disease with pustules, hurting most during the night.

Found in this sense in Hippocrates *Aër.* 3. In Martin's text, the word is quoted from Mead, *De variolis et morbillis liber*, where it is also printed in Greek type, however correctly spelled. Cf. above, s.v. **ANTHRACES**. Found in G, C, and B.

ERYSIPELAS, Bergius 1.8

Gr. ἐρυσίπελας, an inflammatory skin disease, Hippocrates *VM* 19, in Latin known from Celsus 5.28.11b.

ΕΞΑΝΘΗΜΑΤΙΚΟΣ, Martin 1.3, and **EXANTHEMATICUS**, Bergius 1.1; exanthematic

From ἐξάνθημα, 'efflorescence' or 'pustule', Hippocrates *Aph.* 6.9; in Latin Marcellus medicus 19.31(the reign of Theodosius II) (TLL); the adj. seems not to be found in ancient or mediaeval sources, however; nor is it found in any of the four authors of table 2, while the noun *exanthema* is found in G, C, and B. As regards *-icus*, cf. also *lymphaticus, nephriticus, plethoricus, pleuriticus*, and *spasmodicus*, below.

GANGRAENA, Martin 7.2, Bergius 10.2; gangrene
Gr. γαγγραίνα, Hippocrates *Mochl.* 33; in Latin in Celsus 5.26.34. Found in all four reference authors.

HAEMOPTOE, Bergius 2.6; and **HAEMOPTYSIS** Bergius 8.3; bloodspitting
The exact word *haemoptoë* is not found in any of the reference authors, while *haemoptoicus* (adj, also as a noun) is found in GL, and *haemoptoica*, denoting 'remedies for *haemoptysis*' is found in B.

The noun αἱμοπτυϊκός, denoting a person suffering from *haemoptysis* (from Gr. αἷμα, 'blood', + πτύσις, 'spitting'), is found in Dioscorides 2.85.3 (1st cent.); in Latin, the word *haemoptyicus* is known from Marcellus empiricus 16 (L&S). In mediaeval Latin, the form *emoptois* (translated 'blotspiung') is found in Ælfric *sup*, 113 (?–c. 1025) (MLBr). For the relevant period, *haemoptysis* can be found in C and B.

HAEMORRHAGIA, Martin 6.4, Bergius 2.6; a profuse bleeding
Gr. αἱμορραγία, Hippocrates *Art.* 69; in Latin Pliny *NH* 23.7.67. One could note that both Martin and Bergius talk about *haemorrhagia narium*, while a bleeding specifically from the nose seems to be one of the meanings of *haemorrrhagia* in itself, in Greek but also in ancient Latin. Found in GL, with a reference to *sanguis evacuatio*, in G, C, and B.

HYDROA, Bergius 5.4
From Gr. ὕδωρ, 'water', but not found in any Greek or Latin dictionaries; B, who is the only reference author to include the word, says that it is the same as Gr. ἐκζέματα. The *hydroa* of today is, according to Dorland, a skin disease, which is otherwise known as *dermatitis herpetiformis*, and which might or might not be the same as that indicated here.

ICHOR, Bergius 8.7; blood mixed with pus
Gr. ἰχώρ, originally the divine equivalent of blood, *Il.* 5.340, later the blood-serum, Hippocrates *Cord.* 11, or a serous-purulent discharge (lat. *sanies*), Hippocrates *VC* 19; in mediaeval Latin in Burgundio's Galen translation *De complexionibus* 1.4: *subgenerabantur sub cute ycores*, which seems to denote bodily fluids in general. Here probably in the normal modern medical sense. Found in all four reference authors; GL gives a reference to *serum*, while G makes a distinction between *ichor* when present in the body, and *sanies* when external.

ICTERUS, Schröder 16; jaundice
Gr. ἴκτερος, Hippocrates *Aph.* 4.62; in Latin Pliny *NH* 30.11.28, where the word certainly is used about a bird, not about a disease, but as Pliny puts it: *avis icterus vocatur a colore, quae si spectetur, sanari id malum tradunt et avem mori*, there is no doubt that the malady was also known by the same name. Pliny assumes, by the way, that the bird in question in proper Latin would be called *galgulus*.

LARYNX, Bergius 8.23; larynx, throat
Gr. λάρυγξ, Aristotle *HA* 1.12; in Latin the compound *laryngotomia* is found in Caelius Aurelianus *Acut.* 3.4.39, described as *fabulosa arteriae ob respirationem divisura*, but the single word *larynx* does not seem to appear in ancient Latin. It is found in Burgundio's translation of Galen's *De interioribus*, e.g. in 49.29: *larinx idest faux*. Also present in GL, G, C, and B.

LETHARGUS (noun), Bergius 10.18; lethargy
Gr. λήθαργος, Hippocrates *Morb.* 2.65; in Latin Horace *Sat.* 2.3.145. Found in GL, G, C, and B.

LYMPHA, Bergius 3.5; lymph, and **LYMPHATICUS**, Martin 4.6; lymphatic
From Gr. νύμφη, among other things also meaning 'a spring', Athenaios 11.465a (2nd / 3rd cent.), hence 'water', especially in poetical language, as in *Anthologia Palatina* 9.258; in Latin in the more specific sense of 'liquid in the human body' (as a symptom of dropsy) in Serenus 496 (late 4th cent? AD); there is, however, nothing to indicate that Serenus would regard *lympha* in itself as possessing any qualities, different from those of water. The meaning here, apparently close to what is meant by 'lymph' today, is of course not the same as in ancient or mediaeval usage; as we know, the lymphatic system had not been described until mid-17th century scientists Aselli, Pecquet, Bartholin and, above all, Olaus Rudbeck the Elder, put forth their results. The word *lympha* consequently is not found in GL or G, but in both C and B.

MECONIUM, Martin 4.7; faeces of the new-born child
Gr. μηκώνιον, 'opium' (actually, *meconium* as a drug does not seem to have been altogether synonymous to opium at this time; according to Maehle, *Drugs on Trial*, p 142, *meconium* was the pressed and dried juice of the entire poppy plant, while "opium" was, and still is, the dried juice of the seed capsules only); also, probably from the likeness in appearance, in the sense indicated here, in Aristotle *HA* 7.10, where the word however is said to be used by women, not by physicians. The latter sense in Latin, Pliny *NH* 28.4.13. Not found in GL; in G only in the sense of opium. C and B give both denotations; C however with the remark *improprie* for the latter sense.

MELANCHOLIA, Schröder 13; Gr. μελαγχολία, Hippocrates *Aër.* 10; in Latin used by e.g. Cicero *Tusc.* 3.11, but then in Greek letters; first written in Latin letters in Caelius Aurelianus *Acut.* 1.4.42. Found in all four references.

METASTASIS, Martin 6.8; the transference of the seat of a disease
Gr. μετάστασις, 'removal' or 'change'; specifically in the present medical sense: Hippocrates *Aff.* 12; in ancient Latin used mainly of the transfer of e.g. an accusation to somebody else. In the specifically medical sense, however, *metastasis* does not seem to be known from ancient or mediaeval Latin. Found in C and in B, where a reference to μετάπτωσις is given.

MIASMA, Martin 14.1, Bergius 5.11; pathogenic substance
Gr. μίασμα, originally 'dirt' or 'pollution', also metaphorically; in the present sense, however, the word is known neither from ancient Greek, nor from ancient or mediaeval Latin. Found only in B.
According to I. W. Müller, *Iatromechanische Theorie und ärztliche Praxis*, p 150 sq, the meaning of *miasmata* in general was that of poisonous substances, emanating from earth, especially after earthquakes or from sulphuric springs, and which could inflict sickness, e.g. pneumonia and pleurisy, upon less resistent human beings, such as children or old people. Müller further (p 176 sq) refers to Friedrich Hoffmann, who regarded another kind of miasma as responsible for the contagious infectional diseases, like e.g. smallpox, measles, or syphilis. This kind of miasma was produced in human beings, and spread through exhalation. As opposed to the general miasma, this kind would also infect otherwise healthy individuals, thus bringing about epidemics.

NAUSEA, Martin 6.1, Bergius 8.10
Gr. *ναυτία* (from *ναῦς*, ship), 'seasickness', 'disgust', 'nausea', Aristotle *PA* 3.3; in Latin in Cato *Agr.* 156.4. Found in GL, G, C, and B.

NEPHRITICUS(adj.), Martin 6.1; regarding the kidneys
Gr. *νεφριτικός*, Hippocrates *Art.* 41; in Latin Isidorus *Orig.* 4.7. Here probably as an adj. to *dolor* (cf. Zedler, s.v. *Nieren-Weh*), cf. also **COLICUS** and **PLEURITICUS**. In this sense found in GL and C, while B has the noun, and G has the noun *νεφρίτις*.

OESOPHAGUS, Bergius 5.24; gullet
Gr. *οἰσοφάγος*, Hippocrates *Loc. Hom.* 3; not to be found in TLL or duCange. The word used e.g. by Celsus would be *stomachus*, Gr. *στόμαχος*. Found in all references.

PAROXYSMUS, Sundius 0.4; fit of disease
Gr. *παροξυσμός*, in Gr. mainly 'irritation', etc; in the medical sense: Hippocrates *Aph.* 1.11.12. In Latin Oribasius *Syn.* 9.51.2 (c. 4ᵗʰ cent.), which however is a translation from Greek. Found in GL, G, C, and B.

PERIPNEUMONIA, Bergius 5.23; inflammation of the lungs, pneumonia
Gr. *περιπνευμονία* or *περιπλευμονία*, Hippocrates *περὶ ἀρχαίης ἰατρικῆς* 17; known in Latin in the present spelling from Caelius Aurelianus *Acut.*

While *peripneumonia* in modern usage normally means a combination of pleurisy and pneumonia, the old meaning, also in English, as is pointed out in OED, s.v. "peripneumony, peripneumonia", was that of what we today call "pneumonia"; there are examples e.g. from 1634: "Excellent for the pleurisie and Peripnewmony, *i.* the inflammation of the lungs." (Ph. Holland, *Pliny's Historie of the world, commonly called the Natural historie*, II; 167), and from 1752: "The peripneumony under which he laboured … had terminated in an adhesion of the lungs to the pleura." (W. Shenstone, *Works in prose and verse*, 3.191). The Latin term is found in the original sense in all four reference authors.

PHLEBOTOMIA, Bergius 8.5; bloodletting
Gr. *φλεβοτομία*, 'opening of a vein', Hippocrates *Coac.* 288; in Latin Caelius Aurelianus 2. *Acut.* 18. The Latin equivalent being *venaesectio*, the word *phlebotomia* is however found in GL, C, and B. Cf. Latin word list, s.v. **VENAESECTIO**, below.

PHLOGOSIS, Martin 16.1, Bergius 10.24; inflammation
Gr. *φλόγωσις*, 'burning' or 'inflammation', Thucydides 2.49; in Latin not found in Forcellini or duCange. Found in G and C with the remark *olim* = *phlegmone*; in B with the synonyms *phlegmone* and *inflammatio*.

PHRENESIS, Bergius 8.21; frenzy, madness
Gr. **φρένησις*, 'inflammation of the brain', hence the present sense; not found in any Greek sources, but, written in Greek letters, in Celsus 3.18; in Latin, Celsus 2.1.15. Not found in GL or G, but in C and B, in both s.v. *phrenitis*.

PHRENITIS, Martin 6.4; frenzy
Gr. *φρενῖτις*, = *phrenesis*, Hippocrates *Aph.* 3.30; in Latin Fronto *Ver.* 2. The word is found in all four reference authors, in C with the remark: *a Latinis ... introductum est ... phrenesis.*

PLETHORICUS (adj.), Bergius 8.14; overfull (with bodily fluids); plethoric
Gr. πληθωρικός from πληθώρη and πληθώρα, 'fulness'; in Greek medical usage in e.g. Galen 7.578; found, as a noun, denoting *is, qui multo sanguine et succis abundat* in B, while *plethora* is found in GL and in C, with the explanation *sanguinis redundantiam significat.*

PLEURITICUS (adj.), Martin 6.1; pertaining to pleurisy, and **PLEURITIS**, Bergius 5.27
Pleuriticus, Gr. πλευριτικός, 'suffering from pleurisy', Hippocrates *Aph.* 1.12; 'good for pleurisy', Galen 11.711; in Latin Celsus 4.13 and, as a noun for 'patient, suffering from pleurisy', Pliny *NH* 20.15; cf. **COLICUS** and **NEPHRITICUS** above. Found in GL as an adj, and in C as a noun; *Pleuritis*, Gr. πλευρῖτις, Hippocrates *Aph.* 3.23; in Latin Vitruvius 1.6 (the reign of Augustus). Found in all four references.

PODAGRA, Sundius 9.1; gout
Gr. ποδάγρα, originally 'a trap for the feet', also 'gout', *IG4²* 122. In Latin, in the latter sense, Cicero *Tusc.* 2.19.45. Found in this, medical, sense in all four reference authors.

PROGNOSIS, Bergius 5.1; prognose
Gr. πρόγνοσις, 'knowledge beforehand', esp. as a medical term in Hippocrates *Prog,* in Latin Caelius Aurelianus *Tard.* 4.8.112. Found in C, with a reference to *praecognitio*, and in B, while GL has *prognostica.*

PROPHYLAXIS, Martin 19.1
From the Greek verb προφυλάσσω/προφυλάττω 'keep guard', often in a military context; the noun, which is well formed, does not seem to occur in ancient Greek sources. One might note, by the way, that metaphors from warfare still are quite common in the medical field (cf. "Style: Metaphors", below). The exact word is not found in any of the references, but GL, G, and B have *prophylactica/-ce*, and C has *prophylace*, in ancient Greek 'guard in front'.

PTYALISMUS, Martin 6.9, Bergius 5.29; salivation
Gr. πτυαλισμός/ πτυελισμός, Hippocrates *Prog.* 17. This word is not found in ancient or mediaeval Latin, while *ptyelon idest sputum* is read in Burgundio's 12ᵗʰ century Galen translation *De interioribus.* Found in C and B, while G has the verb πτυελίζειν.

SCYBALA (npl.), Bergius 8.17; faeces
Gr. σκύβαλον, 'dung', 'excrement', 'filth', etc, Plutarch 2.352d; used also in Greek medical writing, e.g. by Aretaios (*fl.* 1ˢᵗ cent. AD) in περὶ αἰτιῶν καὶ σημείων χρονίων παθῶν, 1.15: λευκὰ δὲ καὶ ἀργιλώδεα τὰ σκύβαλα (a description of the typical appearance of the faeces of a jaundice patient). Found in C and B.

SPASMODICUS, Bergius 5.20; spastic and **SPASMUS**, Sundius 0.2; spasm, convulsion
From Gr. σπασμός, Herodotos 4.187; in Latin Pliny *NH* 22.8.9. The adj. preferred in ancient Greek seems to be σπασμώδης; no such word as *σπασμοδικός is to be found in L&S, Sophocles or duCangeGr; nor is *spasmodicus* found in Forcellini or duCange. *Spasmus* is found in all four references, but *spasmodicus* only in C, who recommends the spelling *spasmoticus*, and in B, as a noun meaning 'remedy for spasm'. G has σπασμώδης, while *spasmosus* is found in *De interioribus.*

SPHACELUS, Bergius 10.61; gangrene
Gr. σφάκελος, Hippocrates *Aph.* 7.78. Not found in Forcellini or duCange; only occurrence in Bartal is considerably later. However to be found in *De interioribus* spelled <*s*>*facellum* and *sphakelos*, respectively. Found in all four reference authors, with the synonym *sideratio*.

STASIS, Martin 4.7; stoppage
From Gr. στάσις, 'the posture of standing', 'position', etc; apparently not used in the medical sense in ancient Greek, neither found in G nor in GL, while C says that the term, apart from its common meaning, is used about otherwise circulating bodily fluids *quando hi praeternaturaliter subsistant*; of further interest might be that the term, according to C, was introduced in Latin medical language by Stahl, in the dissertation *De motibus humanis spasmoticis*. Not found in B.

STRABISMUS, Schröder 29; squinting
Gr. στραβισμός, Galen 19.436; not found in ancient Latin, whereas *strabonus* (adj.), 'squinting' is found in Petronius 68 (the reign of Nero). *Strabismus* is found in all four references.

SYMTOMA, Martin 6.2; symptom
Gr. σύμπτωμα, Philodemus Ir. p29W (1st cent. BC); in Latin *symptomata, vita S. Guillelmi archiep. Bituric.* t I p 639 (duCange). Found, spelled *symptoma*, in all four references; in B with the addition *sive accidens*.

SYNCOPE Martin 6.7 (footnote g); fainting
Gr. συγκοπή, Aretaios *SA* 2.3 (2nd cent.); in Latin Vegetius 1.35. Found in all four references.

Pure Latin words

General remarks

As is seen from table 1 above, the anatomical word stock of the texts dealt with is, with certain exceptions, pure Latin, while the originally Greek terms still constitute the majority – if not by much – of the pathological and physiological terms.

As is mentioned above, certain readily observable pathological phenomena already had pure Latin names in ancient Roman society – such words are e.g. *tormina*, 'colic', and *tumor*, 'swelling' – while others are early Latin translations of Greek terms; of this kind, several examples are found in, and maybe coined by, Celsus, e.g. *abscessus*, Greek ἀπόστημα, 'swelling', and *inflammatio*, Gr. φλεγμονή/φλόγωσις 'inflammation'. To these two important categories can, for the Neo-Latin period, be added terms denoting newly described syndromes, such as e.g. [*febris*] *scarlatina* (i.e. scarlet fever), dating from 1676, when it was described in Thomas Sydenham's *Observationes Medicae*; such new additions to the terminology were to a great extent Latin, which, by the time dealt with here, had lead to the majority of the Greek terms being rather narrow.

Latin word list

ABSCESSUS, Bergius 5.30; swelling
From *abscedo*, 'to leave'; *abscessus* is used by Celsus: *Ergo tum lippitudines, pustulae, profusio sanguinis*, abscessus *corporis, quae* ἀποστήματα *Graeci nominant* (2.1.6). The Greek term ἀπόστημα as used by Hippocrates in *Aph.* 7.36 seems however not to denote that which is understood by an abscess today (i.e. a large pustule or boil), but appears rather to be some kind of swelling from retention of fluid in the body, in this case due to malfunctioning kidneys. It is of course possible that ἀπόστημα and *abscessus* are used to denote swellings in general, regardless of their contents, a usage which then would include also the abscess of today. There is on the other hand a word, *vomica*, originally denoting the discharge from an abscess, which seems to be used by Celsus about (especially internal?) abscesses, e.g. of the lung: *Dolor etiam pulmonis, si neque etiam per sputa neque per sanguinis detractionem neque per victus rationem finitus est*, vomicas *aliquas intus excitat* ... (2.7.33). The sense in Bergius' text seems to be the same as in Celsus; the *abscessus* are said to be *salutares* ... *si* ... *ad suppurationem redacti*, which would indicate, that pus is not necessarily involved from the start. Cf also **SUPPURATIO** below. Found in B and C, in both cases in the general sense.

BILIOSUS, Bergius 3.5; mixed with bile
In Isidorus *Orig.* 10.30 meaning 'melancholic'; in the present meaning in Celsus 2.6, 2.8. In B used to denote a person, suffering from too much bile. Not found in C.

BULLOSA, Bergius 1.7; a disease with bladders of the skin
From *bulla*, 'bubble' or 'bladder'; the adj, or substantivized adj, as here seems not to be known from ancient or mediaeval Latin; B does not include the word at all, while C has *bulla*, regarded as synonymous to *pustula*. Bergius, for this word, gives a reference to Boissier de Sauvages; the term is not found in the 1759 edition of Sauvages' *Pathologia Methodica*, but the rash, as described in Bergius' text, resembles that of *varicellae* (i.e. chickenpox). The malady *efflorescentia bullosa* is found in *Bene Med.* II.180 (Bartal), which is later however.

CALCULUS, Sundius 9.1; a stone of the urine bladder
A small stone; known in the present sense from e.g. Celsus 7.26. Also in B, where the *calculus* is said to consist mainly of concretions of earths and salts, and in C.

CONTAGIO and **CONTAGIUM**, Martin, passim; infection, contagion
Originally both words mean 'touching' or 'contact' in any sense, good or bad; in the sense of 'infection' *contagio* is found in e.g. Columella 6.5.1, while the npl. *contagia* originally seems to have been the poetical equivalent (cf. OLD, s.v. *contagium*) of *contagio*; it is known from e.g. Lucretius 3.472, and Virgil *Ecl.* 1.50.

For the Neo-Latin period, we might note that Fracastoro, in his *De contagione* (1546) uses *contagio* in the more abstract sense of 'infection', while the "infectious matter" is called *seminaria contagionis*.

As for the texts treated here, there are eleven occurrences of *contagium* to be found in Martin, and one in Bergius, while *contagio* is found in thirteen passages of Martin's text and once in Sundius; even if it is not possible to establish the exact sense in every instance, there quite clearly is a general tendency towards using *contagio* in the more abstract sense, in accordance with the usage of Fracastoro, while *contagium* seems to be used about the infectious matter.

Found in B and C.

DELIRIUM, Martin 6.1, Bergius 5.7

Celsus 2.8, 3.18; in B described as indicating a state of grave delusions; C gives the synonym *insania*.

EXCRETORIUS (adj.), Martin 16.2

From *excerno*, 'separate' or 'discharge'; *excreta* (npl) is the waste matter produced by the body. The present adj. is not known from ancient Latin. Not found in B or C, while C has *excretio*, which is regarded as mainly a synonym of *excrementum*.

The term is frequently used by von Haller in *Primae lineae physiologiae*, e.g. on p 84: [*liquida*] *in proprios ductus excretorios deposita.* Cf. also **INFLAMMATORIUS** and **SECRETORIUS** below.

FEBRIS

Fever, Varro ap. Non. 46.22. Obviously found in both B and C. B also gives a definition: *sanguinis velocitas aucta.*

FLUXUS, Martin 7.1; flow, flux

The word *fluxus* in itself is not necessarily a medical term, but is used in a medical context e.g. in Pliny *NH* 9.79, cf. also DuCange, III.529, *fluxus albus* s.v. fluxus. Found in B in the specific compounds *fluxus alvinus*, ~ *chylosus* and ~ *hepaticus*, while it is not found at all in C. For the Neo-latin period, see also Máty 343 (1762)(Bartal).

FONTANELLA, Schröder 26; fontanel

Fontanella or *fontinella* is known from mediaeval Latin, e.g. Gilbertus Anglicus (d. c. 1250): *cateria maniacis fiant in fontinella colli vel capitis* (II, 106.1) (MLBr), where the sense seems not to be the present one, but rather that indicated in Hyrtl, p 219sq as referred to below.

According to Hyrtl's article, *fontanella gehört nicht der lateinischen, sondern der italienischen Sprache an*; the reason for the name is said to be the originally Arab practice of treating ailments of the head by burning the skin on the fontanel area of the head and keeping the wound running; he also says that good latinists use *fonticulus* or *fons pulsatilis* for the fontanel. In fact, the correct word in medical Latin of today still is *fonticulus* according to Dorland, s.v. "fontanelle". Of the 18th century medical dictionaries, B has, s.v. *Fontanella seu fonticulus*, the modern anatomical sense first, but also mentions the older sense; C has, s.v. *Fonticulus*, the word in its original sense, with a reference to *Fons* for the modern meaning.

The English word "fontanel", on the other hand, is by OED said to originate from Fr. *fontenelle*; in the sense dealt with here, the first occurrence in English dates from 1741: "That Part of the *parietal* and *frontal* Bones, where the *Fontanelle* is in Children" (Monro: *Anatomy of the Bones*, p 71 (OED)).

FRENULUM, Sundius 9.3; the frenulum linguae

Dim. of *frenum*, 'bridle' etc; hence, in a transferred sense, used about several anatomical parts with a more or less 'restricting' function.

According to Hyrtl, s.v. *Frenulum*, this is *kein gutes lateinisches Wort* in Classical Latin, no diminutive form is found, and *frenum* is more frequent in the plural, while the singular form is introduced by Celsus to denote the *frenulum praeputii penis* in 7.25: *si glans ita contecta est, ut nudari not possit ... aperienda est; quod hoc modo fit: subter a summa ora cutis inciditur recta linea usque ad frenum*; Hyrtl further seems to regard the origin of the diminutive form simply as a result of anatomists' liking it better. He also points out that if one were to keep to the Classical Latin usage, such structures as the one treated here would have to be called a *habena* or *habenula*.

The *frenulum linguae*, as it is still called, notwithstanding Hyrtl's opinion, is the fold of mucous membrane which connects the tongue with the floor of the mouth. Not found in this sense in B or C, while Zedler has *frenulum linguae*.

GIBBER, Schröder 20; hunch-backed
Known from e.g. Varro *RR*, 2.5.7. Not found in this form in B or C. B has, however, the form *gibbus*, which is synonymous, while C has the noun *gibbositas*, with a reference to *cyphosis*.

GLANDULA (npl), Schröder 1; glands
In ancient Latin, the common medical denotation seems, specifically, to have been the glands of the throat, *tonsillae*, so in Celsus 4.1. Found in the present general sense in both B and C.

GLOBULUS sanguinis ruber, Martin 7.2, Bergius 8.5; red blood corpuscle
Even if the modern medical notion of the cell would not be formed until the middle of the 19th century, by Rudolf Virchow (1821–1902), the word had been used in its biological sense already by Robert Hooke (1635–1703) in his *Micrographia*, p 112sqq (1665), then pertaining to observations in vegetable material.

The observation also of small particles in the blood was of course possible to the 17th century microscopists, among them Marcello Malpighi (1628–94), and Anton van Leeuwenhoek (1632–1723) – the former a physician and professor, the latter a mechanically skilled amateur, who is said to have made more than 400 microscopes for himself – who, apparently without any notion of each other, studied and described the details of several tissues in the body. Fåhraeus mentions (*Läkekonstens historia*, II, p 134) that Leeuwenhoek used the red blood corpuscle as a measure when describing his observations. *Globulus* is found in C, who also gives a reference to Leeuwenhoek. In B, *Globulus* is also found, but then in the sense of some kind of tumour.

INFLAMMATIO, Martin 5.2, and **INFLAMMATIUNCULA**, Bergius 1.1
Literally a 'burning' of or 'setting fire' to something (e.g. Cicero *Har. resp.* 3). In the present medical sense found in Celsus, e.g. 1. *prooem.* 15: *inflammationem, quam Graeci* φλεγμονήν *vocant*, which might indicate that the word as a technical term has in fact been introduced by Celsus as a direct translation, or 3.10.3, where also the symptoms are given: *notae inflammationis sunt quattuor: rubor et tumor cum calore et dolore.*

Inflammatiuncula is of course a diminutive form, which, even if does not happen to be known from ancient Latin, would be quite easily created when needed.[64] In the present case it denotes the individual, local inflammations of the skin, forming the actual pustules, as opposed to the general state of inflammation, which at the same time affects the entire organism.

INFLAMMATORIUS (adj.), Bergius 5.6
This adj, denoting the quality of bringing about an inflammation, or at least the ability to do so, is not known from ancient Latin. Cf. **EXCRETORIUS** and **SECRETORIUS**.

---

[64] For comparison one might e.g. note that Hoven's *Lexique de la Prose Latine de la Renaissance* lists 557 examples of Neo-Latin diminutives (pp 399–403); cf. also IJsewijn & Sacré, p 382.

INSULTUS [epilepticus], Martin 6.2, Bergius 5.5; fit [of epilepsy]

Insultus is originally (*Carm. de Pass. Chr.* 30, in Lactantius) a synonym to *insultatio*, which in ancient Latin (e.g. Quintilian 8.5.11) means 'scoffing' or 'insulting'. In mediaeval Latin, acc. to DuCange, p 384, s.v. *insultus*, the normal sense seems to be that of a more physical aggression. The sense here, as in the medical language of today, could perhaps be regarded as an example of the military metaphors, which still are quite common in medical language. Found in both B and C.

LUES venerea, Martin 13.2; syphilis

Originally, *lues* means 'plague' or 'pestilence' in general, so in *Carmen Arvale*, and *lues venerea* would then be 'the veneric plague', 'the plague of Venus', i.e. 'syphilis'. This disease was probably unknown in Europe until the late 15th century, when it was transferred from America and then, following the French siege of Naples, spread across the continent, whence the name *morbus Neapolitanus*. Since the disease most notably is spread by sexual intercourse, it was called *lues venerea*. The denomination "syphilis" dates from 1530, when the Veronese physician Girolamo Fracastoro published a didactic poem titled *Syphilis, sive morbus Gallicus*, where the malady is sent by Apollo as a punishment for the impiety of the shepherd Syphilus, who, angry with the hot sun, has abused the god. It might be noted, that the term *lues* today is used only about syphilis, while the meaning 'plague' has altogether vanished. Both B and C mention *lues*; B gives the synonym *siphylis* (sic) *Fracastorii*. Cf also **MERCURIUS vivus** in the pharmacological word list, below.

MEDULLA spinalis, Martin 4.6; the spinal cord

Medulla, meaning the 'marrow' or 'pith' of bones (e.g. in Lucretius 3.250) or plants, or, in general, 'the innermost part' of anything, literally or figuratively, is not necessarily on its own a technical term. The technical term *medulla spinalis*, possibly influenced by Celsus, who has *spinae medulla* (8.1.11) for the spinal cord, is said by Hyrtl, *Onomatologia Anatomica*, p357 to have been introduced by Alessandro Benedetti (1460–1525), thus replacing the earlier, originally Arab name *nucha* (see below, s.v. **NUCHA**); there are however several instances of *spinalis medulla* to be found as early as Burgundio's 12th century Galen translations, e.g. in *De complexionibus*, 1.9: *Spinalis autem medulla humidior quidem, sed frigidior*. Found in B, while C has only *medulla*, in the sense of marrow of bone, without any mention of the *medulla spinalis* in particular; this is however found in Zedler, with a reference to *Rücken-Marck*.

MILIARIA (pl), Bergius 1.3; any disease with millet seed sized rash

From *milium*, 'millet'; nowadays, acc. to Dorland's *Medical Dictionary* (24th ed, p 930, s.v. *miliaria*), a syndrome of skin changes from retention of sweat, which give a rash, resembling the size of millet seeds. B and C both have *milium* in the botanical sense, but not *miliaria*. Zedler has *miliaris herpes*, referring to *Flechte*, where a further reference is found, to *impetigo*. It is probable, that *miliaria* could be used about any rash of millet-seed size, regardless of origin. Cf. **PAPULA**, below.

MORBILLI (pl), Bergius 2.6; measles

This term, a diminutive form of *morbus*, is used to denote the measles; cf. **RUBEOLA**, below.

NUCHA, Bergius 9.4; back of the neck

Originally an Arab word, *nūcha'*, which is used by Rhazes and Avicenna for the spinal cord, while the Arab word used for the back of the neck is actually *nuqrah* according to Hyrtl (p 356). *Nucha* is said by Hyrtl (ibid.) to have been introduced in Latin by Constantinus Afer (1015–87), still in its Arabic sense, which it was to stand until Alessandro Benedetti, striving to clear the medical language of all terms of other than Greek or Latin origin,[65] introduced the term *medulla spinalis* (cf. however above, s.v. **MEDULLA SPINALIS**). *Nucha* is found in B in the present sense, while C has both the original denotation and the later one, as is the case also in Zedler.

OBSTIPATIO, Bergius 8.17, Schröder 32; constipation

The general sense of this word is that of a 'piling up' or an 'accumulation'; the word is known from Laurentius,[66] where it is used about a crowd: *turbarum obsti[r]patione seclusus*. The word is not found in B or C, which might indicate that it still has not become a technical term in itself, but is rather one of several words used to indicate constipation. One might also note, that obstipation in Dorland indicates a more intractable state than constipation does, while Renander (*Medicinsk terminologi*, 1964) regards the two terms as synonymous.

ORIFICIUM ventriculi, Bergius 5.11; orifice of the stomach

The word *orificium*, from *os*, 'mouth', seems to have been used about any opening of the body; for the particular openings of the stomach, the *cardia* and the *pylorus*, cf. Macrobius *Sat.* 7.4.17 *ventris duo sunt orificia*. While the English language still keeps "orifice" in e.g. "cardiac orifice" (i.e. *cardia*), *orificium* has in many cases been replaced by *ostium* in Latin terminology. The term is not found in B, while C gives a reference to Bartholin, *l.1, Anat cap 9.*

PALPHEBRA, Martin 6.6

For *palpebra*, a common Classical word for the eyelid.

PAPULA, Bergius 1.3; bladder, pustule

The word *papula* is known from Celsus, where it, however, is described not as a symptom, but as a particular skin disease, with two varieties:

> *papularum vero duo genera sunt. Alterum est in quo per minimas pusulas cutis exasperatur*
> *et rubet leviterque roditur: medium habet pauxillo levius, tarde serpit ... Altera autem est,*
> *quam agrian (id est feram) Graeci appellant; in qua similiter quidem sed magis cutis*

---

[65] In Benedetti's *Praefatio ad divum Maximilianum Caesarem Augustum* (1503) to his *Anatomice sive de Hystoria corporis humani libri V*, he writes (6v. l.9sqq): *Singulatim praeterea membrorum omnium potentiam cognosces, eorumque nomina tam graeca quam latina, omissis barbaris, percurres, quae Pollux author exquisitissimus, ad Commodum Caesarem summatim persecutus est.* Further, he writes (7r. l.11sqq): *Itaque inter laureas coronas, humanissime princeps hos libellos de historia membrorum hominis, quos latinos pro virili parte fecimus, suscipias, in quibus non sine aliquo labore multa annotavimus, quae a recentioribus praetermissa sunt, qui latinam linguam externis, immo barbaris vocabulis variisque erroribus dedecorarunt, ...* It might be added that the *Pollux* mentioned is the Egyptian-Greek rhetorician and lexicographer Iulius Pollux (fl.c. 170 AD), who edited an *onomasticon* in ten volumes, which was an important source of words to the Atticists, even if Pollux was criticized for incorporating also Homeric and other non-Attic words. The surviving parts of Pollux' *onomasticon* were edited 1900–37 by E. Bethe.

[66] *De Paenitentia* 98[B] (ed Migne)

exasperatur exulceraturque, ac vehementius et roditur et rubet et interdum etiam pilos remittit.(5.28.18).

It might be observed that this word has undergone a change of meaning, which is different from that in most other cases, inasmuch as its meaning has become extended rather than narrowed. The plural is found in B, with a reference to *exanthema*, and regarded as a *species morbillorum*, thus still as a disease rather than as a symptom, while C gives the sense indicated in the present text. In Zedler, the synonym *Hitzblättergen* is given, and several varieties are listed, among which *papula fera*, with a reference to *Flechte* (cf. **MILIARIA**, above). It might be added, that a German synonym of *Hitzblättergen* is *Friesel* (used also in 18th century Swedish, as e.g. in Rosén's *Underrättelser*, p 109) which seems to be an old word for 'millet'; this obviously does not mean, that *miliaria* and *papulae* were regarded as the same disease, but is rather an indication of the main point being the ambition to describe adequately a rash of a specific size and looks as a symptom regardless of the particular disease.

PETECHIAE (pl), Martin 6.5, Bergius 1.6

The Latin form of It. *petecchia*, a spot, which, acc. to Klein, *A comprehensive etymological dictionary of the English language*, II, probably is derived from Gr. πιττάκιον, 'writing-table', 'tablet', or 'label'. The disease named Petechiae is mentioned both in B, where the synonym *pulicharis febris* is given, and in C. Zedler gives a reference to *Flech-fieber*.

PLEXUS nervosus, Bergius 5.12

Plexus in the anatomical sense of a network of vessels or nerves is not known from ancient or mediaeval Latin usage, but would of course be a word close at hand to anatomists from Vesalius on, when describing the internal findings of the human body; it is to be found in B and in C, where it is used mainly about blood vessels however.

PRAECORDIA (npl), Martin 6.1

Praecordia has been used since before the classical Latin period, and in different senses; Plautus uses it in *Merc.* 124: *Genua hunc cursorem deserunt; perii, seditionem facit lien, occupat praecordia*, where the mentioning of other actual parts of the body, likely to react negatively to exaggerated physical exercise, indicates an anatomical sense; comparing Plautus' text to my own, certainly rather limited, experience of running, I would say that what is meant is probably the midriff. The word is also used, especially in poetry, in the sense 'the breast', 'the heart', referring to the aleged seat of feelings and passions, cf. Virgil *Aen.* 2.367 *victis redit in praecordia virtus.* In Pliny, the meaning is more anatomical, albeit rather vaguely defined: *Praecordia ... vocamus exta in homine* (NH 30.42), and in Celsus *praecordia* often seems to be synonymous to *hypochondrium* (i.e. the upper lateral regions of the abdomen, just below the thorax): *si praecordia eius sine ullo sensu doloris aequaliter mollia in utraque parte sunt* (Celsus 2.3); in *De interioribus* two explanations are found: *epigastrium id est precordium* and *ypocondrium idest precordium;* in C, *praecordia* is on the contrary described as *quod utrique hypochondrio interjacet*, while B defines it, in accordance with Pliny, as *viscera omnia in thorace*. Nowadays, the *praecordium* is defined as the region in front of the heart, which indicates a position somewhat higher than that, which seems to be indicated by Celsus; exactly which part of the body Martin aims at, is not possible to ascertain; cf. **SCROBICULUS cordis**, below.

PUS, Martin 5.1, Bergius 8.20

Acc. to Forcellini (IV, 1011, s.v. *pus*) of uncertain origin; probably related to Gr. πύον/πύος (Hippocrates *Aph.* 2.47, *Morb.* 1.15) and known in Latin e.g. from Celsus, 5.26.20:

> *Ex his* [*vulneribus*] *autem exit sanguis, sanies, pus. Sanguis omnibus notus est: sanies est*
> *tenuior hoc, varie crassa et glutinosa et colorata. Pus crassissimum albidissimumque,*
> *glutinosius et sanguine et sanie.*

The passage above from Celsus indicates that even if the word was known to everyone, the medical science had developed a specific notion and a strict definition which turns the word into a technical term.

We might also note that pus is generally regarded as a positive sign, inasmuch as it is regarded as a necessary evacuation of corrupt matter; in accordance with this view, the pus is described as *bonum* e.g. in **Bergius 8.8** and **10.3**; furthermore, where the prevention of pustules appearing is discussed, this is normally brought about by making them appear elsewhere by means of epispastics.

PUSTULA, Martin 6.3, Bergius 2.8; a bladder

In ancient Latin, *pustula* or *pusula* was a vaster concept than it is today, e.g. in Celsus, who seems to use the word in the same sense as *papula* is used in Neo-Latin and modern vocabulary (cf. **PAPULA** above):

> *Earum plura genera sunt. Nam modo ... aspritudo ... fit, similis iis pusulis, quae ex urtica*
> *vel sudore nascuntur: exanthemata Graeci vocant .... Nonnumquam plures similes varis*
> *oriuntur, nonnumquam maiores pusulae lividae aut pallidae aut nigrae, aut aliter naturali*
> *colore mutato; subestque his umor* (5.28.15).

The word has presumably nothing to do with Latin *pus*, but is more likely related to Gr. φυσάω, to 'blow' or 'inflate'.

QUARTANA (noun), Bergius 10.27

Quartana, originally an adjective, is already substantivized in classical Latin; denoting, as here, *febris quartana*, it is used by Cicero: *In quartanam conversa vis est morbi* (Cicero *Fam.* XVI.11), and by Horace: *Frigida si puerum quartana reliquerit* (*Sat.* 2.3.290).

Admittedly, these two occurrences do not say very much about the medical usage of the period, but might just as likely be colloquialisms. However, the noun is also to be found in Celsus: *Quartana aestiva brevis, autumnalis fere longa est* (2.8.42), which provides a stronger case in this respect. Found, as a noun, in both C and B.

QUOTIDIANA (noun), Bergius 10.27

As **QUARTANA** above, a substantivized adjective, denoting a particular variety of fever, apparently one that fluctuated in cycles, comprising twenty-four hours; cf. **AMPHEMERINA** above.

RENES succenturiati, Bergius 3.9; the adrenal glands

These glands have been known under several names since they were discovered by Bartolommeo Eustachio (1524–74), who called them *glandulae renibus incumbentes.*
In Rosén's *Compendium anatomicum* (1738), p 337, the adrenal glands are mentioned as *capsulae atrabiliariae*, while Albrecht von Haller's *Primae lineae physiologiae* (1747), p 414, has *capsulae renales*; the term used here was coined by the Italian anatomist Giulio Casserio (c. 1552–1616); the glands in question are found in B, where also the

synonyms *capsulae atrabiliariae* and *glandulae suprarenales* are given, while C does not mention any of the terms.

RUBEOLA, Bergius 1.4; measles
Not known from ancient Latin, nor from mediaeval Latin in a medical sense. Not found in C, but in B, where it is regarded as a *species variolarum/morbillorum*. The mentioning of Boissier de Sauvages in Bergius' text indicates that he is the main source for the term (Cf. also **BULLOSA** above).[67] In fact, there is still some uncertainty as to what is actually to be meant by *rubeola*; Dorland (1965) gives the definitions 1: Measles; 2: Rubella (i.e. German measles), while the word *rubella* is defined as 1: German measles and 2: Measles. The most common usage among English speakers seems to be, that *rubeola* = measles and *rubella* = German measles; in Sweden, on the other hand, *rubeola* used to be = German measles, which are now called *rubella*, while measles have always been known as *morbilli*.

SALIVATIO, Bergius 8.20
From *saliva*, which is etymologically related to Gr. σίαλον, with the same meaning. *Salivatio* is found in Caelius Aurelianus 3. *Acut.* 2, and then only as a symptom, while it in C is regarded also as a – desirable and intended – result of certain therapeutic measures. B. gives the synonym *ptyalismus* (Gr.)

SCABIES, Bergius 3.12, Sundius 0.3, and **SCABIOSUS** (adj.), Martin 14.2
Scabies, from *scabo*, 'itch', is known from Celsus 5.28.16: *Scabies vero durior: cutis rubicunda, ex qua pusulae oriuntur, quaedam umidiores, quaedam sicciores*, where it is described as mainly a matter of the skin getting rough and hardened. In B it serves as a collective name for *pruritus, impetigo, psora* and *lepra*. C only refers to *psora*. Nowadays the term *scabies* is reserved for the symptoms caused by *Sarcoptes scabiei*, the itch mite.

The adjective *scabiosus* is in ancient Latin used partly about anything that is rough or uneven e.g (of corals): *probatissimum quam maxime rubens et quam ramosissimum nec scabiosum aut lapideum aut rursus inane et concavum* (Pliny *NH* 32.11.22); partly to denote somebody, suffering from scabies, perhaps also as a word of abuse, as possibly in Persius 2.12-14: *Hercule! pupillumve utinam, quem proximus heres | inpello, expungam! namque est scabiosus et acri | bile tumet*. In a more literal sense, it is found in Columella (on the feeding of cattle on acorns): *Nam si paucioribus diebus datur, ut ait Hyginus, per ver scabiosi boves fiunt.* (11.2.83). In Martin's text, where *scabiosus* is used to denote a particular kind of *miasma*, it is likely, that the sense is that of containing/bringing about scabies, rather than that of any more physical feature. The word is not found in C or B.

SCARLATINA, Sundius 6.1; scarlet fever
This disease, caused by the A-type *streptococcus*, had, as we know, not been differentiated from measles until the late 17th century, by Thomas Sydenham, and thus is not likely to be found in any earlier sources. It is mentioned in C and B, in both cases with a reference to Sydenham.

---

[67] In the 1759 edition of Sauvages' *Pathologia Methodica* the author writes (p 276) *Rubeola, vulgo morbilli*, which indicates that *rubeola*, as in modern English usage, is in fact measles; *rubeola SAUVAGES* in Bergius' text might thus, as measles is otherwise called *morbilli* in these texts, be taken to mean simply "the disease which Sauvages calls *rubeola*"

SCROBICULUS cordis, Bergius 5.21

Scrobiculus is a diminutive of *scrobis*, meaning a hole or a pit; a *scrobiculus cordis* is, according to Hyrtl (p 470), only possible to see in those human beings, where the cartilage of the lower ribs protrudes, compared to the cartilage of the sternum, or where the tip of the sternum's cartilage is somewhat bent. Hyrtl says further:

> *Man könnte, um die Trias seiner deutschen Benennungen vollständig zu machen, der Herzgrube, und der Magengrube, noch eine Lebergrube zur Gesellschaft geben. Ich sage dieses nur, um ersichtlich zu machen, wie vag der Begriff der Herzgrube ist.*

The term is found in both B and C; both give the synonym *anticordium*. The sense in my texts, as in general, probably is that of a quite vaguely defined area in front of the heart. Cf. **PRAECORDIA**, above.

SECRETORIUS (adj.), Martin 16.2

From *secerno*, to separate; *secretio* is, in medical language, the production of a gland. Another adjective of the same kind as **EXCRETORIUS** and **INFLAMMATORIUS** above, which is also unknown from ancient Latin, but, like **EXCRETORIUS**, used in von Haller's *Primae lineae physiologiae*, e.g. on p 98: *si multa secretoria organa ex ordine ex arteria secretice provenerint.*

SINCIPUT, Schröder 26

In ancient Latin, *sinciput* (*semis* + *caput*) is used to denote half the head of e.g. a pig: *sincipita verrina* (Pliny *NH* 8.209), especially when used for food.

In medical language of today, however, as in this case, the meaning is 'the anterior and upper part of the head'; this sense is indicated by Petri Gothus, as is the ancient one.

SPUTUM, Bergius 5.29; expectoration

From *spuo*, 'spit', or 'spit out'; *sputum* is in ancient Latin used about spittle in general, e.g. in Seneca *Constant.* 2.1 (about M. Cato):

> *tibi indignum videbatur quod ... a Rostris usque ad Arcum Fabianum per seditiosae factionis manus traditus, voces improbas et sputa et omnes alias insanae multitudinis contumelias pertulisset.*

It is, however, also used in what seems to be a more specifically medical sense by Celsus:

> *In pulmonis morbo si sputo ipso levatur dolor, quamvis id purulentum est tamen aeger facile spirat, facile excreat, morbum ipsum non difficulter fert, potest ei secunda valetudo contingere. Neque inter initia terreri convenit, si protinus sputum mixtum est rufo quodam et sanguine, dummodo statim edatur* (2.8.2),

where the context indicates, that *sputum* here means 'expectoration' rather than 'saliva', thus giving the word the same meaning as in present-day medical language. B treats this word as if it were only a matter of consistency; he defines *sputum* as a *liquor saliva paulo crassior, ab amygdalis &c. in os effusus.*

C. only gives the Greek synonym *ptyelon.*

STUPOR, Martin 6.1, Bergius 5.4
A word, which in ancient Latin could mean a defect or malfunction in any of the senses: *ut quidam morbo aliquo et sensus stupore suavitatem cibi non sentiunt* ... (Cicero *Phil.* 2.45), or a more general stupidity:

> *Tantus igitur te stupor oppressit vel, ut verius dicam, tantus furor, ut primum, cum sector sis*
> *isto loco natus, deinde cum Pompei sector, non te exsecratum populo Romano, non*
> *detestabilem, non omnis tibi deos, non omnes homines et esse inimicos et futuros scias?*
> (*Phil.* 2.26)

In the sense here, probably close to that of today, denoting a state of severe inertia, bordering on unconsciousness, like that found e.g. among deeply depressed patients, *stupor* is found neither in ancient Latin – Celsus seems, e.g, to prefer *torpor* to describe this condition – nor in mediaeval usage. There are however two instances in *De interioribus*, where *stupor* is used to explain the Greek word *coma*, which is close to modern usage. B and C both have the word in its more modern sense, C with a reference to *narche*.

SUPPURATIO, Martin 2.1, Bergius 5.26
Suppuratio, from *pus*, is the production of pus in e.g. a wound, thus normally denoting the process, rather than the result, which would be the *abscessus* or, in Celsus, *vomica*. Forcellini seems however to regard *suppuratio* as synonymous to *vomica* and *abscessus*, which might be true in some cases; there are instances of *suppuratio* probably meaning the result of the aforementioned process, e.g. in Pliny: *Sativae quoque derasae sucus tepefactus auribus medetur, caro eius interior sine semine clavis pedum et suppurationibus quae Graeci vocant* ἀποστήματα (*NH* 20.8) (cf. *abscessus*, above), but Celsus seems to use it about the process, e.g. in 2.8.4:

> *Ex suppurationibus vero eae tolerabiles sunt, quae in exteriorem partem feruntur et*
> *acuuntur. At ex iis, quae intus procedunt, eae leviores, quae contra se cutem non adficiunt,*
> *eamque et sine dolore esse et eiusdem coloris, cuius reliquae partes sunt, sinunt esse,*

where verbs like *procedunt* and *adficiunt* seem to indicate some kind of activity, and in 3.27.4:

> *Suppurationes autem, quae in aliqua interiore parte oriuntur, ubi notae fuerint, primum id*
> *agere oportet per ea cataplasmata, quae reprimunt, ne coitus inutilis materiae fiat; deinde ...*
> *dissipentur. Quod si consecuti non sumus, sequitur ut evocetur, deinde, ut maturescat. Omnis*
> *tum vomicae finis est, ut rumpatur,*

where the process *suppuratio* is mentioned together with the result *vomica*. B has a reference to *abscessus*, while C gives the synonym *purulentia* and a reference to *ecpyema/empyema*.

TORMINA [ventris] (npl), Schröder 31; colic
Tormina, fr. *torqueo*, 'turn', 'wring', or 'torment'; in the sense of pains in the stomach or abdomen found already in Cato's *De agri cultura*, e.g. 126: *Ad tormina et si alvus non consistet et si taeniae et lumbrici molesti erunt, triginta mala punica acerba sumito* ... Found, perhaps in a more specific sense, in Celsus 4.22:

> *Proxima his inter intestinorum mala tormina esse consueverunt: dysenteria Graece vocatur.*
> *Intus intestina exulcerantur; ex his cruor manat isque modo cum stercore aliquo semper*

liquido, modo cum quibusdam quasi muccosis excernitur, interdum simul quaedam carnosa descendunt; frequens deiciendi cupiditas dolorque in ano est.

According to Forcellini *tormina* could also be used about pains from other diseases; his two examples, both from Pliny, seem however both to regard abdominal pains, certainly related to urine problems, but nevertheless not very different from the original sense. It is quite possible, the word obviously having been known well before Celsus' definition, that it has been continously used by laymen in the more general sense of abdominal pains regardless of cause, while physicians have tended to rely on Celsus; B gives e.g. a reference to *dysenteria*. In the medical language of today, the usage has again became more general; in Dorland, *tormina* is defined as 'the colic', while, s.v. "colic", the definition "acute abdominal pain" is given, whereupon no less than thirty-seven different kinds are listed. The sense of *tormina* in the texts treated here, finally, seems to be closer to the modern sense than to that found in Celsus.

TUBERCULUM, Martin 6.8, Bergius 8.12; nodule
Diminutive of tuber, a nodule or tumour; tuberculum could in ancient Latin denote any small tumour, e.g. in Celsus: *In hoc* (sc. *capite*) *multa variaque tubercula oriuntur: ganglia, meliceridas, aetheromata nominant aliisque etiamnum vocabulis quaedam alii discernunt, quibus ego steatomata quoque adiciam* (7.6).

In Bergius' text, the word is used about the smallpox rash, in the stage before that of suppuration; B and C both give references to *phyma*. Hyrtl treats *tuber/tuberculum* together with *tuberositas*, which he regards as being different; while *tuber* and its diminutive *tuberculum* denote smooth nodes, *tuberositas* is said to be a *höckeriger (nicht glatter) Höcker* (Hyrtl, p 577). In present day usage, a tubercle could be either: a) a nodule of the skin, larger than a *papula*; b) the particular kind of node, brought about by the *Mycobacterium tuberculosis*, or c) a more anatomical term, denoting nodules or small eminences of bones, while *tuberculum* is only used about c).

TUMOR, Bergius 5.29; swelling
In ancient Latin *tumor* is used both literally, e.g: *citiusque repentinus oculorum tumor sanatur quam diuturna lippitudo depellitur* (Cicero *Tusc.* 4.37), and figuratively, about the results of vehement emotions in general: *cum tumor animi resedisset* (Cicero *Tusc.* 3.12); perhaps particularly of anger: *nullus tumor indignationis in diis est* (Arnobius 1.28) and presumption: *hinc tumor et vana de se persuasio* (Quintilian 2.2.12). As for medical usage, it is found in Celsus, used to denote swellings in general, e.g. from flatulence in 2.3: *Si inflatio in superiorem partibus dolorem tumoremque fecit, bonum signum est sonus ventris …*; of a presumably more oedematose kind, related to a malfunctioning liver, in 2.7: *tumor in pedibus est, idemque modo dextra modo sinistra parte ventris invicem oritur atque finitur: sed a iocinere id malum proficisci videtur*, but also about more specific varieties. The sense in the present material is thus the same as in ancient Latin, which also is one of the meanings of *tumor* in medical Latin of today; found in C, with references to Gr. *oncos* and *oedos*, and in B.

TUSSIS, Martin 6.1; cough
Known in ancient Latin, e.g. from Terence *Heaut.* 2.3.132: *gemitus screatus tussis risus abstine.* Used also in medical writing, e.g. by Celsus:

Aliud autem quamvis non multum distans malum gravedo est. Haec nares claudit, vocem obtundit, tussim siccam movet; sub eadem salsa est saliva, sonant aures, venae moventur in capite, turbida urina est. Haec omnia κόρυζας *Hippocrates nominat* (4.5).

Found in both B and C; still in use in medical language in the same sense, but hardly to be regarded as a specifically medical term, unless combined with attributes like e.g. *ferina*.

UREDO, Bergius 1.5; some itch or smart, perhaps *urticaria*
From *uro*, 'to burn'; originally, *uredo* is the 'blight', 'rust' or 'mildew' of plants, trees, etc, as e.g. in Columella 3.20:

> *Neque enim umquam sic mitis ac temperatus est annus, ut nullo incommodo vexet aliquod vitis genus: sive siccus est, id quod umore proficit, contristatur; seu pluvius, quod siccitatibus gaudet; seu frigidus et pruinosus, quod non est patiens uredinis.*

Uredo is however also used, by Pliny, in what might possibly be the same sense as here:

> *Sophocles enim poeta venenatum id (sc. trifolium) dicit, Simos quoque ex medicis, decocti aut contriti sucum infusum corpori easdem uredines facere quas si percussis a serpente inponatur* (*NH* 21.88).

In DuCange (8, p 383, s.v. *uredo*) the only meaning given is that of 'the rust', while both meanings are found in Faber Soranus (2680, s.v. *uredo*). In C, the term is, for some reason, explained as *dolor capitis*, while it is not found at all in B. As for modern medical usage, *uredo* is found in Dorland, where it is said to mean 1) an itching or burning sensation of the skin, and 2) urticaria, while it is not found in either Renander nor in Lindskog/Zetterberg.

VARIOLA, Martin, Bergius passim; smallpox
Probably from adj. *varius*, 'mottled', or noun *varus*, a 'blotch' or 'pimple'. According to Barquet and Domingo, the term *variola* was first used by Bishop Marius of Avenches (c. 530–594) in 570; duCange quotes gloss. to Alexander Iatrosophista (13th cent.): *Species turpedinis, quam vulgus Variolas dicit*, and Constantinus Afer: *Variolae sunt multae pustulae in toto corpore, aut ex majori parte dispersae, aut in uno membro, in aliis non* (lib.2. Pantechn. cap. 14). One might also note that Constantinus further says: *Antiqui vocant has ignis carbones* (ibid), which might be a translation of Gr. ἄνθρακες; cf. however Richard Mead's *de Variolis et Morbillis liber* (1747), p 2, where he states that *Frustra enim sunt, qui* ἄνθρακας, ἐπινυκτίδας, *et consimilia in cute* ἐξανθήματα, variolas *nostras esse contendunt*. In Faber Soranus, there is a plural *varioli* (2537, s.v. *varus*), with the translation *die Blattern oder Pocken*, while *variola* is not found. The word is of course found in both B and C, as well as in Dorland and Renander.

VASA, Martin 7.2, Bergius 3.10; (blood) vessels
Vas could denote any kind of vessel or container in ancient Latin, or even, in the plural, household utensils or military package as a collective. In the medical sense of "transporting tubes" for blood or, as perhaps, but not likely, in Martin's text, air, the word is not known from ancient Latin, even if the sense of a container for the blood would not necessarily demand any notion of an actual blood circulation. In mediaeval Latin, *vas* is found in the sense of 'blood vessel' in a Latin translation of Paulus of Aegina (7th cent.), acc. to its editor J. L. Heiberg probably dating from c:a the 10th century: *flebotomare igitur hos oportet a cubito, convenit vero et a naribus, et que sub lingua sunt vasa evacuare sanguine* (Cap. 42). In the same sense, it is found in *De complexionibus*, 1.9: *Et tunice ipse sanguinissimorum vasorum, arterie dico et vene, insanguinee sunt et frigide natura*. In Sweden, *vas* is used in this sense e.g. in Olof Rudbeck the Elder's *Disputatio ... de circulatione sanguinis* (1652): *... sanguis e corde digrediens, per arteriarum obambulat anfractus,*

donec per angustos venarum meatus, tandemque cavae vasa majora, vicissim ad eundem unde discescit (sic) terminum recurrat (Thes. 1). As for more contemporary occurrences, *vas* is found in both B and C, in the sense of blood vessel; the *vasa inhalantia & aperta pulmonum* in Martin's text probably are the pulmonary blood vessels, which are said to "inhale" the smallpox contagion from the surrounding air; *vas* seems never to have been used for any part of the respiratory system; in fact, as recently as in Dorland, *vas* is explicitly said to be "any canal for carrying a fluid".

VENAESECTIO, Martin 18.1

The cutting open of a vein for bloodletting is a very old form of therapy; φλεβοτομία is treated by Hippocrates, and Celsus says, that *Sanguinem incisa vena mitti novum non est: sed nullum paene esse morbum, in quo non mittatur, novum est* (2.10.1). Celsus does not, however, use *venaesectio*, but generally *sanguinis detractio*, e.g. in 2.9.2, or *sanguinem mittere* (2.10, passim). The Greek term *phlebotomia* is used in Latin already by Caelius Aurelianus (c. 5th century): *sed si dolor vehemens fuerit, phlebotomiam convenit adhibere* (*Acut.* 2.18.104); this text is a Latin translation of a work by the Greek physician Soranus (98–138), but *phlebotomia* was soon incorporated also into the Latin medical word stock, and seems to be the normal technical term for the opening of a vein for Burgundio, who, while he often gives short Latin explanations of his Greek loan-words (typically of the kind *idest ~*), uses *flebotomia* without any explanation.

For the Neo-Latin period, *venaesectio* is found in the title of Franciscus Bonafides' *Quaestio subtilis ac clara, de cura pleuritidis per venae sectionem* ... (1533), but not in the text of the book; it could further be noted, that even Olaus Magnus mentions bloodletting in at least two passages in his *Historia de gentibus septentrionalibus* (1555): *Ventosis, seu phlebotomia, uterque sexus pro scabie (ex frigore genita) et intercutaneo pruritu depellendo utitur: seu frequentius phlebotomia* (15.36), where the Greek term thus is used by a non-physician, which might indicate that it was the normal term; likewise: *licet ... ordinaria phlebotomia cum ventosis, aut corniculis inflammatis haud desit* (22.7). It might further be observed that *phlebotomia* is not used by Olaus Magnus as meaning bloodletting in itself, but rather as one of the techniques to perform it; another method, *ventosa* meaning a cupping-glass, is cupping.

Petri Gothus has only *phlebotomia*, while Noltenius says (col 1736) that *SECARE VENAM cum Suetonio in vita Lucani dicunt, qui paullo melius loqui volunt, quam qui Graeco more inscite id per Phlebotomare ... proferunt.*

As for the more important sources for the texts treated here, Richard Mead uses *sectio venae* in one passage of *de Variolis et Morbillis liber*, while his preferred term seems to be *sanguinis missio*. In B and C both *phlebotomia* and *venaesectio* are found; C gives, s.v. *venaesectio*, only a reference to *phlebotomia*. Today, both the Greek and Latin words are used in medical language; they still mean 'incision of a vein' but are probably to be associated more with adding to, than subtracting from, the bodily fluids.

VERTIGO, Schröder 23; dizziness, and **VERTIGINOSUS** (adj.), Martin 6.1

From *verto*, to 'turn' or 'revolve'. Known from Livy 44.6: *rupes utrimque ita abscisae sunt, ut despici vix sine vertigine quadam simul oculorum animique possit.* Not known from any ancient medical authors, thus hardly to be regarded as a technical term; it is found however in both C, with a reference to Gr. *dinos*, and B. The adj. *vertiginosus*, in Martin's text used to further describe a *turbatio*, would mean something like 'with elements of vertigo'; the same word, then as a noun, meaning 'patient, suffering from vertigo' is by Forcellini (VI, p 300) and L&S said to be found in Pliny *NH* 23.28, which, however, is not the case in modern editions.

VESICA, VESICULA, Martin 6.4, Bergius 8.30; bladder

Vesica is, in ancient Latin as well as in medical "Latin" of today, 'a bladder', in ancient Latin chiefly the urine bladder, e.g. in Cicero *Fin.* 2.30: *Tanti aderant vesicae et torminum morbi ut nihil ad eorum magnitudinem posset accedere.* In ancient usage, it could also denote anything made from a bladder, as for instance a purse: *illae autem maritimae piscinae nobilium … magis ad oculos pertinent, quam ad vesicam* (Varro RR 3.17), or, figuratively, 'bombastic speech' etc: *a nostris procul est omnis vesica libellis* (Martial 4.49). *Vesicula* is, quite simply, a small *vesica*. It might be noted that *vesicula* by Albrecht von Haller sometimes is used alone for the *vesica fellea* (i.e. the gall bladder), e.g. in the heading of chapter XXVII of *Primae Lineae Physiologiae* (1747): *HEPAR. VESICULA. BILIS.* Haller's preferred term for this organ is otherwise *vesicula fellis. Vesica* and *vesicula* are found in B and C; for *vesica* C has a reference to Gr. *cystis.* Cf. also **VESICATORIA**, "Drug categories", below.

VISCERA (npl), Martin 6.8; internal organs

In ancient Latin, *viscera* normally are all internal organs of the body, except for those of the digestive system, which are called *intestina*; Celsus writes, after having treated the lungs, heart, liver and kidneys: *Ac viscerum quidem haec sedes sunt. Stomachum vero … intestinorum principium est* (4.1.6). Further proof of there being a difference can be obtained from Celsus 4.18: *A visceribus ad intestina veniendum est.* This difference does not exist today, however, inasmuch as *viscus* can mean "any large interior organ in any one of the three great cavities of the body, especially in the abdomen" (Dorland, s.v. *viscus*), thus also, and in particular, including the gastrointestinal system. One should note that Martin talks about *viscera nobiliora*, which might indicate that the sense of the word is closer to that of today than to that in Celsus, and that *viscera nobiliora* would be the *viscera* of ancient Latin. Both B and C have the word, B with the definition: *organa quae elaborant aliquem humorem in usum publicum*, while C refers to Gr. *splanchna.*

VOMITURITIO, Martin 6.1; impulse to vomit

From *vomo*, to vomit, via the desiderative *vomiturio* (originally from fut ptc act *-turus*, see K-St I, § 217); this noun is not known from classical or mediaeval Latin, but is found in B, where it is regarded as a synonym to *vomitus*, and in C, where the sense is that of an effort or urging to vomit, however without any result. As the noun certainly is formed from the desiderative verb, the definition in C. seems quite probable; perhaps the state indicated is that between *nausea* and *vomitus*?

Pharmacological preparations

Introduction

As is pointed out above, the problems associated with the establishing of a pharmacological word list, such as the one below, are rather different from those one meets when dealing with the regular kind of word list.

The major task, when making a word list to a particular text, is that of ascertaining what was actually understood by the term *when the text was written*. In the pharmacological field, this task is difficult to fulfil for several reasons; the exact meaning of a particular term at a particular time, and in a particular place, is often almost impossible to ascertain, at least when dealing, as is the case here, with a period when every specific preparation was still made on request; the pharmacopoeias of different countries, containing preparations long well-known, described according to established local traditions with respect to ingredients, proportions of those, etc, often give the same, or almost the same, name to slightly different preparations.[68] We also know that the *Pharmacopoeia Holmiensis* (PhHolm) of 1686, which still was the Swedish national pharmacopoeia in the mid 18th century, was edited in a thoroughly revised version in 1752 – an edition which had been in preparation for a long time – and that the pharmacopoeia never had any limiting function in the first place as regards the physician, but rather indicated a minimum of supplies, which the pharmacy was supposed to have in stock. Hence, it is easily understood that the official pharmacopoeias alone do not give sufficient information as to which preparations were actually in use; in addition, I have found that several of the preparations in the short list below are to be found only in the London pharmacopoeia (PhLond).

One must also keep in mind that the dissertations dealt with were written by medical professionals and probably intended to be read in the first place by other medical professionals, furthermore that the extant text of a dissertation was a scientific treatise more than a detailed handbook. These circumstances might lead to the suspicion that not every preparation was mentioned in exactly the same form in the printed dissertation as it would in an actual doctor's prescription; any "real" prescriptions would be indicated by the sign ℞, or the abbreviation *Rc.*, both at this time read as *Recipe!* (i.e. 'Take!'),[69] followed by the exact amounts of the ingredients, while most suggested preparations in this material are only given as a list of ingredients, not necessarily mentioning proportions, etc.

General features of pharmacological texts

First of all, it should be pointed out that writings on these matters are likely to exhibit – apart from terms pertaining to *materia medica* and specific preparations, such as those treated in the word list below – several terms denoting medical weight units and drug

---

[68] See e.g. the preparations **DIASCORDIUM Fracastorii** and **ELECTUARIUM diascordium**, below.

[69] The ℞-symbol is by Bendz, *Latin för medicinare*, 1950, p 339, said to originally have been a somewhat modified symbol for Jupiter (♃), used by early Christians as a symbol for God, and in the physician's prescription as an *invocatio*.

categories; since this is the case also in the texts dealt with here, separate lists for these two groups will be provided here by way of introduction.

Weight units[70]

The Swedish pharmacological weight units, or "apothecaries' weights", were used at least from the 17th century until 1857, and originally based upon the Nuremberg pound, i.e. 356,28 g, which was divided according to the following table:

Latin	English	symbol	Weight		
Libra	pound	℔	12 *unciae*	=	356,28 g
Uncia	ounce	℥	8 *drachmae*	=	29,69 g
Drachma	drachm	ʒ	3 *scrupuli*	=	3,71 g
Scrupulus	scruple	℈	20 *grana*	=	1,237 g
Granum	grain	gr.		=	61,85 mg

Drug categories

The terms used to indicate the *effects* of a drug are generally either *vis* or *virtus* + adj, while *groups* of remedies with specific effects usually have denominations, consisting of a substantivated adjective in the neutre plural, the head-word originally being *remedia*, to denote the group, and in the neutre singular to denote a particular preparation in the group; most names in my list belong to the neutre plural type.

Several more or less detailed systems seem to have existed; as an example one might note that Linnaeus' *Materia medica I* lists 103 categories under *Index virium*;[71] in the following list, however, only those terms will be treated which are actually found in my texts; I have also included terms denoting method of *administration* but not those, which denote method of *preparation*; thus the words *cataplasma*, *clysma*, and *gargarisma* in neutre singular are included, but not e.g. *pulvis*.

ABSTERGENTIA Martin 16.2

The normal meaning of *abstergo* or *abstergeo* is to 'wipe off' etc; *abstergentia* is also mentioned both by Castelli and Blancardus as denoting preparations used to cleanse wounds (is is not found in the *index virium* of Linnaeus' *Materia medica*, however). One might further note that Renander indicates the sense of 'purgatives', which is not found elsewhere in the literature on medical terminology.

ANODYNA Bergius 10.8

Gr. ἀνώδυνος, 'free from pain', 'analgesic' (adj.), found in a general sense in Hippocrates *Aph.* 5.22; specifically about a drug in Plutarch 2.614c; the noun found in Latin in Marcellus Empiricus 25 (fl. 400). Also to be found in GL, C, and B; also in *Materia medica*, where the category, however, has the subheading *Antispasmodica*.

---

[70] Derived from information by Bo Ohlson, certified pharmacist, on the webpage *http://home1.swipnet.se/PharmHist/Artiklar/medicinalvikt.html*, accessed in April, 2003.
[71] P 242sqq.

ANTIPHLOGISTICA Martin 12.1

From *anti* + Gr. φλόγωσις, 'inflammation', Thucydides 2.49 (5th cent. BC); not used in ancient Latin, not to be found in DuCange, MLW or Bartal. *Phlogosis* is found in G, C, and B.

The term in its medical sense (the word was also used in chemistry, in the sense of 'opponent to the phlogiston theory') is found in English from the late 18th century, e.g. in W. Buchan's *Domestic medicine*, 1769: "The plethoric state of the patient … led to the employment of the antiphlogistic … treatment." (XLIII.184), and is still a technical term for 'antiinflammatory remedies'. Cf. OED, s.v. "antiphlogistic".

BALSAMICA Martin 16.2

From Greek βάλσαμον, 'balsam-tree'; in ancient Latin, an originally Greek adj. *balsamodes*, 'resembling balsam', is found in Pliny's *NH* 12.97, while *balsamicus* is not found.

This category is found in Linnaeus' *Materia medica I, Index virium*, p 243, but not in B and C. In Zedler, *balsamica* is said to denote *Artzeney-Mittel, welche voller leimichter und schwefelicher Theilgen sind.*

CARDIACA Bergius 10.18

From Greek καρδιακός, 'belonging to the heart', from καρδία, 'the heart'; not known from ancient Greek or Latin in the present sense of 'preparations to strengthen the heart'; In Zedler, s.v. *Cardiaca medicamenta* the reader is redirected to *Hertz-Stärckende Artzeneyen*, where there is a reference to *Hertz-Stärckende Mittel*, from which entry one is told to read under *Confortativ*, at which point the need for such preparations is urgent.

Another term used for this kind of remedies is *Cordialia* (fr. Lat *cor* 'heart') which is found in *Materia medica* as a synonym to *Cardiaca*; this word is also found in Zedler, however with a reference to *Analeptica*, which term denotes *alle mit spiritu vini oder Wein abgezogene Wasser und Spiritus. Cardiaca* are known both to B and C, as are *Cordialia*.

CARMINATIVA Schröder 13

Preparations for flatulence; not found in this sense in ancient Latin.

The term is, according to C, derived from *carmino*, 'to card', i.e. 'to get rid of something undesired', originally pertaining to the preparation of wool, while B refers to *carmen*, 'a song', which could be used for soothing purposes, as can the *carminativa*. The correct etymology is undoubtedly the first one, which is commented upon in OED: "The object of carminatives is to expel wind, but the theory was that they dilute and relax the gross humours from whence the wind arises, combing them out like the knots in wool". Found also in Linnaeus' *Materia medica*.

CATAPLASMA Bergius 8.33

Gr. κατάπλασμα, 'plaster', Hippocrates *Art.* 40, in Latin known from Cato *Fil.* 4, but also from Celsus 2.33; found in C and B.

CATHARTICA Bergius 8.18

From Gr. καθαρτικός, (adj.) promoting κάθαρσις, 'purging', Hippocrates *Mul.* 1.74 ; in Latin in Tertullian *De pallio* 5 (fl. 2nd/3rd cent.) (L&S)

Found in this sense in C, and B, as well as in Zedler, while G has the adj; cf. **CATHARSIS**, Greek word list, above.

CLYSMA, Bergius 8.6, Schröder 32

Gr. *κλύσμα*, Herodotos 2.77 (5ᵗʰ cent. BC); in Latin *Alphita* I, p 284.5 (MLW). Found in G, C, and B, while GL has *clyster*.

CORRIGENTIA Bergius 8.2

These are, according to Zedler, substances, which are added to a remedy in order to increase its effect; the term is not found in ancient Latin, nor in B or C or in the *Materia medica*.

DEPURANTIA Martin 16.2

Depuratus, most likely in the sense of 'cleansed from pus', is found in *Mulomedicina Chironis*, 571: *vulnera sanabis, sequenti etiam limpida et depurata ... curare incipies*; this meaning would fit in well here, were it not that *Mulomedicina* is less likely to have been read by the author than e.g. the dictionary of Petri Gothus, where *depuro* is derived from *puro*; no translation is provided, but as synonyms Petri Gothus gives *extraho* and *exsicco, unde depuratum dicimus siccatum & mundatum*. In Zedler *depurantia* is found only as a synonym, s.v. *Blut-reinigende Artzeneyen*, and in B and C it is not found at all.

DILUENTIA Martin 18.1, Bergius 8.19

From *diluo*, 'dilute' or 'dissolve'; in the sense here, denoting a specific kind of medical substances, not known from ancient Latin. B has *diluentia*, denoting fluids for diluting other substances, which does not seem to be exactly the meaning here. C does not mention the word at all. In Zedler, *diluens* is however used about any substance that makes the blood more thin (among such substances are listed e.g. tea, coffee, and beer), which also seems to be what is intended here.

EMETICA Bergius 8.9

From Gr. *ἐμετικός* (adj.), 'promoting vomiting', Aristotle *Probl.* 3.18 (4ᵗʰ cent. BC), in ancient Latin as *emeticon* (noun), Caelius Aurelianus *Acut.* 3.4.32 (TLL). Found in C, and B, while G has noun *ἔμετος*.

EPISPASTICA Bergius 8.26

From Gr. *ἐπισπαστικός* (adj.), 'drawing in', 'attractive', Hippocrates *Acut. Sp.* 2; in ancient Latin, the word seems to be known only from translations of the Greek authors Dioscorides and Oribasius (TLL). It does occur in Celsus 5.19.11, but then as a Greek term, written in Greek letters. In mediaeval Latin, (possibly noun, as in the present text), known from *Alphita* 58 (MLBr.), while Burgundio translates Gr. *ἐπισπαστικός* with *evulsivus* (*De interioribus* 153.29). Found in G, C, and B. Cf. also **VESICATORIA**, below.

EVACUANTIA Bergius 8.2

According to Zedler, s.v. *Remedia evacuantia*, a collective term for such preparations as emetics, purgatives etc. Not found in ancient Latin, nor in B or C.

EXCITANTIA Bergius 8.8

Not found in any specifically medical sense in ancient Latin.

In Zedler, s. v. *Anthypnotica medicamenta*, the term *excitantia* is said to denote not only those remedies, which counteract sleep, but also everything that "strengthens the spirits"; the term is otherwise found in *Materia medica*, but not in B or C.

EXPELLENTIA Bergius 8.34

Expello is known, in a medical context, from Celsus 1.3.18, where the sense is roughly 'to relieve the body of something harmful'.

As used here, the *expellentia* seem to be roughly the same as *evacuantia*, above, however with the addition, that Zedler counts also *epispastica* among the external expellents. Found in *Materia medica* and in C.

GARGARISMA Martin 17.3, Bergius 8.31; 'gargling fluid'

From Greek γαργαρισμός, 'gargling', known from Alexander Trallianus 5.4 (Li&Sc); in Latin, *gargarizo*, 'to gargle', is found in Celsus 4.2.8.

A *gargarisma* is by Zedler defined as *ein fliessend, äusserliches Artzeney-Mittel, den Mund, Halß und beyliegende Theile auszuspielen und auszugurgeln*; for his examples, however, Zedler does not use the form *gargarisma*, but rather *gargarismus*, to denote a single preparation.

B lists as synonyms *gargarismus, collutio oris* and διάκλυσμα, while C says that *gargarisma* is sometimes used *late pro omni collutione oris ... proprie vero est hujus saltem species*; the *gargarismata* are only those *collutiones* which are specifically intended to cure maladies of the mouth and throat.

LAXANTIA Martin 16.3, Bergius 8.17

Purging preparations; from *laxo*, which means 'stretch out', 'extend', but also 'open' or 'relax'. In the sense of purging or loosening the bowels in Pliny *NH* 8.129 (of bears) *herbam quandam ... laxandis intestinis ... devorant.* Found in B, while C uses *Laxativa*; *Materia medica* has a reference to *eccoprotica*.

PAREGORICA Bergius 10.25

From Greek παρήγορος, (adj.) 'comforting', etc; *paregoricum* in the sense of 'analgesic preparation' is found in Latin in Soranus p 66.16; found in Zedler, in B and C, and in *Materia medica*.

PURGANTIA Schröder 13

While *purgatio* is found already in Cato *Agr.* 157.13, this particular form is not known from ancient Latin; found in Zedler as synonymous to *cathartica*; found also in B, in C, and in *Materia medica*.

REFRIGERANTIA Bergius 8.8

These are cooling or refreshing remedies, most notably juices of various fruits, but also such preparations as diluted acids; found in Zedler and in *Materia medica*.

SAPONACEA Bergius 8.22

For this group, Zedler provides the synonyms *salsa remedia* or *salzigte Mittel*, found also in *Materia medica*, but not in B or C.

TOPICA Bergius 8.25

From Gr. τοπικός, 'having to do with a place', from τόπος, 'place', etc; known in Greek in a medical sense from e.g. Hippocrates *Aph.* 2.46; neither found in Burgundio's Galen translation nor in the 1541 Latin Galen, while the Latin term in both these cases is *localis*; in C, the *topica* are also treated under *localis*, while the entry *topicos* consists only of a reference to the Latin term.

C also mentions that *localis* can be used either *late* or *stricte*; in both cases, however, the term pertains to locally effective remedies, the only difference being that the more narrow sense refers to externally applied remedies only.

The distinction between these two meanings does not seem altogether clear, since probably a vast majority of all locally effective remedies would be applied externally anyway; even such preparations as *gargarismata* or *clysmata* are included in the category by Zedler, while C does not provide any examples; B, on the other hand, says explicitly that these remedies *sunt medicamenta externa* which also are specifically effective in certain cases; as an example he has *emplastra* for wounds.

One might note, that Bergius talks about *topica externa*, which perhaps indicates that the wider sense of C was the normal meaning at the time.

VESICATORIA Bergius 8.8
The adjective *vesicatorius* or the substantivized adjective *vesicatorium* is not known from ancient or mediaeval Latin, while its Greek equivalent, *epispasticum*, is found in Celsus 5,19,11, then in its Greek form, which might indicate, given Celsus' general method for dealing with Greek terms (cf. Langslow, pp. 118–121), that there was no Latin term readily available. Found in both B and C. For the adj. *vesicatorius*, cf also EXCRETORIUS, INFLAMMATORIUS and SECRETORIUS in the Latin word list, above.

The preparations

ACETOSA Bergius 8.22
The *Rumex acetosa*, which originally was believed to contain acetic acid, whence the name; in 1784, however, Scheele established that the acidous component of this herb is actually oxalic acid.

ACETOSITAS citri Bergius 8.6
Since citric acid was not discovered until 1784 (by Scheele), this probably means "sourishness from lemons" – lemon juice, quite simply – or something similar; cf. *Zwölf Schlüssel Fratris Basili Valentini*, ch. 8: *so bleibt/ durch offtere Distillation eines gemeinen Wassers/ wol abgesüsset / daß die acetositas aller wider davon kommet/ So hat man ein süsses Pulver*, where *acetositas* probably means just 'sourishness' in general; cf. also Sw. *syrlighet*, used about matters consisting of, or containing, acids, e.g. by Urban Hiärne, 1706: *Spiritus vitrioli och salis fräsa starckt medh alcali, så wäl fixis som volatilibus urinosis. Spiritus nitri något sachtare medh urinosis än de förra; ändå sachtare medh ättickia och andra förbrutna syrligheter* (Cf. SAOB, s.v. *Syrlighet* 3).

ACIDUM vi[c]trioli
Cf. SPIRITUS victrioli, below; sulphuric acid, by Zedler also called *acidum universale*. According to Sch (Schneider, *Lexikon zur Arzneimittelgeschichte*) VI, p 26, this acid was first used in alchemy, and sold in pharmacies at least since the late 16[th] century.

AETHIOPS mineralis Martin 15.1
Mercury sulphide, a mixture of mercury with the equal weight of flower of sulphur, as e.g. in *Pharmacopoea Svecica* I (PhSuI), or, according to Zedler, eight parts of mercury and six parts of sulphur; C further says that the mixture is to be ignited, and that the *aethiops mineralis* is the substance that remains when the sulphur has been consumed.

According to Sch (VI p 126) the matter has been used in India since the Middle Ages and known in Europe since ca. 1600, but not found in pharmacopoeias until c. 1740, when it was prescribed for tumours, fistulae, and quartan fever; also used externally in skin diseases, e.g. scrofula. Found in PhLond.

ALUMEN crystallinum Bergius 8.32

Στυπτηρία (sc. γῆ), which denotes 'adstringent earth', consisting probably of alum and/or ferrous sulphate (i.e. vitriol; cf. **VITRIOLUM martis**, below), was used in Greek medicine, e.g. to cleanse ulcers (Hippocrates, Περὶ ἕλκων, 14); under the name of *alumen* this substance is also mentioned by Pliny, e.g. in *NH* 35.52, where a light and a darker variety are said to exist; the lighter of these varieties would probably be a natural form of what we call alum, while the darker variety would contain ferrous sulphate.

According to Zedler, *alumen* – still, probably no clear distinction was made between alum and vitriol – was used e.g. in a paste, made with earthworms, to cure cancer, further to cleanse wounds and as an adstringent, which also is the major medical use for the alum today.

ANTIMONIUM Martin 13.1

This is antimony trisulphide, or stibnite (also known as *stibium*, whence the chemical abbreviation *Sb* for what we today know as "antimony", but which in this period would be called the *regulus antimonii*). The word seems to be derived from the Arabic *ithmid* (perhaps ultimately from Greek στίμμι), mlat *athimodium, atimonium*. Popular etymology, however, derived the word from fr. *antimoine*, meaning '[poison] against monks', which is also referred to in Zedler:

> *Der Name Antimonium soll vornemlich aus der frantzösischen Sprache, von dem*
> *griechischen Wörtlein ἀντι; contra, wider, und dem frantzösischen Moine, Monachus, ein*
> *Mönch, herkommen, daher es auch im frantzösischen Antimoine heisset.*

Powderized stibnite had been used in cosmetics already in ancient Egypt, but also as an external remedy; the internal usage apparently has its origin in Paracelsus' early iatrochemical practice (Maehle, *Drugs on Trial*, p 2; L&G II, p 244), which by the traditionalists was regarded with suspicion; so did e.g. the resistance from the Medical Faculty in Paris lead to a prohibition of the use of antimony between 1566 and 1666 (Maehle, ibid).

In Germany, however, antimony was used e.g. to cure scabies, hydrops, and various intermittent fevers (Sch VI p 43), even if the main feature of the substance was its ability to induce vomiting; one might note the *poculum vomitarium*, a cup designed for the curing of alcoholics, where wine was left overnight and then, when drunk by the addict on the next day, made him throw up, thus, hopefully, arousing disgust with drinking (Sch VI p 44; L&G II p 248).

AQUA alexiteria spirituosa Londinensis Bergius 8.8

The adj. *alexiterius* is a slight ortographical distorsion of Gr. ἀλεξητήριος, helping or healing; the preparation is made from leaves of *Mentha crispa*, leaves of *Angelica archangelica*, flowering tops of *Artemisia maritima*, diluted alcohol and water, which mixture is then distilled.

In PhSui, the *Aqua alexiteria* consists of leaves from *Mentha*, flowers of *Sambucus nigra*, and seeds of the *Angelica*, which are distilled with water.

Cf. also *Pulvis alexiterius*, acc. to Th. Dover,[72] this preparation consisted of antimony, opium, and ipecacuanha. Regarded as a means to provoke sweating.

AQUA bryoniae Martin 15.2
Made from *Bryonia alba*, which had been used from ancient times for epilepsy, palsies, gout, dropsy, etc; Sch (V:1 p 198sq) also gives references to 16th century sources which recommend the *bryonia* internally for the plague, and for snake poison; externally it was regarded as useful for abscess and fractures, but also as an ingredient in ointments for paralysed limbs. In Zedler, a recipe for making an *Aqua bryoniae composita* is given, while the preparation is not found in PhSuI.

AQUA cinnamomi Martin 15.2, Bergius 8.25
Basically water, distilled with *Cinnamomum verum*; the *Cinnamomum* family includes several plants of medical interest, among others the *Cinnamomum aromaticum* (*cassia*), the *Cinnamomum camphora* and the *Cinnamomum verum*. The *Cinnamomum* was in ancient Greece regarded as a useful diuretic, but also, when applied externally combined with *Myrrha*, as an andidote against the bite of venomous animals; cf. Sch V:1 p 306sq. Found in PhLond and in PhSuI in slightly different versions.

AQUA floris acaciae Schröder 31
This is not water, distilled with flowers of *Acacia*, but rather water, distilled with flowers of *Prunus spinosa*, which, according to Linnaeus' *Materia medica* I, was known in Sweden as *Acacia nostra*, while the genuine *Acacia*, of which, according to PhSuI, the fruit juice, but not the flowers were used, would be *Acacia vera*.

AQUA mineralis Seidlizensis Sundius 7.4
A solution of Seidlitzer salt (magnesium sulphate) in carbonated water, named after Seidlitz (in Bavaria, Germany), where magnesium sulphate had been found in 1717, reputedly by Friedrich Hoffmann; cf. also **SAL catharticum**, below.

AQUA picis navalis Martin 17.2
Pitch-water, made from *pix navalis*, 'pitch' ('tar' is known as *pix liquida* in the Swedish pharmacopoeias up to PhSuVII, where the name is changed to *pyroleum pini*), not found in PhHolm or PhLond, but, as *aqua picea* – without distinction between *pix navalis* and *pix liquida* – in PhSuI; the preparation was made by mixing pitch or tar with water, which was left for twelve hours, whereupon it could be used; Rosén recommends the use of *Tjär-Watten* ('tar water') to prevent smallpox in *Underrättelser*, p 155, with a reference to "the late Bishop in Ireland, Mr. Berkley" (George Berkeley (1685–1753), famous philosopher, bishop of Cloyne from 1734): *Så snart Koppor begynna at gå, dricker man däraf ... hwar morgon och afton, så länge, til dess man antingen får Kopporna, eller Farsoten afstannat* ("As soon as Pox start spreading, one drinks of this ... each morning and evening, until one either gets the Pox, or the Epidemic has stopped").

AQUA stillatitia Bergius 8.33
Apparently synonymous to *aqua destillata*, distilled water.

---

[72] Dover started his career as an assistant of Thomas Sydenham's but later became a privateer, known as the captain who rescued Alexander Selkirk, who to some extent was to serve as a model for Defoe's Robinson Crusoe.

AQUA vitriolica caerulea Bergius 8.32
Water made with cupric sulphate (called *vitriolum* from *vitrum*, glass, as the crystals of this sulphate are glass-like), alum, and sulphuric acid; used as a styptic.

BALSAMUM embryonale Bergius 8.25
This is maybe equal to the *spiritus aromaticus* of PhSuI, which is also called *balsamum embryonum sive Aqua vitae mulierum*, and which consists of, among other things, leaves of *Mentha piperita*, bark of *Cinnamomum culilawan*, peel of *Citrus aurantium*, seeds of *Angelica* and brandy.

BALSAMUM stomachale Schröder 35
This is equal to *balsamum aromaticum*, of which the variety found in PhSuI, also called *Balsamum cephaelicum Scherzeri*, contains oil from the seed of *Myristica fragrans*, mixed with the oils of *Syzygium aromaticum* and of *Lavandula angustifolia angustifolia*, and with amber oil. Two varieties of *balsamum aromaticum* are also found in Zedler – however with slightly different formulas – as is the *balsamum Schertzeri*, which is described thus: *Nehmet destilliert Rauten-Lavendel-Dosten-Muscaten Oel, jedes ein Quentgen und vermischet es wohl mit einander.*

BERBERIS Bergius 8.22
Juice of the berries from, probably, the *Berberis vulgaris*, at this time used mainly as a flavouring, even if the drug earlier seems to have been prescribed for diarrhoea and liver ailments (Sch V:1 p 170sq).

CALOMELANUM Martin 16.2
From Greek καλός + μέλας; mercurous chloride, seems originally to have been used in a preparation to cure hereditary syphilis in children, but also as a purgative. Also known, e.g. in PhSuI, as *mercurius dulcis*. Cf. **MERCURIUS dulcis** below.

CAMPHORA Martin 15.2, Bergius 8.23
Camphor, made from the oil of *Cinnamomum camphora*.

   Camphor was often recommended to prevent the smallpox, e.g. by Rosén in his *Hus- och Rese-Apotheque*, 1772

CASSIA Bergius 8.18
At this time probably the *Cassia fistula* (Sch V:1 p 247), used mainly as a mild purgative, while *cassia ligna* still was wood from the *Cinnamomum aromaticum*.

CASSINE Martin 17.3
The two plants known as *cassine*, the *Ilex cassine*, used in pharmacology as *folia cassinae*, and the *Cassine peragua*, used as *folia peraguae*, were, according to J.D. Schoepf's *Reise durch einige der mittlern und südlichen vereinigten nordamerikanische Staaten …*, 1788, both used as substitutes for tea in South Carolina, where they are indigenous; neither of them is found in PhLond or PhHolm, however.

CERASUS niger Bergius 8.6
This is 'black cherry', i.e. the fruit of the *Prunus cerasus*, used as a refreshing flavouring.

COCCINELLA Martin 15.3

An alternate spelling of *coccionella*, the dried bug *Coccus cacti*, indigenous in Central America, and introduced in Europe in the early 16th century; the Württemberg pharmacopoea (1741) prescribes *coccionella* for fever, but also as a diuretic remedy; otherwise it was mainly used as an analgesic. According to Zedler, the question whether this matter actually consisted of seeds from a *Ficus* or of insects was still debated in the early 18th century; cf. Sch I p 31.

CONFECTIO seminum anisi Sundius 7.4

A *confectio* was made by coating a drug, often the seeds of certain herbs, with sugar; PhHolm also points out that *Confectiones saccharatae ad fallendos prudenter aegros inventae sunt*, which applies mainly to *confectio seminum cynae*, which was not made from the seeds, but rather from the flower buds of the *Artemisia cina* and used for intestinal worms; the other kinds of *confectio* listed are made from seeds of *Carum carvi*, *Cuminum cyminum*, *Foeniculum vulgare*, and *Pimpinella anisum*, respectively, which probably would have been regarded mainly as sweets, which also is the modern meaning of "confectionery"; according to PhSul, *Confectiones siccae ... rarissime si unquam a Pharmacopoeis parantur.* Cf. also **SEMEN anisi**, below.

CONSERVA flavedinis corticum aurantiorum Schröder 35

A *conserva* is, according to PhHolm, a preparation made by grinding the drug with fine-grained sugar, and with the optional addition of sulphuric acid; another kind of preparation made with sugar is the *conditum*, which however seems to have been boiled.

The *conserva* dealt with here is a preparation of peel of *Citrus aurantium aurantium*, believed to strengthen the stomach and also used for its flavour. Found in PhLond, while PhSul has only a *conditum corticis aurantiorum*.

CONTRAYERBA Bergius 8.8

'Counter-herb' (Sp. *yerva* from Lat. *herba*), the root of the *Dorstenia contrajerva*, used as a universal antidote.

CORTEX chinae Martin 12.4, Bergius 8.8

Also known as *cortex cinchonae*, *cortex Peruvianus*, or *chinchina*, the bark from South american *Cinchona*-trees.

The usage of this drug – the "prototype", as Maehle puts it, "of a 'specific' remedy" – seems to have its origin in confusion between *Cinchona* and *quina-quina* or *quinua-quinua*, the bark of the *Myroxylon peruiferum* (*Myroxylon balsamum*), which was used by the native inhabitants of Peru to cure fevers, but also collected by Jesuit missionaries and sent to Rome, where it, after the first shipment had been examined and approved of by Gabriele Fonseca (?–1688), physician-in-ordinary to the Pope Innocentius X, was spread throughout Europe with jesuits, travelling from Rome (cf. *polvo de los jesuitas*, another name under which the drug was known).

The *Cinchona* tree seems however also to have been known to the jesuit missionaries as early as in mid-17th century, even if the name *Cinchona* was not established until about one hundred years later by Linnaeus; according to A.W. Haggis (*Bulletin of the History of Medicine*, vol X, nr 3, 1941, p 439sq), a description of what is called *Arbol de Calenturas* by the jesuit Bernabé Cobo in a manuscript finished on July 7, 1653, pertains to the *Cinchona*.

En los términos de la ciudad de Loja, diócesis de Quito, nace cierta casta de árboles grandes, que tienen la corteza como de canela, un poco más gruesa, y muy amaro; la cual, molida en polvos, se da a los que tienen calenturas y con sólo este remedio se quitan …Son ya tan conocidos y estimados estos polvos, no sólo en todas las Indias, sino en Europa, que con instancia los envian a pedir de Roma. (Historia del Nuevo Mundo, in Haggis, p 591)

It seems as though the *Cinchona* bark – or Loxa bark, under which name it was also known – was also collected and sent to Europe, however not as a remedy in its own right, but rather as an illicit addition to, or even substitute for, the *quina-quina*, and under the same name. Since the *Cinchona* tree was considerably more common, the drug did soon consist only of the *Cinchona* bark, while the original name of *quina-quina* was kept (one might note that the *Cinchona* is actually more efficient as a remedy for intermittent fevers, which however was yet to be discovered).

As for the use of the drug in other diseases than intermittent fevers, one might note the discussion in the *Philosophical Transactions* (cf. **Bergius 10.62–65** with commentary), regarding the china treatment of gangrene, introduced by surgeons; even if the use of china bark in smallpox therapy had been suggested already in the late 17th century by Richard Morton in part two of his *Pyretologia* (cf. **Bergius 2.2**), it seems as it was not until the reports of the effect in gangrene – which was believed to consist mainly in promoted suppuration, which as we know was considered essential – that the bark began to be important in the treatment of smallpox; cf. Maehle, pp 247–258, w. notes; Maehle points out, however, that the drug probably would have no specific effect on a gangrene, but that the treatment might have been promoted by the surgeons as a way to get to practising internal medicine, which otherwise was the physician's privilege.

Cf. also S. Jarcho (ed): *Tractatus simplex de Cortice Peruviano*, 1992; Lindgren & Gentz, s.v. *Kinabark*.

CROCUS Bergius 8.25

Crocus, Gr. κρόκος (cf. also Arab/Persian *kurkum*, sanskr. *kungkuma*), i.e. saffron, the stigma tips from *Crocus sativus*; this drug, and the *Crocus* plant, have been used for its colour, its fragrance and its (alleged) medical qualities throughout the history of western civilization; the flower is mentioned by Homer (*Il.* 14.348), and Pliny treats the drug in *NH* 21.31–34, where he among other things also points out that nothing is subject to as many forgeries (*adulteratur nihil aeque*), and in 21.137–139, where he recommends it for all inflammations, especially those of the eyes, but also of the chest, kidneys, liver, etc, as well as for ulcers of the gullet or maybe stomach (*stomachi exulcerationes*). Pliny also states that wreaths of crocus is useful against drunkenness (*coronae … ex eo mulcent ebrietatem*), while he on the other hand says in 21.33 that such wreaths are not in use (*usus eius in coronis nusquam*).

As regards the 18th century usage, the drug is considered a strong *resolvens* by Linnaeus; he regards it as a poison if not used in sufficiently small quantities, but says also that it might be of use for those, who lead a sedentary life (*Diaeta naturalis*, p 84), and as a means to promote menstruation (*Dietetik* p 184); otherwise, the drug was not used much in medicine.

DECOCTUM album Londinense rhabarberinum Bergius 9.3

This decoction, used mainly for diarrhoea, is made by boiling burnt hartshorn with *gummi arabicum* (i.e. the dried sap of several different *Acacia*-trees) and water, here added with rhubarb (cf. below, s.v. **PULVIS infantum**). This preparation is taken from

PhLond, but in PhSuI an almost identical *decoctum album* is found, added, however, also with *pasta amygdalina*, a paste made from sweet and bitter almonds, seville orange water, and sugar.

DECOCTUM tamarindi cum senna Bergius 8.18

The pulp from the fruit of *Tamarindus indica* was used as a mild laxative, as was the *senna*, leaves from various *Cassia* plants.

The origin of the name *senna* is the Arab *sanā* or *senā*, and the drug seems also to have been used first among Arab physicians; with the introduction of Arab medicine in Europe, the *senna* – also spelled *sena* – was of course also included, and from the 16th century, the plant was cultivated in Europe, mainly in Italy, but also as far north as in Germany.

The Egyptian *senna*, obtained from *Cassia senna* and *Cassia angustifolia*, and known as *sena alexandrina*, *sena levantica* or *sena orientalis*, was however regarded as better than the European *sena vulgaris*, which consisted of leaves from *Cassia italica*.

DIASCORDIUM Fracastorii Bergius 9.3

Diascordium, or *Electuarium e Scordio Fracastorii*, is found in PhSuI, where it is said to consist of the resin from the *Acacia catechu*, leaves of *Teucrium scordium* – which, according to Sch V:3 p 330sq, hade been used in ancient Greece for dysentery and strangury, but also as an antidote for snake poison – seeds from the *Nectandra puchury major* (in the pharmacopoeia known as *faba Pechurim*), root of *Potentilla erecta*, opium, Spanish wine and syrup of rose petals.

The word *diascordium* has its origin in a Greek construction of διά with the genitive, used to denote the matter out of which something is made (cf. also **ELECTUARIUM diascordium**, below), but where the prepositional expression has been regarded as one word; the phaenomenon is discussed by Maria Fredriksson in her doctoral thesis *Esculapius' De stomacho*, 2002, p 91, and by Léon Rippinger in "Les noms de médicaments en *dia-*", in *Latomus* 52,2 (1993), pp 294-306; *scordium*, from Gr. σκόρδιον, is the *Teucrium scordium*.

In Zedler, where the preparation is described as a *schmerztreibende Lattwerg*, the ingredients amount to about twenty different ones, including most of those found in the Swedish variety.

ELECTUARIUM diascordium Schröder 13

This preparation is also known as *diascordii electuarium* or *electuarium e scordio*.

An *electuarium* – or, as in PhLond, *electarium* – is a viscose preparation of the pulverised active substance with e.g. honey or syrup.

This electuary consisted among other things of opium, petals of rose, root of *Potentilla erecta*, *Cinnamomum*, *Zingiber officinale*, honey and no fewer than two different kinds of clay.

ELIXIR paregoricum Londinense Bergius 10.29

An *elixir*, from Arab *el-iksir*, 'the powder' – originally in Latin usage meaning 'the philosophers' stone', later used of several preparations – is, according to Zedler, *eine aus vielen einfachen Sachen mit einem tüchtigen Menstruo aufgelösete flüssende und an Farbe dunckele Artzeney.*

The *elixir paregoricum* was originally named by Paracelsus, and was known in more than twenty more or less different varieties; in later pharmacopoeias several names were used for the same preparation, e.g. *tinctura opii camphorata*, and *tinctura thebaica benzoica*. In this case, the preparation is made in accordance with the London pharmacopoeia, and thus consists of oil from *Pimpinella anisum*, camphor, benzoic acid, opium and undiluted alcohol; an identical preparation is found also in PhSuI. For *paregoricum*, see **PAREGORICA**, "Drug categories", above.

EPITHEMA aromaticum Schröder 35
From Gr. ἐπίθημα, a lid or cover, in the medical sense a poultice or lotion. *Aromaticum* means only that the poultice is made with aromatic substances.

EXTRACTUM aloes Martin 16.2
The dried sap of different varieties of *Aloë*-plants; several preparations existed, most notably the *aloe hepatica*, which, according to L&G I p 6, was exsiccated at a low temperature and came out opaque and brown, and the *aloe lucida*, dried at a high temperature, which was clear as glass; according to Sch (V:1 p 72) the process consisted in boiling the cut leaves in water, which was then distilled, to produce the *aloe lucida*, while *aloe hepatica* was produced by pressing the leaves and leaving the sap to dry. Out of the different preparations, the Indian aloe was regarded as the most efficient by Pliny and Dioscorides. It was in ancient times recommended as a purgative and, mixed with vinegar, as an haemostatic. Used in northern Europe since the 10th century. An *extractum* seems, according to PhHolm and PhLond, to have been made by boiling the drug in water or alcohol, whereupon the filtered fluid was boiled down to the desired consistency; the *extractum aloes aquosum* of PhSuI is made from *aloe hepatica*, water and lemon juice.

FLOS sambuci Bergius 8.8
The flower of *Sambucus nigra*.

FLOS sulphuris Martin 15.2, Bergius 9.2
Sulphur sublimatum, a yellow powder, made by sublimation (cf. my commentary to **Martin 14.2** s.v. *sublimatus*) of crude sulphur. Used mainly for diseases of the respiratory organs, but also in unguents for scabies. *Sulphur* is found in PhLond, however without any further indication as regards its form; *flores sulphuris* are included in PhSuI, however with the remark *Vix umquam a Pharmacopolis parari solent*.

HERBA rutae Martin 15.3
Herba is the pharmacological term for the leaves and flowering tops of a plant; *ruta* is the *Ruta graveolens*, which was known as a medicinal herb – most notably a universal antidote – even in ancient Greece (cf. also below, s.v. **THERIACA Andromachi**), and which still was much used in the 18th century, often as a preservative for the plague.

JULAPIUM acidulum Bergius 10.24
Originally from Pers. *gul-ab*, rose-water, via Arab. *julab*, here a mixture of sugar, aromatics and salt or, as in this case, *acidulum* meaning 'sourish', acid.

LIQUOR cornus cervi succinatus Schröder 16
Found in PhSuI, and made by mixing *spiritus cornus cervi* (obtained by destillation of hartshorn) with succinic acid; the preparation is recommended by Rosén in his *Hus-och Rese-Apotheque*, p 21, as a remedy for e.g. convulsions and flatulence.

The medical use of *cornu cervi* seems to be of very old age; Sch (I p 34) refers to papyrus Ebers (c. 1500 BC), where the preparation is prescribed as "dispelling poisons".

MACIS Schröder 33
Mlat. from *macir*, originally an Indian spice mentioned by Pliny (*NH* 12.16).

The drug, *arillus myristicae*, is the involucre of the *Myristica fragrans*, and was used mainly to "strengthen" the stomach; Linnaeus also mentions (*Dietetik* p 184) the drug as a means to provoke menstruation and, when applied to the temples, to promote sleep.

MAGNESIA alba Schröder 35
Magnesia; magnesium carbonate, a white powder, used as an antacid and, in larger doses, as a mild laxative. Cf. *magnesia nigra*, which is not a magnesium compound, but rather manganese dioxide.

MANNA Sundius 1.1, Schröder 31
The dried sap of mainly the *Fraxinus ornus*, used as a mild laxative.

MASTICHE Schröder 34
The secretion from the *Pistacia lentiscus* var. *chia*. Used in the Orient as incense, and as a "chewing gum"; the name *Mastiche*, Gr. μαστίχη, was derived from Gr. μαστιχάω, late Latin *mastico*, 'to chew'. M. has an irritating effect upon mucous membranes; it's medical use has often pertained to the mouth and stomach (cf. Pliny *NH* 12.72; Dioscorides 1.70).

MEL Bergius 8.22
Honey, which at this time probably was used mainly as a flavoring or as a vehicle in unguents, has nevertheless long been regarded as a medically active substance; Pliny mentions its ability to keep a body from putrefaction, and further regards it as useful e.g. for ailments of the throat; for pneumonia and pleurisy he recommends a decoction of honey, while *mulsum*, honey wine, should be used for paralysis (*NH* 22.107–115); Celsus (5.22.2a) recommends honey, mixed e.g. with lentils, to correct decaying flesh; he also regards it as useful when applied to ulcers of the ear (6.7.4a).

MENTHA crispa Bergius 8.31
This was the most common variety of mint in 18th century pharmacology; it was used mainly as a carminative.

MERCURIUS dulcis Martin 14.2, Bergius 8.18
'Mild mercury', calomel (see above s.v. **CALOMELANUM**), as opposed to sublimate, mercuric chloride, which is even more poisonous.

MERCURIUS vivus Martin 13.3
Mercury; in ancient Latin known as *argentum vivum*, e.g. in Pliny *NH* 33.64: *aes inaurari argento vivo aut certe hydrargyro legitimum erat*, where it further should be noted that the term *hydrargyrus* (Gr. ὑδράγυρος) at the time was used to designate mercury obtained from cinnabar, which was regarded as different from the natural *argentum vivum*.

Even if mercury has been known to humankind at least since ancient Egypt, it was in Greek and Roman medicine generally regarded as dangerous to the organism; Pliny says (*NH* 33.124) that one at most could use this substance as an unguent on the head or stomach, but not take it orally, since it would then bring about ulcers in the intestines; this opinion was to prevail through the Middle Ages, thus preventing the use of mercury, even in cases where it would have been efficient.

In mediaeval alchemy, on the other hand, mercury was to play an important part due to its unusual properties as compared to other metals; its volatility rendered it the name *Mercurius* after the "quickest" planet.

The medical use for mercury in Europe began to increase after its introduction by the Arabs in the 11th century; it was used mainly in an unguent for several skin diseases, and when syphilis started spreading throughout the continent in late 15th century (cf. above, Latin word list, s.v. **LUES venerea**), this disease was also, quite naturally, treated with the mercury unguent, which turned out to be quite an effective remedy.

Following the introduction of *lignum guaiaci* (cf. below, s.v. **RESINA guajaci**) in 1508, physicians generally tended to side either with the mercury or the guaiac treatment – Fracastoro's *Syphilis* (1531) includes both, however – one of the arguments against mercury being its toxicity, leading to hypersalivation, loss of teeth, etc, while the mercurialists rather regarded the symptoms of intoxication as signs of the cure being effective; a less rigid view upon the matter, however, grew more common during the 17th century, and the French physician and chemist Nicolas Lémery (1645–1715) writes: *Le vis-argent est un des plus grands Remedes que nous ayons dans la Medecine … mais il est tres-dangereux lors qu'il se rencontre entre les mains des Charlatans qui s'en servent pour quelque maladie que ce soit …*(*Cours de Chymie*, 1675, p 141).

MORA Bergius 8.22
The fruit of *Morus nigra*, used for flavour and refreshment.

MORSULI citri Bergius 8.6
A *morsulus*, from Mlat *morsellum*, a 'morsel' or 'small bite' (cf. Lat. *mordeo*, to bite), is a small square consisting of sugar and an effective agent or an aromatic, in this case oil of *Citrus limon* and citric acid; in PhSuI, the preparation is found as *saccharum citratum*.

MOSCHUS Bergius 6.2
Gr. μόσχος, etymologically unrelated to the purely Greek μόσχος, 'calf', but rather related to Pers. *mušk*, Sansk. *muska*, 'testicle'; originally 'small rat'. Musk, the secretion from a gland of the *Moschus moschiferus*, was used as a stimulant, and in perfumes; according to Sch (I p 52sq) the high price led to forgeries, and to prevent these, the musk was sold in its original gland. It was also used, together with amber, *Cinnamomum verum*, *Syzygium aromaticum*, benzoin, etc. in amulets carried for protection against e.g. the plague.

MYRRHA Martin 15.2, Bergius 10.4
Gr. μύρρα. The dried secretion of various *Commiphora* plants. Used as incense, also as an expectorant and stimulant.

OLEUM amygdalinum Bergius 10.44, Schröder 31
Also known as *oleum amygdalarum* or *oleum amygdalae*, oil from the seed of *Prunus dulcis dulcis*, used internal as a mild laxative, and as a vehicle in several preparations.

OLEUM essentialium ex seminibus cymini Schröder 33?
Made by distillation of seeds from *Cuminum cyminum* with water. Found in PhLond.

OLEUM liliorum alborum Bergius 11.2
This preparation is, according to Zedler, s.v. *Oel (Lilien-)*, made by macerating flowers
of white lily in olive oil. Zedler mentions that this oil is used e.g. on burns and plague
boils. Not found in PhHolm or PhLond.

OXYMEL Bergius 8.22
From Gr. ὀξύς, 'sharp', + μέλι, 'honey', according to Pliny *NH* 23.60 made by boiling
honey, vinegar, sea salt and water; in PhLond a combination of acetic acid and honey,
which was boiled to a viscous consistency; found also in PhSuI.

PHILONIUM Romanum Schröder 22
Philonium might be derived from the Greek physician Philo, who is mentioned in
Celsus 6.6.3 regarding a preparation for inflammations of the eye.
   Philonium Romanum is, according to Zedler, a name used for several analgesic
preparations; the common ingredients of the three recipes communicated by him are
seeds of *Piper nigrum*, opium and hyoscyamine, which are also ingredients of the
electuarium philonium Romanum of Ph Holm. In PhLond the corresponding preparation
is called *philonium Londinense*, and consists of *Piper nigrum*, opium, and seeds of *Zingiber
officinale* and *Carum carvi*.

PHLEGMA victrioli Martin 17.2
According to Zedler (with further reference to Lémery), this is the result of a slow
distillation of vitriol. The *phlegma* was, according to Zedler, used for ailments of the
eye.

PULVIS e alumine crystallino & vitriolo martis Bergius 8.32
A powder made from alum and ferrous sulphate; see **ALUMEN crystallinum**, above,
and **VITRIOLUM martis**, below.

PULVIS e chelis cancrorum & coccinella Martin 15.3
A powder made from crayfish shell and cochineal; Sch says (I p 25) that the ashes of
burnt crayfish were used in ancient Greece for e.g. stones of the bladder and cancer;
the Württemberg pharmacopoea recommends the shell, as well as the *oculi cancrorum*,
as an absorbent, and as a diuretic.

PULVIS e nitro purificato crystallino Bergius 8.6
A powder of crystalline saltpetre; *purificatum* means only that the matter has been
purified by the pharmacy.

PULVIS infantum Sundius 2.3
This preparation is found in PhSuI, with the remark *Vulgo pulvis puerorum Rosensteinii*
(commonly: Rosenstein's baby powder); the powder of PhSu differs slightly from the
one in Sundius' text, inasmuch as it consists of magnesium oxide, *confectio seminum
foeniculi*, and the root of *Rheum* (Gr. ῥᾶ, ῥῆον; cf. Dioscorides 3.2: ῥᾶ· οἱ δὲ ῥῆον
καλοῦσι) *palmatum palmatum*, which originates from China and Tibet.
   The Greek name ῥᾶ is, according to Ammianus Marcellinus, taken from the river
Ra (the Volga): *huic Ra vicinus est amnis, in cuius superciliis quaedam vegetabilis eiusdem nominis*

gignitur radix…(22.8.28); according to Lindgren & Gentz, s.v. *Rabarberrot*, however, it is probably derived from the Turkish word *rävend* (Arab *rēvend*, Persian *rīvend*), while the term *rhabarbarum* is Gr. ῥᾶ + *barbarum* (cf. also *reubarbarum*, Isidorus *Etym.* 17.9.40).

The original drug was probably not the root indicated above, but rather that of *Rheum rhaponticum*, which grows in the Black Sea-area; when the Chinese root reached Europe in the late antiquity, both varieties were provided as *rheum* – Alexander Trallianus (6th century) talks about ῥέον βαρβαρικόν (9.2) and ῥέον ποντικόν (e.g. in 12), respectively – and used mainly as purgatives.

After the discovery of America, several newly introduced purging drugs were called *rhabarbarum*, while the original *rha barbarum* became *radix rhei sinensis*; in the early 18th century, all import to Europe of the Chinese root went through Russia, and the drug then received the name *radix rhei moscovitici*.

For the period dealt with here, we might note, that Linnaeus' *Materia medica* lists two drugs under *Rhabarbarum*; *rhabarbarum verum*, which is the root of *Rheum palmatum*, and *rhabarbarum monacis*, which is a *Rumex* root. There is also another drug known as *rhaponticum*, which is not a rhubarb root at all, but the root of *Centaurea centaurium*, and which was used as a substitute for the *Rheum*.

PULVIS nitrosus & camphoratus Bergius 10.6, Schröder 16
Pulvis nitrosus is found in PhSuI, where it consists of saltpetre, tartar and sugar. This particular powder would thus be the *pulvis nitrosus* added with camphor.

PULVIS pro nutrice Sundius 2.3
Probably identical to *pulvis nutricum*, which is a powder consisting of magnesium oxide, peel of *Citrus aurantium aurantium*, seeds of *Foeniculum vulgare* and sugar, prescribed to wet-nurses to neutralize acidity of the stomach, to better the appetite and thus to promote lactation.

PULVIS radicis ireos florentinae Schröder 31
The pulverized root of *Iris germanica* var. *florentina*, used to mitigate the pains of dentation, by Linnaeus also used as an expectorant and a diuretic; perhaps the preparation intended is the *pulvis pectoralis* of PhSuI, which consists of the *Iris* root, of *Zingiber officinale*, saffron, and sugar.

RADIX enulae Campaniae Martin 15.2
The root of the *Inula helenium* (*inula*, which is the name used by Pliny, e.g. in *NH* 20.38, is probably derived from Gr. ἐλένιον), which was much grown during the Middle Ages in Campania, hence *Campaniae*. This preparation was much in use since ancient times; in Hippocrates' περὶ γυναικείης φύσιος ("On the nature of woman"), ἐλένιον is mentioned together with several other preparations suitable for women's maladies (Hippocrates ed Littré, VII.358.3). Pliny says (*NH* 19.91) that the drug is harmful to the stomach on its own, but most beneficial when mixed with something sweet. It is also mentioned by Horace, who regards it as a remedy for an overladen stomach (*Sat.* II.2.44). In the 17th century it was prescribed mainly to cure skin maladies, and for bites and swellings. In popular medicine, the *inula* was to be used into the 20th century.

RADIX hellebori nigri Schröder 13
Root of *Helleborus niger*, a herb, possessing a purging effect, and which in ancient times was prescribed as a major remedy for mental illnesses, for instance by Dioscorides

(IV.149); Otto, *Sprichwörter*, p 124, mentions the proverbial use, as e. g. in Plautus *Pseud* 1185: *Elleborum hisce hominibus opus est*, to indicate lunacy; cf. also Horace *Sat.* II.3.82f, where the herb and its major exporter, the Greek city Anticyra, are mentioned.

RADIX ipecacuanhae recens pulverificata Bergius 8.15
Pulverized fresh root of *Cephaelis ipecacuanha*.

RADIX verbenae Sundius 9.4
Root of verbena, which at this time, as nowadays, is a specific plant, the *Verbena officinalis*; Originally *verbena* was used about several herbs of ceremonial and medical usage (cf. Celsus, 2.33).

The particular herb intended here was otherwise known as *aristereon*, from Gr. ἄριστος, 'best' or 'noblest', but Pliny mentions that this herb, which is the most appreciated among Romans, in Latin is called *verbenaca* (*nulla ... Romanae nobilitatis plus habet quam hiera botane. Aliqui aristereon, nostri verbenacam vocant* (*NH* 25.105)), which indicates a more specific denotation; in Pseudo-Apuleius *Herb.* 65, the same herb, here *herba peristereon*, is also called *Ferraria* or *Ferranea*, which could be conferred with Germ. *Eisenkraut* or Sw. *järnört*. As for the name *peristereon*, Dioscorides says (4.59), that it reputedly is derived from the fact, that pigeons (Gr. περιστεραί) like to stay by the plant. Another, perhaps more probable, origin of this name would be a corruption of *aristereon*.

RESINA guajaci Martin 16.2
The resin of the *Guajacum officinale*, the wood of which for the first time in Europe was prescribed for the curing of syphilis in 1508 (cf. also Fracastoro's *Syphilis*, where the final passage is a homage to the guaiac tree), as was the bark of the same tree; the resin was also prescribed for the same disease, and later for gout and headaches; cf. Sch V:2 p 146sq.

RIBES Bergius 8.22
Fr. Arab *ribas*, Pers *riwas*, a sourish and bitter plant. Denoting several of the *saxifragaceae*, e.g. the alpine currant, the currant and the gooseberry.

ROB sambuci Bergius 10.47
Rob (from Arab and Pers. *rubb*, a thick juice) *sambuci* is the juice of the berries from *Sambucus nigra*, boiled down, sometimes added with sugar, into a viscous consistency.

RUBUS idaeus Bergius 8.6
Used for flux and diarrhoea and to strengthen the heart.

SAL absinthii vere alcaline Bergius 8.33
A salt, made by dehydrating a suspension of water and the ashes of burnt *Artemisia absinthium*, or of some other bitter plant; in PhSul known as *sal herbarum fixum*.

SAL ammoniacum Bergius 8.6
In an 18th-century context, like today, this is ammonium chloride; originally, however, the name seems to denote rock salt from Egypt, according to Pliny (*NH* 31.78–79) known as *hammoniacum*, since it was found under the sand (Gr. ἄμμος or ἅμμος).

The ammonium chloride, on the other hand, was probably not known in Europe until the 7th century (L&G II p 202), when it was introduced by Arab scientists as *sal armeniacum*.

According to L&G, the substance was, due to confusion, generally known as *sal armoniacum* well into the 17th century; L&G also points out that Egypt was the major source for the ammonium chloride, which might have facilitated the confusion between the two salts; from c. 1750, *sal ammoniacum* is the normal denomination.

The substance is recommended for fever by the Württemberg pharmacopoeia (Sch VI p 39); otherwise, it has mainly been used as an expectorant, and as flavouring in liquorice candy.

SAL catharticum Bergius 8.18
Magnesium sulphate, a purgative, cf. **AQUA mineralis Seidlizensis**, above.

SALVIA Bergius 8.31
The *Salvia officinalis*, Dioscorides (3.33) mentions a herb called ἐλελίσφακον, which the Romans call σάλβια. According to L&G, II, p 206, the *salvia* used by the Greeks is not likely to have been the *S. officinalis*, which is said to be very rare in Greece, while it probably was the variety used by the Romans; from Italy the plant was spread throughout Europe, and during the Middle Ages it was one of the most common herbs in monastery gardens.

In popular belief, the herb seems also to have possessed magical (among other things the ability to make pools of water dry up) and aphrodisiacal qualities (L&G, II, p 208).

As regards the medical use of *salvia* in the 18th century, Linnaeus lists the herb under three categories, viz. *adstringentia*, *stomachica* and *tonica*, in the *Index virium* of the *Materia medica*.

SEMEN anisi Schröder 13
The seeds of *Pimpinella anisum*, which seem to have been used in ancient Greece; Pliny notes, in *NH* 20.185–195, that it is one of the few drugs approved of by Pythagoras.

Pliny further mentions the usefulness of anise as a flavouring, but also lists several ailments where the drug could be used; as its main virtue, however, he regards its ability to cure flatulence.

SEMEN carvi Schröder 13
The seeds of *Carum carvi*; the only medical usage was the one prescribed here, as a carminative.

SERPENTARIA virginiana Bergius 8.8
The root of the *Aristolochia serpentaria*; promotes the activity in all secretory organs.

SINAPISMUS Bergius 8.28
Probably the same as *cataplasma sinapinum*, a poultice, made either from seeds of *Brassica nigra* and water only (*~fortius*), or with ¼ of the seeds substituted with rye flour (*~mitius*). Used to irritate the skin in different ailments and cramps.

SPECIES emollientes Bergius 8.28
Species emollientes are found in PhSul, where they consist of *Malva* leaves, flowers of *Chamomilla recutita* and seeds of *Linum usitatissimum*; used for making emollient plasters.

SPIRITUS salis Martin 14.2, Bergius 9.6
Hydrochloric acid, used e.g. (diluted!) as a cooling drink for fever patients.

SPIRITUS victrioli Martin 17.2
Diluted sulphuric acid, used as the previous item, and as a diuretic; cf. **ACIDUM vi[c]trioli**, above.

STIBIUM Martin 13.1
See above, s.v. **ANTIMONIUM**.

SYRUPUS acidi Bergius 8.6
This is maybe identical to the *syrupus aceti* or *syrupus acetosus simplex* of PhSuI, which is a syrup, made from vinegar and sugar; otherwise, it might be just any combination of a syrup with some sour substance.

SYRUPUS baccarum sambuci Martin 15.2
A syrup with juice of the berries from *Sambucus nigra*, in PhSuI as *syrupus sambucinus*. A mild diuretic.

SYRUPUS cichorei cum rheo Sundius 1.2
In PhSuI a *syrupus rhei* is found, with the alternative name *syrupus cichorii cum rheo*. This syrup, however, does not contain any *Cichorium*, but rather root of *Taraxacum*. A mild purgative.

SYRUPUS e meconio Londinensis Bergius 10.29
Syrup of opium, basically; also known as *diacodion* (as regards *dia-*, cf. **DIASCORDIUM Fracastorii**, above) or *syrupus papaveris albi*. According to J.G. Wallerius' *Praelectiones pharmaceuticae*, 1754, there were actually three varieties, of which the *syrupus simplex* was made by decoction of seed capsules from *Papaver somniferum* in water, to which then sugar was added; the *compositus* variety also included the fruit of *Ceratonia siliqua*, while the *syrupus crocatus* was added with *Crocus*. In PhSuI, there is a *syrupus papaveris*, which is equal to the *syrupus e meconio* of PhLond.

SYRUPUS floris papaveris rhoeadis Martin 17.2, Schröder 6
Syrup, made from the petals of *Papaver rhoeas*, also known as *Papaver erraticum*.
  According to Sch (V:3 p 26), the use in European pharmacology goes back at least to the 16th century; the drug was prescribed as an analgesic and hypnotic, but also in diseases of the throat and chest; the syrup is found in the Württemberg pharmacopoeia, where it is called *syrupus papaveris erratici*; cf. also **TINCTURA florum papaveris erratici**, below. One might note that *Papaver rhoeas* is not included in the *Materia medica* of PhSuI.

SYRUPUS quinque radicum aperientium Martin 15.2
In PhHolm, there is a *syrupus de quinque radicibus*, which might be this preparation.
  The PhHolm preparation is made from roots of *Apium graveolens*, *Foeniculum vulgare*, *Petroselinum crispum*, *Asparagus* and *Ruscus aculeatus*, with seeds of the *Apium*, *Petroselinum* and *Foeniculum*, which are boiled in water, which then is boiled again, with sugar and vinegar.

In PhSuI, on the other hand, there is a *syrupus aperiens, vulgo syrupus e quinque radicibus*, which actually is made from only four roots, namely those of *apium, foeniculum, petroselinum* (as above), and *Taraxacum vulgare*, which are boiled and sugared.

THERIACA Andromachi Bergius 8.23, Schröder 22

Theriaca, Gr. θηριακή (sc. ἀντίδοτος), originally, θηριακή denoting something pertaining to venomous animals, means an antidote for bites from such creatures as vipers. The origin of the theriac seems to have been the reputedly universal antidote used by Mithridates, the famous king of Pontus in Asia Minor (1st century BC), the composition of which was brought to Roman knowledge following Pompey's victory over Mithridates; acc. to Pliny (*NH* 23.149) the ingredients of this original preparation were walnuts, figs, and leaves of *Ruta graveolens*, with a pinch of salt added. Elsewhere (*NH* 29.24), Pliny mentions the *excogitata compositio* of *theriace*, but also states, that the *mithridatium antidotum* is composed by no less than fifty-four ingredients.

Quite naturally, the prospect of a universal antidote would be of great interest to the ruler of any empire, and one of the many physicians-in-ordinary to experiment with improved compositions was Andromachos, physician of the emperor Nero, who is said to have introduced the meat of viper as a part of the composition (Galen *Antidot.* I:6); among the other ingredients were opium and several spices.

After the fall of the Roman empire, the manufacture of theriac became an Arab specialty, and intricate ceremonies, with the prospective purchasers of the preparation invited from all Europe, as a means to promote sales, seem to have been developed around the process of manufacture (L&G II p 300).

When Arab medicine in ca. 900 AD became known in Europe, especially in Italy, several Italian cities, most notably Venice, started their own theriac fabrication, and the *Theriaca Veneta* was, from 1295, sold only in officially sealed packages, which lead to its being regarded as a reliable preparation; the penalties for forgery of theriac were also severe.

Also in other European countries, such as France, England and Germany, theriac was made from ca. 1500 on, and the manufacturers often continued to "improve" the compositions, which lead to such preparations as e.g. *theriaca coelestis*, invented in 1693 by D. Hoffstadt in Hanau, Germany, which contained 184 different ingredients (L&G II p 304).

In the Swedish PhHolm, both *electuarium Mithridatium* and *theriaca* are to be found, having a few features in common: the number of ingredients is large in both cases; mithridate contains forty-nine, and theriac sixty-five different ingredients, several being common to both preparations (only the theriac contains meat of viper and asphalt, though). The prescriptions regarding the actual mixing together of the ingredients are also similar; in both cases, the ingredients should first be divided into a number of groups, or classes, which then were prepared individually, the final step being the mixture of all classes into the complete remedy. One remarkable difference between the preparations of PhHolm is, by the way, that the ingredients of the theriac often seem to be of more choice quality; when mithridate contains *terebinthina*, for theriac *terebinthina Venetiana* is specifically prescribed; mithridate has *cassia ligna*, while theriac has *cassia ligna vera*, etc. This might of course be due only to the two prescriptions being excerpted from different sources with slightly differing names for the ingredients, but might otherwise indicate, that mithridate at the time was used as a low-budget theriac, as it were.

In PhSuI the theriac no longer contained any meat of viper, but was still included in the PhSuVI, 1845. From 1869 it was no longer in the pharmacopoeia, and after the opium had been excluded due to new legislation in 1876, the popular demand for the preparation rapidly decreased.

As for the *theriaca Andromachi*, this preparation is found in PhLond and consists of sixty-one ingredients, basically the same as that of PhHolm, while the *theriaca* of PhSul has only eight ingredients, and the *theriaca diatesseron* ('[made] from four [ingredients]' fr. Greek δια + gen. of τέσσαρες; cf. *diascordium* s.v. **DIASCORDIUM** Fracastorii, above) of the same pharmacopoeia has actually not four, but five.

TINCTURA florum papaveris erratici Martin 17.2
A tincture, i.e. an extraction with e.g. alcohol, of the flowers in question; cf. also **SYRUPUS floris papaveris rhoeadis** above.

TINCTURA rhabarberi Schröder 35
There are two varieties of this tincture to be found in PhLond, one made with white wine, the other made with alcohol; besides the fact that they both contain, in addition to the rhubarb (cf. above, s.v. **PULVIS infantum**), the fruit of *Elettaria cardamomum* and *Crocus*.

TINCTURA rosarum Martin 17.2
A tincture, according to PhLond made from the buds of red roses, macerated in diluted sulphuric acid, and then sugared; there is also a *tinctura rosarum rubrarum* found in PhHolm, which contains some other herbs as well.

ULMARIA Bergius 9.2
The *Filipendula ulmaria*, earlier known as *Spiraea ulmaria*, also as *Regina prati* (Blancardus), which contains a preliminary stage to salicylic acid, and thus would have an antiinflammatory effect; according to Sch (V:2 p 100sq) it seems however to have been used mainly as a diuretic. Not mentioned in PhSul.

VINUM Canariense Martin 15.3
This is, according to Zedler, *Canarien-Sect*, a strong and sweet white wine from the Canary Islands; Orrelius' *Köpmans- och Material-Lexicon* says, s.v. *Secht*, that one distinguishes between *Canarie-* or *Palme-Sect*, which is the best, *Malaga Sect*, which is the sweetest, and *Xeres-* or *Seres-Sect*, which does not taste as good, but which is no more harmful than the other two kinds. While PhSul mentions *vinum album Gallicum*, *vinum Hispanicum*, *vinum Rhenanum* and *vinum rubrum Gallicum*, this wine is not included.

VINUM ipecacuanhae Bergius 8.15
Wine with peel of *Citrus aurantium* and root of *Cephaelis ipecacuanha*, probably introduced in Europe by Jesuits in the late 16th century (Sch V:1 p 264), and prescribed mainly for dysentery. The *ipecacuanha* is for some reason not mentioned by L&G, but has obviously been sufficiently well known in Swedish medicin to be included in Linnaeus' *Materia medica*. Found in PhLond.

VITRIOLUM martis Bergius 8.32
Ferrous sulphate, used much for the same purposes as alum, and often, in early medicine, confused with the latter; cf. **ALUMEN crystallinum**, above. In PhSul as *sal martis*.

Style

This part will examine, in addition to the four edited texts, fifteen other medical dissertations from Uppsala, constituting a representative selection of dissertations, defended under some of Sweden's most renowned professors of medicine during a period of just over one hundred years, namely:

De corporis humani ... divisione, 1634,
    praeses J. Franckenius, *respondens* N.E. Osander (Os)
De febribus, 1641,
    praeses J. Franckenius, *respondens* O.E. Lithselius (Lit)
De sero eiusque vasis, 1661,
    praeses O. Rudbeck the Elder, *respondens* O. Figrelius (Fi)
De concoctione, 1677,
    praeses P. Hoffwenius, *respondens* S. Poppelman (Po)
De flatibus, 1681,
    praeses P. Hoffwenius, *respondens* J.J. Fahlström (Fa)
De functionibus corporis humani primariis, 1695,
    Praeses O. Rudbeck the Younger, *respondens* J. Dalin (Da)
De passione hypochondriaca, 1697,
    Praeses O. Rudbeck the Younger, *respondens* M. Detterberg (De)[73]
De foeda lue venerea, 1705,
    praeses L. Roberg, *respondens* J. Linder (Lin)[74]
De erroribus in curandis febribus ..., 1738,
    praeses L. Roberg, *respondens* G.F. Voigtlender (Vo)
De tussi, 1, 1739,
    praeses N. Rosén, *respondens* E. Rosén (Ro1)
De tussi, 2, 1741,
    praeses N. Rosén, *respondens* E. Rosén (Ro2)
Amphimerina catarrhalis, 1750,
    praeses N. Rosén, *respondens* J.G. Wahlbom (Wa)
De dentitione difficili, 1757,
    praeses S. Aurivillius, *respondens* J. Petri Halenius (Ha)
Lepra, 1763,
    praeses C. Linnaeus, *respondens* I. Uddman (Ud)
De doloribus, 1765,
    praeses S. Aurivillius, *respondens* E.O. Rydbäck (Ry)

Excerpts from these dissertations are printed in a smaller size throughout this chapter.

It should also be pointed out, that "Style" might not be a fully adequate heading to label the contents of the present chapter, since I also include phaenomena which otherwise perhaps could be dubbed "genre conventions". It should further be noted

---

[73] This is one of the two known Swedish medical dissertations *pro gradu* from the period before 1738, even if the *respondens* seems never to have had the degree conferred upon him.

[74] Linder's dissertation differs from the rest in some respects; not only had he, according to his preface, achieved a degree in humanities (1702) at the university of Åbo by a dissertation *De pomis Hesperidum*, but he was also a Latin poet of some importance (cf. Ihre/Wåhlberg: *De poetis in Svio-Gothia latinis*, 1739, p 39sqq); this background might explain the fact, that Linder's dissertation gives a more "literary" impression than medical dissertations in general; among other things, he refers to, and quotes extensively from, ancient literature considerably more often than any other *respondens* in this material.

that when I write e.g. "Voigtlender ... assures the reader", this does not implicate that I regard it a verified fact that Voigtlender, and not *praeses*, Lars Roberg, is the actual author of his dissertation; it is merely a matter of convenience.[75]

General remarks

Firstly, one might consider the various ways to organize the factual matter in the dissertations, in which respect there are some differences; thus, out of the altogether nineteen dissertations dealt with in this chapter, seven consist of relatively short theses,[76] while the rest are texts of a considerably more continuous character, albeit divided into longer or shorter chapters.[77]

If we then consider the disposition of each singular dissertation of the more coherent type – always keeping in mind, of course, that the material is far too small to allow any general conclusions – we note that the differences are rather small; generally, the texts start out with a *definition* of the disease or phaenomenon dealt with, whereupon the *subspecies*, if any such are known, are given, together with the *causes*; the treatise is then concluded by suggesting a *cure*. No one would dispute that this is a logical order in which to present the matter.

Of greater interest, however, are the small differences which nevertheless *do* exist; some of the authors provide us with short *introductions* where e.g. the reasons for their choice of subject are given: Martin believes that the physician should concentrate on the most fatal diseases to fulfil his duties; Uddman says that he has chosen to write about *lepra* since this disease is common in his home district of Österbotten, Finland; Voigtlender, who treats erroneous fever therapy, assures the reader that his goal is not to criticize his colleagues, but that he wishes to contribute to the public good; in Linder's case, he uses his introduction to, *inter alia*, apologize for naming the bodily parts *quas vestes celant* (i.e. those, 'which the clothes cover'), which he does *non ex quadam animi prurigine* ('not from sensual lust'), but only since the subject demands it.

There are also differences as regards the profundity of treatment; a notable example of a very detailed treatise is Eberhard Rosén's sixty-six page dissertation *de tussi*,[78] which was submitted in two parts, and which begins with a rather thorough relation of the anatomical and physiological aspects of coughing; this dissertation also devotes two pages to "risk categories", and no fewer than twelve pages to prognosis, as regards the various subspecies of cough.[79]

---

[75] The authorship of a dissertation is often quite difficult to ascertain; in some cases, we have contemporary testimonies, or even extant drafts, to prove the authorship, while we, in other cases simply cannot with certainty establish the author; cf. e.g. Anna-Lena Pehrsson, p 89, Östlund, p 16.

[76] None of these (Os, Lit, Fi, Po, Da, De and Schröder) is a dissertation *pro gradu*, which of course might be a coincidence.

[77] There also exist examples of dissertations organized into a more table-like form; one of these is J. Schröder's doctoral dissertation *Genera morborum*, 1759, defended under the direction of Linnaeus; no such dissertation has however been included in my material.

[78] It is possible that the fact that the *respondens* was the younger brother of the *praeses* has led the former to show off a bit; another possibility is of course, that E. Rosén was an unusually competent physician (he was, after all, to achieve a professorship, albeit at Lund).

[79] Even if doctoral dissertations at this time generally are considerably shorter than Eberhard Rosén's, we cannot draw any certain conclusions regarding the quality of the doctoral candidate's efforts, since the dissertations which we have left have been put forth as the basis for an oral defence, of which we do not know very much; the amount of knowledge

This chapter, however, will deal mainly with two important elements of the texts, viz. (1) *Rhetorical tropes and figures* and (2) *The interaction with the reader*, which seems to be a characteristic feature of the dissertational discourse.[80]

Rhetorical tropes and figures

As one might expect from an epoch, when the rules of classical rhetoric were still studied, and still considered an ideal pattern for certain literary genres, these texts, even if not particularly intent on form, contain elements of traditional rhetorical embellishments; it is of course also possible that such tropes and figures in some cases are the result, not of any deliberate stylistic aim, but rather of the method by which Latin was learnt (cf. "Language", above).

Metaphors

These are very frequent, and taken from several fields; the two major categories, however, are the *Metaphors of travel and movement* and the *Military metaphors*.

Metaphors of travel and movement

As is pointed out by Östlund, this category of metaphor is a typical feature of the dissertational genre,[81] used to describe the act of discussing the subject, of writing and defending a thesis, as a *journey* or a *walk* or a *voyage* at sea:

> Propero *jam ad generalem illam indicationem* (Martin 12.1)

> *Eum* tramitem insistam, *quem … apperiit medicus* (Martin 12.4)

> *ut ordine* procedamus (Da thesis 7)
> *Ad prognosin itaque* properamus (De thesis 20)

This kind of metaphor can also be used to indicate a digression:

> *omnium quidem primum ad ea* recurrendum est *tempora, a quibus … morbi hujus vestigia repeti possunt* (Martin 3.1)

or, more often, the intent to avoid digressions, i.e. to pass something without stopping:

> *Merito vero* praeterimus *alias aliorum opiniones* (Martin 4.7)

> *Hoc … obiter tantum et* tanquam in transitu, *tangam* (Martin 12.2)

> *Ultra limites vero* excurremus, *si singula conquireremus prognostica signa* (Bergius 5.1)

> *Eam … silentio* praeteriimus (Sundius 9.3)

---

communicated by any doctoral candidate through his dissertation plus its defence might well have been of about the same weight as that of his colleagues.

[80] Cf. Östlund, p 69sq.

[81] Östlund, p 65sq.

> *Caeteras ... species* sicco pede praeterimus (Lit thesis 30)[82]
> *ne simus adeo prolixi, eos* sicco transimus pede (Fi thesis 12)
> *Multa ... sciens in hoc negotio* praeterii, *ne excresceret Dissertationis moles* (Lin, p 2)
> Festinanti *et respicienti ad crescentis Dissertationis molem* praeterire *liceat* (Lin, p 45)

A subspecies of the metaphor of movement is the *sailing metaphor*, which has often been used to describe the course of life as a journey across an often rough sea towards a safe haven.[83]

This particular category of metaphor was used already in ancient Latin, e.g. in Cicero's *Cato maior de senectute*, 71: *tam iucunda est, ut, quo propius ad mortem accedam, quasi terram videre videar aliquandoque in portum ex longa navigatione esse venturus*, and in Horace, *Carmina*, 2.10;[84] one might also compare this usage to the frequent use, during the Renaissance, of the ship as an emblematic element; cf. Henkel and Schöne (ed): *Emblemata: Handbuch zur Sinnbildkunst des XVI und XVII Jahrhunderts*, 1967/1978, col. 1453sqq.

In dissertations as well as in other scholarly texts, the sailing metaphor, facilitating also the hinting at difficulties, is rather frequent as a means to visualise the process of discussing a matter in a turbulent environment, filled with stormy debate and opposition, abounding in erroneous theories and hypotheses; there are examples also in this material:

> *Dicas mihi ad* quam ... sacram *confugiendum* anchoram (Bergius 10.34)

> *Hoc certe ...* pelagus *nemo facile sine* naufragii periculo *transibit* (Lin, p 16)
> *ut* scopulos et syrtes, *quas observasse memet mihi visus sum, indicarem amicis et artem adamantibus, inter eosdem mecum fluctus forte* navigantibus agitatisque (Vo, p 1)

Military metaphors

Very frequently, metaphors in a medical context are taken from the field of warfare; today, the findings of modern microbiology would make such metaphors more or less accurate descriptions in many cases, but the comparison of illness to an attacking enemy has obviously been close at hand early in history; there are e.g. three instances in Celsus of *invadere* in a metaphorical sense: *Diutius saepe et periculosius tabes eos male habet, quos invasit.* (3.22); *At si simul ea utrumque oculum invaserunt* (6.6), and *Si quando autem ulcera oris cancer invasit* (6.15); cf. also Thomas Campanella's (1568–1639) discussion of the nature of fever in his *Medicinalium ... libri septem* (1635);[85] likewise, *impetus* is known from Celsus: *in ipso acuti morbi impetu* (2.4), and *occurro* is used – about the disease, not about the physician – e.g. by Soranus.

---

[82] Cf. Östlund, p 72.

[83] The metaphor of travel and movement in general has of course also been used about the life of man; cf. e.g. John Bunyan's (1628–88) *The Pilgrim's Progress*.

[84] There are also examples from Greek literature, e.g. in Plato (c. 429–347 BC), νόμοι, 803 b; cf. Nisbet & Hubbard, *A commentary on Horace: odes book II*, p 158sq, with further references.

[85] Campanella's text is treated by L.J. Rather and J.B. Frerichs in *On the Use of Military Metaphor in Western Medical Literature: The* bellum contra morbum *of Thomas Campanella (1568–1639)* (in *Clio Medica*, vol 7, No 3, 1972, pp 201–208.).

The phaenomenon is still very common in the period dealt with here:

Of the disease

Constat, hunc morbum ... fatalem fuisse ... ejusque non minus periculosum quam maturum adventum salutem hominum ... oppugnare (Martin 2.2)

in procinctu *variolas esse possis praedicere* (Martin 6.2)

Cum jam in primo stadio rigor calor et dolores ... aegrotum invaserunt (Martin 7.1)

apparuere 4 die ... tubercula denso agmine (Bergius 8.12)

pustulas faciem reliquisse, ingentem ... earum copiam pedes occupasse *videbat* (Bergius 8.30)

illud tempus ... quo ... invaserat *Epilepsia* (Sundius 3.3)

certum est nullam Febrem non satellitibus stipatam *humanum genus* invadere (Lit th 48)
hae febres plerumque horrore quodam invadunt (Vo p 6)
*Homines ...*aggreditur *Amphimerina* (Wa p 12)

Of the physician and his remedies

Solis luce clarius est ... qua via maxime conveniat morbo occurrere (Martin 8.1)

contagium ... , virtute [antimonii] virus quodcunque debellante, *destrui ... videtur* (Martin 13.3)

[Medicus] debet enim ... symptomatibus maturo occurrere *auxilio* (Bergius 8.23)

Purgantium ... in hac febri debellanda *usum ... demonstravit J.* FREIND (Bergius 10.30)

In casu adeo ancipiti ... ad Corticem Chinae propinandum ... nos accinximus (Bergius 10.53)

Modus ... quo ... occurrere *huic malo ... queamus* (Sundius 4)

Contra primam caussam pugnare *possumus Rhabarbaro ... Secunda* superatur *mellitis ..., tertiae vero* opponimus *oleosa* (Schröder 31)

nec remedia, laude quidem sua digna, sed tamen non sine ... violentia venenum debellatura (Lin p 32)
Hoste *interim relicto* infensissimo pugnant (Vo p 9)
Cortex Peruvianus ... victoriam reportare *solet* (Wa p 15)
symptomatibus profecto obviam ire *convenit* (Ha p 15)
ejusmodi arma *difficilis dentitio ejusque symptomata requirere non videantur* (Ha p 17)

The military metaphor can also be used with regard to the patient:

> *Contagium hoc … infecturum mox illos, qui hoc morbo antea non* occupati *fuerunt*
> (Martin 9.4)

or to describe the entire situation:

> *Scire vero licet hoc modo* inducias *tantum factas esse,* bellum non compressum
> (Schröder 35)

Other metaphors

Apart from the two major groups treated above, our texts also contain metaphors from other areas of life; as might be expected, some of the common expressions, pertaining to the act of *methodically treating a subject,* and which are mentioned by Östlund[86] are also found here, e.g. from *textile work;* methodical and logical analysis is depicted as weaving:

> *definitionem rei essentiam …* subnectimus (Lit th 8)
> *Dum … coeptam* telam pertexere *aggredior* (Ro1 p 3)
> *Duceret nunc tractationis* filum *… ad perstringendas differentias* (Ro1 p 12)
> Telam *… pro viribus* perteximus (Wa p 20)

As for *theatrical metaphors,* there are also examples:

> *Febris sane denuo mutata, & loco inflammatoriae, putridae scenam ludere visa*
> (Bergius 10.33)

> *Tussis … incipit,* malorumque scenam *infantibus quos invadit* aperit (Ro1 p 15)
> *non semper* eandem ludit scenam (Wa p 10)

Linder makes use of this kind of metaphor with some extra refinement, as, in his description of syphilis symptoms, he treats the entire progress of the disease as a theatrical performance; he is stageing the illness with the intention, as he puts it, to give a relation of the symptoms *eo ordine, quo venenum et agere primo incipit, et tandem luctuosam scenam absolvit* (Lin p 23); he then proceeds with a description of the primary infection, which ends: *estque primus … hujus fabulae actus* (Lin ibid). After treating the second stage[87] he concludes his reasoning in very much the same way: *Estque hic secundus actus fabulae* (Lin p 24), whereupon the tertiary symptoms are dealt with, leading to the final remark: *Adeoque hic tertium fabulae Actum … habemus.* (Lin p 26).

Linder also uses metaphors from another area, where action takes place under the eyes of spectators, namely athletics:

> *sequor autoritatem Helmontii … adferentis non omnes morbos simul venisse* in palaestram (Lin p 3)

He also uses the personification of an abstract:

> *nonnulla* fidissima *semper* comes paupertas *denegavit.*

Apart from those treated above, there are of course several other rhetorical figures to be found in the material, such as:

---

[86] Östlund, p 66sq.
[87] "Stage" is NOT intended as a theatrical metaphor here.

Litotes
An affirmation by negation of its opposite:[88]

> *Patronos* haud paucos *invenies* (Martin 3.3)

> haud inconsultum *ducimus … illa stadia … persequi* (Martin 5.2)

> haud rari *casus probant* (Bergius 4.1)

> non inconsultum *arbitramur refrigerantia adjungere* (Bergius 8.6)

> *Humores acres … prodibant,* haud sine *aegri* solatio (Sundius 5.2)

> *haec* … haud inepte *jungimus* (Schröder 31)

> haud raro *quoque evenit* (Schröder 34)

> *quaestio discursu* non indigna *sese offert* (Lit thesis 50)
> *hoc* non sine causa (Fig thesis 2)
> nec male *haec vox convenire videtur* (Po thesis 1)
> non ultimo loco *numerandus dolor ille capitis* (Fa p 51)
> *id certe* non raro *contingit* (Lin p 22)
> *Contingere autem haecce … observamus* haud raro (Vo p 9)
> *Epidemica tussis vergente in autumnum aestate* haud raro *incipit* (Ro1 p 15)
> Haud ignoro … *Phthisin subinde contagiose propagari* (Ud p 101)[89]
> Non inepte *vero comprehendi omnes possunt* (Ry p 3)

Hyperbaton

This figure, consisting in the emphasizing of a word or phrase by a word order, diverging from the expected,[90] is a very common rhetorical figure at this time (which probably would have considerably diminished the emphasizing function):

> *ea, quae* praesentissimam *afferre videntur* noxam (Martin 1.1)

> *[fermentum] quod …* tantum *in corpore excitare dicitur* motum (Martin 4.2)

> Deglutitionis *sentitur* molestia (Martin 6.3)

> *Memoria* dictos *tenenti* characteres (Bergius 1.1)

> *Si … sanies* salsum *praebeat* saporem (Bergius 5.28)

> *morbum hunc Epilepsias* genuinam *esse* speciem … *facile patet* (Sundius 0.1)

> *Nutrix vero* illis *uti debet* remediis (Sundius 3.3)

---

[88] Cf. Sz, *Stilistik,* § 32.

[89] The pagination as regards Ud is in every instance in accordance with the edition in *Amoenitates academicae.*

[90] Cf. Sz, *Stilistik,* § 2.

praecepta quae sequentes *proponunt* canones (Schröder 4)

nullum *omnino excitare debet doloris* sensum (Schröder 8)

Cerebrum sublimem *corporis occupavit* sedem (Os thesis 39)
unaquaeque suam *postulat* descriptionem (Lit thesis 8)
Causae *quippe* contrariae, contrarium *edunt* effectum (Lit thesis 49)
angustissimos *transit* meatus (Fi thesis 5)
alimenta digeruntur magnam*que subeunt* alterationem (Po thesis 1)
Dolendi *praeterea* modi … *indicant* (Fa p 48)
Sunt & aliae *hujus affectus* species (Fa p 52)
Divinum *inter animalia* miraculum (Da thesis 1)
ne corpus … nimiam *suae substantiae* jacturam *faceret* (Da thesis 20)
famosa *illa mulierum* passio (De thesis 2)
pro … ordinario *tunc temporis Gallorum in militia* pabulo (Lin p 8)
nulla *fere videtur esse* differentia (Vo p 3)
tussis cognitioni lucem *affundant* majorem (Ro1 p7)
summa *Auctorum in scribendo* inconstantia (Ud p 94)
sensum, qui corpori … situm *negat* quietum (Ry p 3)

Chiasmus

As will be seen, this figure, as opposed to those above, is rather uncommon; it is not
to be found in every dissertation, and in noone there are more than two or three
instances:

Salivatio in adultis, in infantibus diarrhoea (Martin 6.9)

nominare nominibus et coloribus describere liceat Oratori (Lin p 2)
post varias migrationes gentium et Imperiorum mutationes (Lin p 3)
ex pectoris oppressione et dolore pulmonum (Vo p 6)
forma variantior, atque difficilior curatu (Ud p 95)
placent alia, alia displicent (Ry p 8)

Exclamations

Extensive use of exclamations is made in Bergius' thesis:

En itaque curam variolarum … paucis tradendam momentis! (Bergius 6.1)

Quanta saepius non excitatur febris! (Bergius 10.32)

Quid putredinis! (Bergius 10.32)

Dicas mihi … et magnus mihi eris Apollo! (Bergius 10.34)

Sed quam subita metamorphosis! (Bergius 10.44)

Apart from these, the only exclamations found in this material are

Horribile dictu! (Lin p 9)
proh dolor! (Wa p 20)

Rhetorical questions

As regards these, too, the usage among the authors varies; Martin and, to some extent, Bergius use this means of expression rather frequently – the following examples constitute only a selection – while it is not found at all in Sundius and Schröder:

quid aliud consequi potest …? (Martin 7.2)

quid propius ad similitudinem accedit …? (Martin 7.2)

Nonne optime ab initio procederes …? (Martin 8.3)

Et quo, quaeso, successu judicia sua … interponunt autores? (Martin 9.2)

Sed quid ad propriam experientiam provocemus? (Bergius 10.8)

Quid enim in praxi frequentius …? (Bergius 10.32)

Out of the remaining ten dissertations, rhetorical questions are found in Lin:

Num Morbi nunc plures quam olim? (Lin p 3)
nonne conspectum frequenter Medicis est …? (Lin p 19)

and in Ud (also a mere selection):

Nonne Dr. Schreiber exercitum Russorum …a peste liberavit? (Ud p 101)
quid magis verosimile, quam …? (Ud p 101)
numne Micrographi … ingentem vim vermium detegunt …? (Ud p 102)

This stylistic device, trying to convince the reader through "asking" questions without expecting any answer – least of all in the negative – may be regarded also as a *means of involving the reader* in the argument, which leads us to

Interaction

Interaction with the reader
The inclusion of the reader in the discussion by direct address is sometimes used; the reader is generally addressed as *Benevole lector* or *Candide lector.*

tuae, Candide lector … (Martin 2.3)

Mirum tibi non videbitur …(Lit thesis 36)
Haec sunt, Lector benevole, quae … congere licuit (Po thesis 22)
Haec itaque sunt, Benevole lector, pauca illa …(Vo p 14)
jam subsisto, finemque huic Dissertationi, tua Benevole lector, indulgentia fretus (Vo ibid)
Tuum erit, Benevole lector, aequi bonique consulere (Lin p 2)
per Te intelligis, Lector Benevole …(Ud p 95)

The mentioning of the reader in 3rd person as a means to include him in the discussion is also used in some cases:

exempla …inveniet B. L. apud Galen. Lib. 2 (Fa p 39)

84

Interim meretur, ut ...Iguana Benevolo Lectori hic suam speciem ostendat (Lin p 9)
Sed ne Lectori prolixitate displiceam (Lin p 11)
Quae spectant ad morbi historiam ...recensui, ut prodessem Benevolo Lectori (Lin p 29)

Interaction with the *praeses*

The *praeses* is also sometimes referred to in the text; as is pointed out elsewhere,[91] Östlund has shown that this might be the case even if the *praeses* himself is the author of the dissertation, in which instances the phaenomenon must be regarded as a mere convention:

missa jam facio testimonia aliorum ... ad unius Nobilissimi Domini Praesidis experientiam provocaturus (Martin 16.1)

Vaporem ... adhibuit Illustris Dominus PRAESES (Bergius 10.14)

Julapium refocillans Illustris PRAESIDIS (Bergius 10.46)

Occurras Electuario ...juxta quae ... a Nobilissimo Domine Praeside allata sunt (Sundius 1.1)

Quod ... laborare possit evidenti experimento Nobilissimi Domini Praesidis constitit (Sundius 2.1)

drachmam dimidiam sumat Pulveris pro nutrice Nobilissimi Domini Praesidis (Sundius 2.3)

Prolixiorem ... descriptionem a Nobilissimo Domino Praeside expectamus (Sundius 7.4)

Ut haec elegantissime nos omnia docet Clarissimus Dominus Doctor Praeses (Fa p 57)
videtur mihi ... sufficiens hypothesis, quam debere me CLARISSIMO PRAESIDI lubens profiteor (Lin p 47)

Interaction with the opponents

Linder is the only *respondens* to mention the opponents:

Cum ... statuendum mihi aliquid sit, saltem in Dominorum Opponentium gratiam (Lin p 13)

Here, one might wonder why this passage is at all included in the printed dissertation; normally, the imaginary dialogue with the reader could probably replace the dialogue with the opponent when the text was read; perhaps this passage is due to some mistake in editing the manuscript before printing?

Interaction with the audience

Also in this case, there is only one occurrence:

hanc ... materiam ... huic celeberrimo Auditorio proponere ... voluimus (Lit thesis 59)

---

[91] My commentary to **Bergius 10.14**.

Modifying expressions

These expressions partly correspond with those which Östlund labels *modifying expressions*;[92] since the affirmation however seems to be a far more common feature in the dissertations which are examined here than is the assumption, and since thus only the former phaenomenon will be dealt with, a more adequate caption would perhaps be *affirmative expressions*.[93]

One possible way to group these expressions might be the following:

Appeal to common sense

    Citra controversiam est (Martin 8.3)

    non difficile est existimare (Martin 12.1)

    nemo facile negaverit (Martin 14.2)

    nemo dubitare posse videatur (Martin 16.2)

    inficias iverit nemo (Bergius 3.1)

    ultro patet (Bergius 8.14)

    Ratio in promtu est (Bergius 8.20)

    dubium non est (Schröder 14)

    In eo tamen omnes fere conspirarunt (Da thesis 2)
    cuivis facile patet (Vo p 5)
    Nemini non constat (Ud p 100)

Appeal to more or less well-tested experience

    Experientia ulterius constat (Martin 11.2)

    Jam experientia patet (Martin 13.2)

    experientia docet (Martin 14.1)

    experientia quotidie edocet (Bergius 8.10)

    Sed quid rei, tot … observationibus, extra controversiam positae, diu immoremur? (Bergius 10.66)

    Experientia probat haec vera esse (Fa p 19)
    usque ab incunabulis experti sumus (Da thesis 3)

---

[92] Östlund, p 74sqq.

[93] It is of course an interesting question, which might be worth a separate investigation, whether the predilection for this kind of assertions is more common among medical writers *in genere* than it is among scholars of the humanities.

Quantum … unicuique medicinae perito, judicandum relinquo (Vo p 11)[94]
multiplici constat observatione (Wa p 12)
experientia de hac re nos satis reddit convictos (Wa p 13)
Cernimus quotidie infantes … facile dentibus sensim ornari (Ha p 10)
Observationes & experimenta monstrarunt (Ry p 5)
Ex qvotidianis tamen observationibus … discitur evidentissime (Ry p 7)

or to a – true or alleged – consensus among earlier authors

plerique Medici Statuunt (Fa p 14)
ut Hippocrates, Galenus, … & alii multi confirmant (Fa ibid.)
quod recentiores & maxime nostri aevi Scriptores confirmant (Fa p 23sq)
Medici omnes aperte fatentur (Lin p 40)
Uno fere ore confiteantur Auctores (Ud p 105)

Reference to a supporting discussion (within the dissertation or elsewhere)

Sed ex iis, quae postmodum afferentur, perfacile erit existimare (Martin 4.1)

Ex his omnibus indiciis … quivis … facile colliget (Martin 7.1)

Inde satis elucet (Bergius 8.11)

Ex iis quae dicta sunt, haud difficulter constat (Sundius 1.1)

Facile quivis ex jam dictis eruere potest (Fi thesis 12)
ab hac causa deducimur (Fa p 18)
venia illius viri, affirmare audemus …(Fa p 20)
Ex hisce allatis facile patet (Vo p 12)
Ex his datis principiis … definire possumus (Ro1 p 5)
Ex cognita … structura … patet (Ro1 p 12)
Ex illis … intelligi queat (Ro1 p 24)
Quod ut credamus eo firmius, sequentibus … rationibus inducti sumus (Ud p 104)

Modesty of the author

One feature, finally, found in these texts is the more or less sincere apology for not treating one's subject exhaustingly enough, or for not being competent enough (expressions, bordering upon those listed below, might of course also be found among e.g. the metaphors of travel and movement above):

Equidem tenuitatis meae conscius probe perspicio viribus meis hoc onus minus respondere - - - benevolentiae haut diffidendum crediderim, si in re ardua omnem movere non valeam lapidem (Martin 2:3)

Quam … difficilem … ingredior disputationem, cum, in hac virium mearum tenuitate eam rem propugnandam suscipio (Martin 8.2)

---

[94] Which, by the way, also might be regarded as an example of interaction, albeit not as direct as those listed above.

Cum tamen & temporis & aliis premar angustiis (Martin 17.1)

Allatas vero species propius considerare, instituti non sinit ratio (Bergius 2.10)

Prolixiorem quippe curationem postulat, quamque describere loci angustia non permittit (Sundius 9.3)

video fateorque non pauca hic aut omissa, aut pro exigentia argumenti, minus accurate tractata esse, quae omnia huc pertinentia, ob temporis angustiam, institutique rationem, hic colligere mihi non fuit permissum. Accedit rerum amplitudo & difficultas, quibus me adolescentem … longe imparem agnosco (Po thesis 22)

intelligis … mearum non esse vrium neque experientiae argumentum hoc summe arduum atque huc dum vix satis extricabile ad liquidum perducere (Ud p 95)

His omnibus assentior (Author's remark).

De variolis praecavendis, resp Roland Martin,
text and translation

Adjuvante Deo

DISSERTATIO MEDICA
DE
VARIOLIS
PRÆCAVENDIS
QUAM
SUFFRAGENTE AMPLISSIMO ET EXPERIENTISSIMO REGIAE
ACADEMIAE UPSALIENSIS SENATU MEDICO,
PRAESIDE
VIRO NOBILISSIMO
DOMINO DOCTORE NICOLAO
ROSÉN,
Sacrae Regiae MAJESTATIS ARCHIATRO,
MEDICINAE ET ANATOMIAE PROFESSORE REGIO ET ORDINARIO
REGIARUM ACADEMIARUM SCIENTIARUM STOCKHOLMENSIS
ET UPSALIENSIS MEMBRO
PRO GRADU DOCTORIS
SUMMISQUE IN MEDICINA HONORIBUS OBTINENDIS,
VENTILANDAM SISTIT
AUCTOR,
STIPENDIARIUS STIEGLERIANUS
ROLANDUS MARTIN, PETRI FILIUS,
UPLANDUS.
IN AUDITORIO CAROLINO MAJORI,
AD DIEM XXIII FEBRUARII ANNI MDCCLI,
HORIS ANTE ET POST MERIDIEM CONSVETIS

———

UPSALIAE

With the Help of God

A MEDICAL DISSERTATION
ON
THE PREVENTION
OF SMALLPOX,
WHICH
BY PROMOTION OF THE GREAT AND EXPERIENCED MEDICAL FACULTY
OF THE ROYAL UNIVERSITY OF UPPSALA
UNDER THE PRESIDENCY OF
THE HONOURABLE
DOCTOR NILS
ROSÉN,
ARCHIATER to Their Sacred Royal MAJESTIES,
PROFESSOR REGIUS ET ORDINARIUS OF MEDICINE AND ANATOMY,
MEMBER OF THE ROYAL ACADEMIES OF SCIENCES
OF STOCKHOLM AND UPPSALA,
IS PUT FORTH FOR DISCUSSION
FOR THE DOCTOR'S DEGREE
AND FOR THE ACHIEVEMENT OF THE HIGHEST RANK IN MEDICINE
BY THE AUTHOR,
THE HOLDER OF THE STIEGLER SCHOLARSHIP
ROLAND MARTIN, SON OF PETER,
FROM UPPLAND,
IN THE MAJOR CAROLINE AUDITORIUM,
ON FEBRUARY THE 23RD 1751,
AT THE USUAL TIME AM AND PM

UPPSALA

KONGLIG MAJESTÄTS
HÖGTBETRODDE MAN OCH PRAESIDENT
UTI DESS OCH RIKSENS
CAMMAR-COLLEGIO,
RIDDARE OCH COMMENDEUR
AF KONGLIG MAJESTÄTS ORDEN
~~SAMT~~
HÖGVÄLBORNE GREFVE,
HERR
CARL
FREDRICH
PIPER,

Hvad. Som. Än. I. Dag.[95]
Underhåller.
Den. Ärefulla. Högacktning.
SVEA. RIKE.
Med. Detta. Hundradetalet.
Fattat.
För. Det. PIPERSKA. Namnet.
Är.
Icke. Mindre.
Et. Djupt. Förstånd.
En. Ogemen. Oväldughet.
Och.
En. Medfödd. Mildhet.
Som.
NÅDIGE. HERRE.
Dag. Ifrån. Dag.
Pryda. EDERT. Höga. Väsende.
Än.
Den. Äros. Högd.
Hvilken.
Alle. Svenske. Män. I. Gemen.
Och. Hvar. Redlig. I. Synnerhet.
Ei. Utan. Nitfull. Vördnad.
Tillstå.
Att. Herr. GREFVEN. Och. PRESIDENTEN.
Så. Värdigt. Besitter.
Desse. Lysande. Egenskaper.
Hafva. Under. En. Sådan. Allmän. Värkan.
Jämväl. Upeldat. Mitt. Hopp.
Ej. Allenast.
Om. Nådigt. Tillträde.
Hos. Herr. GREFVEN. Och. PRESIDENTEN.
Utan. Ock.

---

[95] As regards the contents of the gratulatory texts, see my commentary, p 124sq.

Om. Den. lyckliga. Påfölgd.
Att. Mitt. Ringa. Academiska. arbete.
Af. EDERT. Höga. Namn. Må. Förädlas.
Att. Det.
Under. Så Kraftigt. Beskydd.
Vinner.
Hos. Allmänheten.
Hvad. Det.
Genom. Min. Oförmögenhet.
Saknar.

HÖGVÄLBORNE HERR GREFVENS
Och PRESIDENTENS
SAMT
RIDDARENS Och COMMENDEURENS
AF KONGLIG MAJESTÄTS ORDEN

Allerödmjukaste tjenare
ROLAND MARTIN

KONGLIG MAJESTÄTS
TROMAN OCH ÖFVERSTE,
SAMT
RIDDARE AF KONGLIGA SVERDS-ORDEN,
HÖGVÄLBORNE BARON,
HERR MAURITZ
POSSE

HERRE, mannamod med vett
Och ett väsend rikt af heder
Er hos Höga vänskap gett
Och de lägres nit bereder
När jag vördsamt lägger ner
Desse blad, ehuru ringa;
Vill jag, under skydd af ER,
Dem till högre värde bringa.
HÖGVÄLBORNE HERR BARONS
Och ÖFVERSTENS
SAMT
RIDDARENS AF KONGLIGA SVERDS-ORDEN

allerödmjukaste tjenare
ROLAND MARTIN.

In Nomine Dei

CAPUT PRIMUM
De natura & indole variolarum.

§**1.1** In iis incommodis, quae, naturae quadam necessitate, homines infestant, ea principe loco reponantur, quae praesentissimam afferre videntur noxam. Quin morbi & vitae humanae spatium comminuant & jucunditatibus obicem ponant, tanto minus dubitare convenit, quanto magis id experientiae, quamvis deplorandae, consentaneum est. **1.2** Nihil itaque praestantius est eo medico, qui morbos non modo cavere, sed etjam tanquam in exilium proscribere valet. Is vero si officii sui numeros explebit, non tam id agat, ut iis se opponat morbis, qui minus humano generi sunt funesti, quam iis praecipue, qui maximum cladis & perniciei afferunt. **1.3** Huc merito referas eam morborum catervam, quos graeco nomine ἐξανϑηματικούς vocant. Idque eo magis, quo certius est, cum iis non modo gravissimas accessiones conjunctas esse, sed etiam vitae spem ancipitem. Sic autem commodissime definiuntur: *sunt morbi febriles, cum efflorescentia cutis.*

§**2.1** Horum vero non unum est genus; quidam enim suppuratione terminantur, quidam non. Illorum numero, & quidem maxime periculosorum Pestis & Variolae habentur. Illam, tanquam scelerum & flagitiorum vindicem, a Deo mortalibus immissum, rimandi & penitius cognoscendi facultatem medicis denegatam esse, apud plurimos est in confesso. **2.2** Variolae autem utpote non tam praecipitis exitii plenae, copiam sui dederunt majorem. Jam cum experientia duce constat, hunc morbum plurimis hominibus, quam alium quendam, fatalem fuisse, ejusque non minus periculosum, quam maturum adventum salutem hominum, Pestis instar, oppugnare, non operam perdidisse is censendus est, qui non modo naturam morbi sed & qua ratione obviam ipsi eatur, ex accuratis & diu institutis observationibus, exposuerit. **2.3** Equidem tenuitatis meae conscius probe perspicio viribus meis hoc onus minus respondere, at cum in magnis etiam aliquid tentare pulcrum sit, non committendum putavi, ut difficultas operis ab incepto me deterreat; praecipue cum Tuae, Candide Lector, benevolentiae haut diffidendum crediderim, si in re ardua omnem movere non valeam lapidem.

In the Name of God

THE FIRST CHAPTER
On the nature and character of smallpox

§**1.1** Among the inconveniencies which, according to some law of nature, plague mankind, the foremost place must be given to those, that seem to bring the most obvious harm. The more we must agree upon this experience, even if regrettable, the lesser we should doubt that diseases both diminish the length of human life and put up obstacles for pleasure. **1.2** Nothing, thus, can surpass the physician, who is able, not only to avoid illness, but also to condemn it, so to speak, to exile. But, if he wants to fulfill all his duties, he should not concentrate on fighting those illnesses, which are less fatal to mankind, as much as those, especially, that bring about the most death and danger. **1.3** Among those one could well-deservedly count the troup of diseases which, by a Greek term, is called $\varepsilon\xi\alpha\nu\vartheta\eta\mu\alpha\tau\iota\varkappa o\iota$, even more so, as it is quite sure that with these are connected not only serious complications, but also endangerment of life. They are suitably defined thus: *they are fever diseases with skin eruptions.*

§**2.1** But they are not of only one kind: some end up in purulence, some do not. To the former kind, and, for that matter, the most dangerous of that kind, are assigned plague and smallpox. According to the prevalent opinion, the permission to examine, and more thoroughly get to know the former of these has been refused to the physicians, as it were a disease sent by God as a punisher of sins and atrocities. **2.2** Smallpox, on the other hand, as they do not bring about such a quick death, have given us better opportunities. As it is already clear, from experience, that this disease has brought about the death of more humans than any other, and that its arrival, just as dangerous as it is quick, attacks the health and safety of man just about as much as the plague does, the opinion must be that he, who has put forth, from exact, and long approved of, observations, not only the nature of this disease, but also by which method it is combatted, has not wasted his exertion. **2.3** Even as I, aware of my insignificance, quite clearly understand that this task does not very well suit my capacity, since it is fair, in great issues, at least to try, I have wished, not to be guilty of letting the difficulties of this task deter me from my purpose, especially since I would believe that I could hope for your indulgence, My Sincere Reader, if I, in such difficult conditions, should fail to do my utmost.

§3.1 Ut itaque ab ovo, quod ajunt, incipiam, omnium quidem primum ad ea recurrendum est tempora, a quibus longissime morbi hujus vestigia repeti possunt. Videntur quidem hujus rei nulla certa afferri testimonia posse; alii enim non ante seculum septimum apud Arabes invaluisse hunc morbum contendunt, alii ingentibus istis rei medicae, inter antiquos, statoribus, *Hippocrati & Galeno,* olim innotuisse eundem perhibent, & quidem nomine τωυ ἐξανθημάτων. **3.2** Priorem illam sententiam strenue inprimis tuetur illustris *Werlhof,* cui suum etiam calculum addit summus Angliae Medicus Illustris *Mead,* qui, cum in libris de variolis, veterum ἀντράκας & ἐτινυκτίδας parum cum variolis affinitatis habere persvasus sit, in ea est opinione, ut *Rhazes* Arabum Medicorum quidam, qui locum de variolis egregie pertractavit, primum auctorem adtulerit nomine *Aaron,* qui materiam hanc enodavit. Hinc suspicatur Celeberrimus *Freindius* originem morbi ab Ægypto repetendam, qvum ibi lucem *Aaron* iste primum aspexerit. **3.3** At simul observatur *Johannem Reiske,* adhuc antiquiores reperiisse variolas & morbillos, cui sententiae verba, in exemplari manuscripto Leidensis Bibliothecae inventa, occasionem dederunt[a]. Posterioris autem sententiae Patronos haud paucos invenies, qui morbi hujus peritiam nec Patribus graecis defuisse existimant. **3.4** Ut alios taceam, illustre hujus rei documentum dabit Nobilissimus *Linderstolpe,* Medicus nostras celeberrimus, cujus haec est sententia: morbi hoc genus, ab ipsis mundi initiis, primordia sumsisse, veteribusque Medicis non ignotum fuisse, licet per simplicitatem alimentorum non tam sevierint, uti nostrae aetatis luxu[b]. Idem in notis paginae 310 confirmat *Stenzelius,* qui opinionis suae fautorem adducit *Zacutum Lusitanum: Medicorum principorum historia, pag. 164* **3.5** Neque nos videmus, qua specie veritatis negaveris, idem veneni antiquissima memoria in orbe sparsum fuisse, hocque progenuisse malum. Quod reliquum est, de antiquitate variolarum, eruditissimum Hahnii scriptum rotunde dilucideque exponet[c].

§4.1 Cum iam ordinis servandi ratio jubeat, in caussas variolarum inquirere, congruens quidem esset, primo loco de proxima, deinde de sic dictis προκαταρτικοίς & προηγουμένοις disserere. Sed ex iis, quae postmodum afferentur, perfacile erit existimare, quid de prima sit statuendum. **4.2** De reliquis autem cum nihil certi quid affirmem, habeam, breviter tantum percurram dissentientes auctorum, de hoc genere, opiniones. Inter eas autem primo referendae sunt conjecturae, de *fermento innato,* quod, accedente caussa epidemica externa, tantum in corpore excitare dicitur motum, tantamque fermentationem, ut inde humores, naturali sangvinis cursu vitiato, in eam putredinem abirent: atque ejusmodi placitum est, antea laudati *Rhazes,* in commentario de variolis & morbillis, Cap. 1, cujus haec sunt verba: **4.3** *mustum aliquod est, quo sangvis puerorum assimilatur, in quo nondum inccepit fieri coctio, & cui nondum competit motio ad fermentationem. Juvenum autem sangvis assimilatur musto, cum quo effervescentia fit & vapores erumpunt. Ipsas autem variolas dicit esse fervescentiam & ebullitionem, quae excitari solet in musto, in illo fervoris tempore.*

---

[a] *haec vero sic se habent:* Hoc demum anno conparuerunt primum in terris Arabum variolae & morbillae. *Fuit autem annus post Natum Christum 572 de quo ibi loquitur: idem scilicet, quo Mahomet natus erat.*

[b] *confer Nobilissimi* Linderstolpe *libri de venenis Cap. VI Thes 4.*

[c] *id quod etiam citat Celeberrimus* SCHULTZ *in appendices pathologiae specialis de morbis infantum § 168.*

§3.1 Thus, to start, as it were, *ab ovo*, I will first of all return to those times, when the earliest traces of this disease can be found. It seems, indeed, as though no certain evidence could be produced; some assert that this disease did not grow strong until the seventh century, among the Arabs; others maintain that the same disease was known in antiquity, to those great founders of medical science, *Hippocrates and Galen*, and then by the name τά ἐξανθήματα. **3.2** The main advocate of the former opinion is the distinguished *Werlhof*, to whom even the foremost English physician, the distinguished mr. *Mead*, gives his support. As in his book on smallpox he is convinced that the ἄνθρακες and ἐπινύκτιδες of the ancients had little to do with smallpox, he assumes the opinion that a certain *Rhazes*, one of the Arab physicians, who brilliantly deals with the subject of smallpox, has brought forth as the first source someone named *Aaron*, who has explained the matter. Hence the famous *Freind* conjectures that the origin of this disease should be sought in Egypt, since this *Aaron* was born there. **3.3** But it is also noted that *Johannes Reiske* has found even older cases of smallpox and of measles, an opinion supported by certain statements, found in a manuscript in the Leiden library.[a] One can also find not so few supporters of the latter opinion, who believe that not even the Greek Fathers lack experience of this disease. **3.4** Not to mention others, the right honourable *Linderstolpe*, our most famous physician, has given a clear statement of this view, his opinion being this: that this kind of disease can trace its origin back to the very beginning of the world, and has not been unknown to the physicians of ancient times, although, because of the simplicity of provision, it did not rage to the same extent as in our luxurious age.[b] The same statement is made by *Stenzelius*, who brings forth, in notes on p. 130, as witness to his point of view the Portugese *Zacutus' Medicorum principorum historia*, p. 164. **3.5** Neither do I understand, under what pretext one could deny that the same poison has been spread out over the world in ancient times, and that it has created this evil. What remains to say about the old age of smallpox, Hahn's learned treatise explains in a well-rounded and quite distinct manner.[c]

§4.1 As the traditional method of a dissertation demands an investigation into the causes of smallpox, it would be suitable to deal, first, with the nearest cause, then with the so-called προκατάρτικα and προηγούμενα. But from that which briefly will be put forth, it will be most easy to understand what is to be said about the first cause. **4.2** As for the rest, though, as I do not have anything definite to say, I will just briefly rush through the different opinions of the authors in this respect. Among these should be reported first of all the conjectures of an *inherent ferment* which, when an external cause of epidemic is added, is said to bring about such disturbance in the body, such fermentation, that hence the fluids, as the natural course of the blood is destroyed, end up festering in this way. An opinion of this kind is that of the above-mentioned *Rhazes*, whose words in his commentary on smallpox and measles, chapter 1, read as follows: **4.3** *There is a kind of must, which the blood of boys resembles, where not yet any warming up has started, and to which no motion has yet given the impulse to fermentation. But the blood of young men is like a must that is foaming, and where vapours burst forth.* But smallpox itself, he says, are *the foaming and bubbling* which *usually is brought about in a must during the period of fermentation.*

---

[a] *These are the actual words:* This year the smallpox and measles appeared for the first time in the Arab countries. *The year dealt with here is AD 572, which is the year, in which Mohammed was born.*
[b] *Cf the Honourable* Linderstolpe, *liber de venenis, Chapter VI, Thesis 4.*
[c] *Which also the famous SCHULTZ quotes in the appendices to Pathologia specialis de morbis infantum, § 168.*

4.4 His accedunt, qui caussis variolarum *reliquias sangvinis menstrui* adjiciunt, cujus sententiae socius est *Alexander Petronius Trajanus*, quem Nobilissimus *Linderstolpe* adducit & *Stentzelius* refutat p. 311. Haec etjam hypothesis fusius, in *actis Breslaviensibus ad annum 1721 mensis martiae die 4.* exposita est.

4.5 Tertio loco nominanda est eorum opinio, qui verminosam quandam pullitiem hujus morbi caussam esse volunt, cui suffragantur *Kircherus, Hauptman, Langius, Rivinus,* inprimis *Laneisius & Chesneau,* qui argumentis quibusdam huic rei lucem foenerari conantur.

4.6 Tanquam malum Haereditarium quarto etjam habitus est morbus hic, a qua sententia non abhorret *Lister*, qui, suffragante *Bergero*, ex esu vel morsu venenati cujusdam animalis, primam morbi originem derivandam censet.

Quinto denique non omittendam duxi opinionem Magni *Hoffmanni*, in Operibus Physico-Medicis tom. II, p. 5, qui caussam hanc non tam ponendam esse in ipsa sangvinis & humorum massa contendit, quam potius in succo quodam chyloso lymphatico impuro & corrupto matris; hunc vero humorem viscositate quadam involutum firmiusque tubulis aliquibus impactum tamdiu delitescere, donec ab aliis caussis in motum deducatur. Hoc autem latibulum verisimili quadam ratione medullae spinalis tubulos obstructos praebere censet.

4.7 Merito vero praeterimus alias aliorum opiniones, ut quae de reliquiis meconii[d] & praecipue de noxio pulmentorum esu[e] feruntur. Operae pretium non ducimus allata variorum judicia convellere, cum rationis momenta satis idonea non adsint; nam si darem, teneris infantum humoribus fermentum aliquod inesse, nonne tum ex rariori & extenuato aëre elastico, qui a fermentatione nunquam abest, stasis & obstructio sangvinis in trunco quodam vasorum cito oriretur, unde praesens afferretur interitus.

4.8 Dicant mihi, ubinam loci in Corpore Humano servarentur reliquiae sangvinis menstrui, vel meconium non penitus eductum, usque dum variolae se proderent? Qua ratione verminosa pullities gigneretur? & quis ante suppurationem simile quidquam vidit? An rationi consentaneum est, alios etjam morbos exanthematicos malo cuidam haereditario natales suos debere? at utriusque rei eadem esset ratio, variolarum nimirum &, quos diximus, morborum. **4.9** Ex quibus omnibus efficitur, nos in caussis afferendis certam rei veritatem assequi non posse. Neque tamen dissentionem opinionum inutilem esse scitu judicavi, ut perspicuum inde evaderet, quam nihil certi, in caussis remotis eruendis, constitui possit, quamque deliberate id agam, ut, omissis incertis opinionibus, ea saltem, quae ex indubitatis morbi phoenomenis deducuntur, sequar & adferam.

---

[d] *vide Medici olim ad Provinciam Dalecarliam nomine* Fhalstrom *dissertationem pro gradu Doctoris Parisiis habitam anno 1685.*

[e] *inde est, quod Guido Patinus parentibus suis gratiam habeat, qui interdicto usu hujus cibi, a variolis eum immunem praestiterunt.*

4.4 Kindred to these are those who add *residue of menstrual blood* to the causes of smallpox; an opinion of which one of the followers is *Alexander Petronius Trajanus*, whom the Honourable *Linderstolpe* brings up, while *Stentzelius* refutes him, p. 311.

This hypothesis is also expounded at length in *Acta Breslaviensia* for the year 1721, March 4th.

4.5 In third place shall be mentioned the opinion of those who think that some brood of worms is the cause of this disease, and who are supported by *Kircher*, *Hauptmann*, *Langius* and *Rivinus*, and, first and foremost, by *Lancisius* and *Chesneau*, who with certain arguments try to shed some light on this matter.

4.6 Fourthly, this disease is also regarded as an hereditary evil, an opinion from which *Lister* does not shrink back, who, supported by *Bergerus*, supposes the original cause of the disease to be the eating of some poisonous animal, or the bite from such an animal.

In fifth place, finally, I do not want to omit the opinion of the great *Hoffmann*, who, in *Opera physico-medica*, tome 2, p. 5, says that this cause is to be located not so much in the mass of blood and fluids itself as in some chylose and lymphatic, impure and corrupt fluid of the mother, and that this fluid, as soon as it has invaded some minor vessels and because of its sticky nature got stuck there, hides there until it is driven into motion by other causes. Its hidingplace he thinks, for reasons of verisimilitude, that the closed canals of the spinal cord offer. **4.7** There is good reason to pass by other opinions of other men, like what is said about residue of meconium[d] and, especially, about the danger of eating porridge.[e] I do not regard it worthwile to refute the opinions of various authors which I have quoted, when rational arguments are lacking, for, granted there were some kind of ferment in the thin bodily fluids of children, would not, then, stoppage and impediments to the blood soon arise in some branch of the blood vessels, from the thin and diluted elastic air, which is always present in a fermentation, whence immediate death would be brought about? **4.8** Perhaps they could also tell me in what place in the human body the residue of menstrual blood, or the not severed meconium would be kept until the smallpox shows up? In what way would that brood of worms arise? and who has ever seen anything like it before purulence? Or is it consistent with reason, that other exanthematic diseases owe their origin to some hereditary evil as well? for both things would have the same explanation, of course, smallpox and the other diseases that I mentioned. **4.9** From all this the result is, that, by suggesting the causes, we cannot obtain with certainty the truth of the matter. On the other hand, I have not regarded it as unfruitful to know about the divergences of opinions, so that it would become quite clear from them, to what extent nothing is possible to ascertain through digging for those remote causes, and that it is after careful deliberation that I omit uncertain speculations in order to pursue and bring forth only those facts which are derived from incontestable appearances of the disease.

---

[d] *See the doctoral dissertation by a former physician in the province of Dalecarlia, by the name of* Fhalström, *put forth in Paris, 1685.*

[e] *This is why Guido Patinus is grateful to his parents, who, through prohibiting this kind of food, preserved him from smallpox.*

§5.1 Ut itaque propius ad propositum veniam, antequam signa morbi separatim notare possim, dividendi rationem, ab auctoribus receptam, explicare visum. Generatim itaque duas variolarum species notamus, quarum alteri *spuriae*, alteri *verae* nomen dederunt. Illae, in quas saepius homines per vitam incidunt, quaeque, vel lymphaticae, vel duriores sunt[f], rarius in pus abeunt, sed aut exhalat liquidum in iis contentum; aut alio modo exarescit, quo fit, ut sua sponte decidant. Has, a proposito nostro alienas, missas facimus, in altera specie exponenda operam collocaturi. **5.2** Sunt autem *verae*, vel *discretae*, vel *confluentes*, quarum diversitas gradu tantum & intensiori vi cernitur, id quod diligentius explicabitur, cum infra utriusque varietatis signa & accessiones recencebimus. Haec autem curatius enodaturi, haud inconsultum ducimus separatim quatuor illa stadia, ab auctoribus dimensa, persequi, quae, praeeunte experientia, haec sunt; scilicet: *1:um status contagii, 2:dum inflammationis, 3:um suppurationis, 4:tum exsiccationis seu prolapsus.*

§6.1 In primo stadio haec exstant indicia, qua *distinctas*. Post meridiem plerumque incidunt, tumque adest rigor & horror vagus, calor intensus & vertiginosa turbatio, nausea & vomituritio, dolor circa praecordia, inprimis si manu premantur, dolores capitis & dorsi tensorii & leviter punctorii, accedunt colici, nephritici, pleuritici; propensio in sudores, praesertim in adultis, oculorum splendor, lacrimatio; Interdum sternutatio, tussis, oppletio pectoris, febris, continuata saepe deliria, haud raro narium & mensium fluxus, stupor & somnolentia; Alvus stricta in adultis, in infantibus saepius diarrhoea. **6.2** Non numquam in iisdem insultus epileptici, quibus si corripiuntur dentitione peracta, in procinctu variolas esse, possis praedicere, sub his quoque non raro eruptio fieri solet. Qua *confluentes*, eadem quidem, sed atrociora adsunt symtomata. Febris enim, anxietas, dolor & vomituritio immanius saeviunt, licet rarior sit adultorum in sudores propensio; sed in his frequens diarrhoea nonnumquam eruptionem praecedens & diutius protracta, id quod in discretis vix observes.
6.3 Secundum stadium aliis in discretis, aliis in confluentibus internoscitur signis; scilicet *in discretis*, quarto inclusive ab invasione die, non numquam serius, raro ante illum erumperunt pustulae sparsim primum in facie collo & pectore prodeuntes, leviterque supra cutis superficiem elevatae, tenuissimarum acicularum puncta aequantes. Accessiones febris tum vel minuuntur, vel plane desinunt. Successive per universum corpus pustulae augentur; ante haec tamen fauces dolent & deglutitionis sentitur molestia. **6.4** Pustulae in vesiculas elevantur circiter octavum ab insultu diem, jamque earum intervalla rubescere incipiunt doloreque tensivo affici. Vesicularum liquor primum tenuis & pellucidus, de die in diem flavior evadit & ad puris indolem accedit. Palpebrae extenduntur &, ut vesica inflata, oculos claudunt. Proxime a facie intumescunt manus, distendunturque digiti. In *confluentibus* pustulae tertio die, aut citius, raro tardius erumpunt, ac quo citius, eo magis confluunt. Ob gravius autem quoddam symtoma, vel dolorem vehementiorem, ad quartum, quandoque ad quintum diem eruptio differtur.

---

[f] *vide Celeberrimus* Johannis Osterdyk Schacht *Institutiones Medicinae Practicae, Cap XIII §2*

§**5.1** In order to come closer to my designs, then, before I can specify the symptoms of this disease separately, I think I should explain the method of division, as recieved from the authors. Generally we speak of two kinds of smallpox, of which one is called *the false*, and the other *the genuine*. The former, with which humans more often fall ill during their life, and which are water-clear or harder,[f] more seldom end up purulent, but either excrete their liquid or dry up in some other way, whereby they spontaneously fall off. These, as not belonging to my subject, I will leave aside to concentrate my labour upon exposing the other kind. **5.2** There are, of *the genuine* smallpox, two types: *the distinct* and *the confluent*, the difference being discernible only as a matter of degree and through the more violent nature; which will be more elaborately explained as I below will treat the symptoms and attacks of both. To explain these more precisely, I thought it wise to deal separately with the four stages, which the authors have distinguished by means of empirical experience, i. e. *1ˢᵗ the stage of infection, 2ⁿᵈ the stage of inflammation, 3ʳᵈ the stage of suppuration* and *4ᵗʰ the stage of drying up or of collapse.*

§**6.1** In the first stage, the following indications are to be seen in the *distinct* smallpox: Mostly, they break out in the afternoon, with rigidity and general ague, intense heat with giddiness and confusion, nausea and impulses to vomiting, pains in the chest, especially when pressed by the hand, tensive and moderately stinging pains in the head and back. To these are added pains of colic, nephritis and pleuritis, tendency to sweat, especially among adults, glossy eyes, tears: sometimes sneezing, coughing, obstruction of the chest, fever, often a prolonged state of delirium, not seldom running nose or menstrual flux, unconsciousness and sleepiness: among adults constipation, among children more often diarrhoea. **6.2** Among the latter also quite often epileptic fits, from which, when they occur after teething, you could predict the outbreak of smallpox. Quite often the smallpox also breaks out during a fit. The symptoms present in *confluent* smallpox are the same, only more grave. This means that the fever, the ague, the pain and the nausea rage more vehemently, even if the tendency towards sweating is less frequent among adults: among those, however, diarrhoea is often a portent of the outbreak, and also lasts longer, which you hardly will see at all in distinct smallpox.

6.3 The second stage is distinguished by different symptoms in confluent and distinct smallpox respectively; in *distinct*, on the fourth day, including the day of outbreak, or often later, though seldom sooner, pustules erupt, scattered first over the face, neck and chest, slightly elevated above the skin surface, looking like pinpricks. The attacks of fever at this stage are either diminished or altogether extinct. Gradually the number of pustules increase throughout the body: before this, however, the throat is aching, and difficulty of swallowing is felt. **6.4** The pustules rise into blisters in approximately the eighth day, and also, during this interval, begin to redden and to be afflicted by pain of tension. The liquid of the blisters is at first thin and clear, but becomes, day by day, more yellow and approach the state of pus. The eyelids swell, and close the eyes as an inflated bladder. Then, after the face, the hands become swollen, and the fingers are stretched apart. In *confluent* smallpox, the pustules erupt on the third day or earlier, but seldom later, and the quicker the eruption, the more they flow together. But, from more grave symptoms or from more vehement pain, the eruption may be retarded to the fourth, or once in a while to the fifth, day.

---

[f] *See the Famous* Johann Osterdyk Schacht's *Institutiones Medicinae Practicae, Chapter XIII, §2.*

6.5 Accessiones heic graviores, aut multos etjam post eruptionem dies aegrum discruciant, aut ad summum remittere videntur, raro tamen cessant. Majores quidem de die in diem evadunt, nunquam autem molem discretarum adtingunt. Facies maturius quam in discretis elevatur, pustulaeque sibi invicem implicitae, tanquam vesicula rubra vultum omnem contegunt. Diarrhoea eruptionem praecedens in unum vel alterum ab eruptione diem protrahitur. Salivatio in adultis saltem non semper adesse observatur, inciditque primo hujus stadii die. Hic autem saepe quoque invadunt phrenitis, coma, petechiae, nigredo variolarum, narium haemorrhagia, mictus cruentus, sangvinis sputum, fluor menstruus & urinae suppressio. Vide Schachti institutiones Medicinae Practicae, Caput XIII.

6.6 Tertia *distinctarum* periodus hisce notatur phoenomenis. Octavo ab invasione die facies tumidissima citius stadium hoc attingere & absolvere videtur, quam ceterae corporis partes. Pustulae antea leves & rubrae jam asperae (quod, observante *Sydenhamo*, primum maturationis indicium est) & *subalbidae* apparent. Palphebrae inflatissimae: Manuum pedumque tumor. Interstitia papularum colorem exhibent floridum & rosarum Damascenarum aemulum. Ipsa quaelibet papula liquore flavo purulento turgidissima maximeque supra cutim elevata, crassiorem quandam materiam summitati suae adhaerentem exprimere incipit. Haec de die in diem augeri sensimque detumescere videtur. Reliqui corporis pustulae indies quoque conspiciuntur, minus quidem asperae, albae magis. **6.7** Febris sub fine stadii prioris rediens, quae interdum etjam semper continuavit, jam exacerbari consuevit. *Confluentes* variolae periodum hanc aliquando die demum undecimo, decimo quarto, immo decimo sexto attingunt & sic *distinctis* serius, quo autem diutius hoc protrahatur, eo pejus. Pustulae ad instar pelliculae vultui adglutinatae, cutis superficiem non admodum superantes paulatim magis exasperantur colore fusco, perfectissimum autem pus raro continent[g]. Intensior est dolor cutis. Salivatio autem parcior evadit, obque tenacitatem & visciditatem vix faucibus aliquid excernitur; tandem penitus desinit, unde anxietas summa, manuum insignis tumor, urinae copiosissimae, febris gravissima.

6.8 Quartum variolae emetiuntur stadium, & quidem *distinctae*, hisce indiciis: die undecimo recedunt faciei tumor & inflammatio, & crusta densa, sub qua variolae teguntur & pus fluctuat, exarescit amplius, jamque pustulae rumpuntur & decidunt. Pus saepe in viscera nobiliora per metastasin deponitur, periculosissimosque morbos creat. Decimo quarto, vel decimo quinto die pereunt funditus pustulae faucium, manuum autem pertinaciores adhuc albae sunt & recentes. Inter haec crustae faucium decidere incipiunt, quibus elapsis rubicunda primum apparet cutis, deinde desquamantur, hisque squamulis furfuraceis foveae succedunt. Non raro tubercula hinc inde enascuntur, spuriaeque variolae, secundariae dictae.

---

g Lommius *in Observationum Medicinae Libro 2 p 294 de hujus generis variolis sic habet: Ceterum mala sunt, scilicet exanthemata, quae lente prodeunt, magisque si violacea sunt, sub his enim frequens sit syncope. Commoda quoque non sunt, quae vel lividi coloris, aut viridis, aut atri sunt, quaeque iteratis vicibus modo emergunt, modo occaluntur.*

6.5 The attacks are then more grave, they either torment the patient for several days, even after the eruption, or, having reached a peak, seem to abate: very seldom, though, they do recede. The pocks get larger day by day, but never get close to the size of the distinct. The face gets swollen sooner than in the distinct kind, the pustules, connected with each other, cover the whole face like one red blister. The diarrhoea which precedes the eruption is prolonged one or two days after the eruption. Salivation is, at least among adults, not always present; it comes about on the first day of this stage. At this stage, also, there are often attacks of frenzy, of unconsciousness, of petechiae and blackening of the pustules, bleeding from the nose, blood in urine and in expectorations, menstrual discharge and difficulty to pass water. See Schacht's *Institutiones Medicinae Practicae*, chapter 13.

6.6 The third phaze of the *distinct* pox is distinguished by these symptoms: on the eighth day, the swollen face seems to reach and complete this stage earlier than the rest of the body. The pustules, which first have been smooth and red, now already appear rough (which, as *Sydenham* notices, is a first sign of maturation) and *whitening*. The eyelids are very inflated. There is swelling of hands and feet. The skin between the pustules show a bright colour, like that of *rosae Damascenae*. The pustule itself is swollen with a yellow, purulent liquid and very much raised above the skin: they start to secrete a thicker substance that sticks to their summits. This substance seems to increase day by day, and the swelling to recede. On the rest of the body as well, more pustules are to be seen for every day, less rough, however, and more white. **6.7** The fever reappears towards the end of the first stage. In some cases the fever has been constant, and at this stage it begins to be more intense. The *confluent* smallpox sometimes do not reach this stage until the eleventh day, the fourteenth day or even the sixteenth day, and thus later than the *distinct* kind; the more this stage is delayed, however, the worse. The pustules are agglutinated into something like a membrane covering the face, only slightly raised above the skin surface, and gradually become more rough, with a dark colour; they seldom contain fully developed pus, however.[g] The pain in the skin is more intense. Salivation, though, becomes less profuse, and, because of its clamminess and stickiness, hardly anything is excreted through the throat. Finally, it completely ceases, which causes vehement anguish, a prominent swelling of the hands, large quantities of urine and a violent fever.

6.8 The smallpox pass through the fourth stage, as far as the *distinct* type is concerned, showing these symptoms: on the eleventh day the swelling and inflammation of the face recede, and the thick coating, by which the pocks are covered, and under which the pus floats, dries up even more, and soon the pustules burst and recede. Pus is often deposited in the upper internal organs by metastasis, where it brings about most dangerous diseases. On the fourteenth or fifteenth day, the pustules of the throat dissappear altogether, but those of the hands are more long-lasting, still white and recent. About this time the crusts on the neck begin to fall off; when they have disappeared the skin at first appears red, then is abraded. Scars follow these bran-like flakes. Not seldom are boils brought about by this procedure, and false, so called secondary smallpox.

---

[g] Lommius *writes about this kind of smallpox, in Observationes Medicinae, book 2, p. 294, thus: Furthermore, those are bad—i.e.rash— that arise slowly, the more if they are violet, since with such often goes fainting. Neither are those convenient, that are either livid, or greenish, or black, and that repeatedly now emerge, now are hidden.*

6.9 *Confluentes* autem sic se habent: Intentior est dolor cutis, donec tandem in truculentiori morbo, non nisi post diem vicesimum pustulae latioribus laminis desquamantur. Observatu dignum judicat *Sydenham* quod quanto pustulae maturescentes propius ad colorem subfuscum vergant, eo deteriores lentius abscedant, quo magis autem flavescunt, eo minus confluxerint & ocyus se proripiunt[h]. Vultus nulla scabritie afficitur, quando pelliculae primum decedunt; statim vero squamulae furfuraceae apparent indolis corrosivae, quae foveas profundiores & cicatrices relinquunt. Interdum dorsum & collum cuticula denudantur. A frequentia vero & numero pustularum in facie periculum est aestimandum. Confluentes saepe concomitatur salivatio in adultis, in infantibus diarrhoea, quae non ita mature ac ptyalismus advenit. Cessanti ut plurimum salivationi, nisi faciei intumescentia aut manuum succedunt, mors instare videtur.

§7.1 Ex his omnibus indiciis, quae in memoratis stadiis observantur, quivis, cujus cognitio a firmis initiis progressa est, facile colliget variolas ad morbos inflammatorios esse referendas. Ut autem melius de hac re convincamur, videamus quousque haec criteria cum iis consentiant, quae de inflammatione constituta sunt. Cum jam in primo stadio rigor calor & dolores, cum nausea febrique continua conjuncti aegrotum invaserunt, fit, ut sanguis, cujus alias aequabilis est cursus, vehementius ad superiora extremaque corporis pellatur, ubi sensim in reticulares arteriarum distributiones intruditur. Et quid aliud produnt oculi lacrimantes, splendentes, tussis, sternulatio & pectoris oppletio? quid aliud narium fluxus & mensium. **7.2** Qvum haec symtomata, usque ad eruptionem variolarum vim suam continenter, aut servent, aut etjam augeant, indicio sunt febrim majori attritu globulorum sanguinis in vasorum minimorum tunicas ingravescere, corde saepius ad contractionem irritato, unde sanguis etjam a tergo magis urget, omniaque ea concurrunt, quae ad inflammationem producendam faciunt. Absoluto jam primo stadio, cum liquida ad ea confluxerunt loca, quae ipsis continendis natura non sunt destinata: quid mirum, si ad cutis superficiem erumpant, ibique stagnando cohibeantur. Hac ratione reditu ad cor occluso, quid aliud consequi potest, nisi quod liquores leviter putrescant, solida tenera atterant, solvant, fluidisque misceant in unum similem, album, spissum, glutinosum, pinguem humorem, pus dictum? & quid propius ad similitudinem accedit alterius illius rationis, qua, ex mente *Boerhavii* inflammatio terminatur? **7.3** Et quid aliud sunt id genus variolae, quas confluentes vocant, nisi intensior inflammationis gradus cum febri graviore, vehementiori sangvinis motu obstructioneque majori conjunctus? Ut adeo liquida magis inflammata & malignitate symtomatum magis dein corrupta, quaeque his indiciis majori copia effunduntur, hic tanquam in massam quandam congerantur. Hinc cum & solida & liquida corporis gravius afficiantur, facile perspicitur, quid sit, quod imminuantur vires, resolutio aegrius tentetur, visque resistendi in minimis arteriolis debilitetur, unde eruptio praeceps, & justo vehementior, quominus acriora liquida blandius solida atterere possit, non modo impedit, sed vel citissime in gangraenam abit, vel puris generationem protrahit, accessionesque omnes porrigit & extendit.

---

[h] *Vide Sydenhami process. intgr. de variolis.*
[i] *Aphorismi 387.*

6.9 The *confluent* pox, though, behave thus: the pain in the skin is more intense, until, finally, in the most savage cases of the disease not until after the twentieth day, the pustules are abraded in large leaves. Noteworthy is the opinion of *Sydenham* that the closer the mature pustules get to assuming a dark colour, the less well and more slowly they will recede; the more yellow they are, however, the less they will flow together and the quicker they will become mature.[h] The face will not be affected by any roughness when the membrane has first fallen off: at once, though, bran-like flakes will appear, with a corroding nature, which leave rather deep pits and scars. At times the back and neck are abraded. From the multitude and number of pustules in the face, the risk can be estimated. The confluent kind is often accompanied by salivation among adults, among children by diarrhoea, which does not come about as early as the salivation. If the interruption of the salivation is not followed by the swelling of face and hands, death seems imminent in most cases.

§7.1 From all these signs which are to be seen in the above-mentioned stages, anyone, whose knowledge is founded on a firm ground, could easily understand that smallpox are to be classified among the inflammatory diseases. To be even more convinced in this matter, however, we will see, to what extent these criteria agree with those, that are established as regards inflammations. As already in the first stage stiffness, heat and pain, accompanied by nausea and constant fever afflict the patient, the result is that the blood, the course of which otherwise is even, is driven more vehemently towards the upper and outer parts of the body, where it gradually intrudes into the artery network. And what else is revealed by the watered, glossy eyes, the cough, the sneezing and the obstruction of the chest? What else by the running nose and the menorrhoea? **7.2** As these symptoms keep, or even increase, their intensity right to the outburst of pocks, they show that the temperature rises because of the increasing attrition among the blood corpuscles against the membranes of the smallest blood vessels, and the heart receives more frequent impulses to contraction, whence the blood urges even more from behind, and all this concurs to bring about an inflammation. Already the first stage is completed, as the fluids have flowed to places which were not naturally intended to lodge them. What wonder, then, if they erupt at the skin surface and are kept there by this overflow? As the way back to the heart is thus closed, what else could follow, than that the fluids rot slightly, that the more solid bodies tear away the softer, dissolve them, mix them with the fluids into just one homogenous, white, thick, gluey, greasy liquid, known as pus? And what could come closer to be like that other mode, by which, according to *Boerhaave*,[i] the inflammation ends? **7.3** And what else is the kind of smallpox that is called the confluent, than a more intense stage of inflammation, with higher fever, accompanied by more vehement motions of the blood, and greater obstruction? so much that the fluids, more inflamed and, by the malignant symptoms, more ruined, which, according to the signs, are effused in larger quantities, gather here like some kind of mass. From this, as both the solid and the liquid parts of the body are affected, it is easy to see, why the strength is failing, why the resolution is more difficult to bring about, and that the resistance of the minor vessels is weakened, whence the sudden, and extremely violent, eruption not only prevents the more aggressive liquids from wearing out the softer of the solid tissues, but also ends up in gangrene or prolongs the production of pus, and make all attacks longer and worse.

---

[h] *See Sydenham: process. integr. de variolis.*
[i] *Aphorismi, 387.*

§8.1 Jam vero perspecta magna illa convenientia, quae indolem hujus morbi naturamque inflammationis intercedit, solis luce clarius est, non modo cui classi morborum variolae sint subjectae, sed & qua via maxime conveniat morbo occurrere, ejusque curationem praescribere. Merito itaque in antecessum tenenda est generalis illa perceptio, quam *Boerhavius*[k] apponit, quippe quae tutissima omnium, rationique maxime consentanea videtur. Ita vero ille: *stimulo inflammatorio ablato, sanetur status praesens, & impediatur ulterior ejus progressus, & proinde caveatur futura suppuratio, gangraena.* **8.2** Quam vero difficilem periculique plenam ingredior disputationem, cum, in hac virium mearum tenuitate, eam rem propugnandam suscipio, quam tot eruditi convellere conantur? Faciendum vero non puto, ut secus sentientibus non occurram, iisque praecipue, qui vana victoriae spe adducti Magno *Boerhavio* dicam scribere sunt ausi. Quorum numero primo accensendus est *Censor Anglus*, qui cum saepius epistola sua, diario anglico inserta, dogmata *Boerhavii* perstringat, tum haec quoque in re tanto viro se opponere non verecundetur. Hujus autem argumentum eo nititur fundamento, quod nullus esse possit variolosus morbus sine erumpentibus variolis, quodque unica, qua hoc malum tollitur, via, suppuratio habeatur, quae adeo, magis crisis ex natura morbi dependens, quam accessio quaedam morbi censeatur. **8.3** Non est autem quod ad objectionem multis respondeam, cum celeberrimus *Richter* hoc in negotio otium me fecerit[l]. Id saltem jam afferam me intelligentia consequi non posse, cur non suppuratio molestior terminus inflammationis caveatur, resolutioque tentetur, magis naturae conveniens. Citra controversiam est, suppurationem non symtoma esse morbi, irritaque resolutione tentata variolas optime & felicissime terminare. Sed quot quamque periculi plena symtomata alia huic affinia sunt? Nonne optime ab initio procederes, optimaque caperes consilia, si hanc evitares? **8.4** Quemadmodum in febribus intermittentibus, licet calor frigus excipiens cum dolore, nihil aliud fit, quam crisis, seu nisus naturae in materia morbi expellenda; tantae tamen ejus sunt admonitiones, ut cortice peruviano omnia haece mala optime caveantur. Et cum ante *Boerhavium* Magnus ille *Sydenham* expertus fuerit, non modo variolosas febres sine variolis exstitisse[m], sed etjam suppurationem, quoad fieri potest, diminui debere[n], non video, quare non modo prius illud hodieque contingere, id quod revera contigisse demonstrabitur, sed etjam e mitiori suppuratione plane nulla evadere possit, cum fieri potuerit, ut gravior in leniorem converteretur, id quod ipsi dissentientes haud negant. Itaque tantum abest, ut *Censoris Angli* argumenta mihi probentur, ut potius mirer, quo jure *Fischerus* hac in re *Boerhavium* hallucinatum miretur[o].

---

[k] *Aphorismi 1388.*

[l] *Vide Ejus programma pro vindiciis Boerhavii.*

[m] *Vide Ejus Opera ed Leiden 1741 p 130—131 162 170.*

[n] *Loco Citato p 356.*

[o] *Confer Ejus Commentarios de remedio Rusticano variol. Balneo aqua dulci curandi in praefatione.*

§8.1 According to what I have shown we have now seen quite clearly the conformity between the nature of this disease and that of inflammation; it is self-evident, not only under which class of diseases the smallpox are to be ranged, but also by what method it would be most appropriate to fight it, and to prescribe the cure of it. One should, thus, regard as the foremost the general notion, which *Boerhaave*[k] puts down, as this seems to be the most safe and that which most agrees with reason. He says: *When the inflammatory stimulus has been removed, the present state of disease should be cured, and its further progress should be stopped, and in the same way the suppuration and gangrene should be avoided.* **8.2** But what a difficult and hazardous disputation am I not entering, undertaking as I am, by my tenuous powers to defend a thing, which so many learned men try to criticise? I do not think, however, that I can avoid meeting the arguments of those who have dissentient ideas, and especially those who, led by a vain hope for victory, have dared, so to speak, to bring a juridical action against the great *Boerhaave*. To the first rank among them can be referred *Censor Anglus*, who not only often in his letters, inserted in his English journal, criticizes *Boerhaave*'s opinion, but also in this matter does not hesitate to object to such a man. His argument is founded, however, on the principle that there could be no smallpox disease without the eruption of the pocks themselves, and that the only way to the curing of this evil is the suppuration, which, according to him, should be regarded as a crisis depending on the nature of the disease itself, rather than as a complication of it. **8.3** There is no need to say much against this, however, since the famous *Richter* has relieved me of this task.[l] I will only state that I cannot understand why suppuration, being a more troublesome end of the inflammation, should not be avoided, and a recovery should be aimed at, which is more in accordance with nature. It is beyond doubt, that suppuration is no symptom of the disease, and that it, when an attempted cure has failed, makes an end of the smallpox in an excellent and most successful way. But how many symptoms, and how dangerous, are there not, that are related to suppuration? Would you not make the best progress, make the best decisions, if you could avoid this? **8.4** Just as in intermittent fevers – even as the heat that follows upon the freezing, accompanied by pains, is nothing else than a crisis, or nature's labour to drive out the matter of disease – his advice in this field is only that all these kinds of evil should be avoided by means of the cortex peruvianus. And as, prior to *Boerhaave*, the Great and famous *Sydenham* had experienced, not only that the fever of smallpox does appear without the pustules,[m] but also that suppuration, as far as possible, should be diminished,[n] I do not understand, not only why it should not be possible even today to achieve the former of these things – which, as will be shown, has, indeed, been achieved – but also why a state of no suppuration at all could not develop from a lenient, as it has been possible for the grave suppuration to change into a more lenient one, which not even those who disagree can deny. Consequently, it would be so far from me to agree with the arguments of *Censor Anglus*, that I rather wonder by which right *Fischer* should be astonished that *Boerhaave* is talking idly in this matter.[o]

---

[k] *Aphorismi, 1388.*

[l] *See his Programma pro vindiciis Boerhavii.*

[m] *See his Opera, Leiden 1741, p 130-131, 162, 170.*

[n] *ibid, p 356.*

[o] *Cf. his Commentarii de remedio Rusticano variolas Balneo aquae dulcis curandi, in the preface.*

§9.1 Postquam jam superioribus ex ipsa natura variolarum brevi ostendimus, morbum hunc ad febres referri debere inflammatorias, eumque ad earum indolem recte currari (*sic*), & eam adeo indicationem, quam *Boerhavius* praescripsit, genuinam esse: id mihi jam negotii datum intelligo, ut quo pacto ea peragi curatio debeat ulterius disquiratur. Denuo autem non modo antea nominatum censorem Anglicum, pariter & *Fischerum* sententiae meae adversari video, sed etjam alios, inque iis summum Angliae Medicum, illustrem *Dominum Mead*, qui nescio quibus adductus rationibus eorum damnat consilium, qui indicationi *Boerhavii* assensu suo comprobant. Nihilo tamen secius, duce sana ratione & praeeuntibus postmodum nominandis auctoribus inquirere lubet, quousque modus a Boerhavio praescriptus morbo tollendo sufficiat. **9.2** Cum itaque stimulum inflammatorium primo auferendum jubeat, quaeret in antecessum quispiam, quid rei hic stimulus sit, & in quo consistat? Sed quemadmodum in caussis nihil certi & deliberati adduci potuerit, ita etjam heic me respondendo sustinere vellem. Et quo, quaeso, successu judicia sua hac in re interponunt autores? Mihi quidem suffecerit, ea exponere, quae fonte experientiae hausta, jamque dudum a Celeberrime *Lobb* solide observata sunt[p]. Quae omnia eo recedunt, ut stimulus iste producatur ab effluviis sui generis, quae contagione serpente per aërem propagantur, & a contaminato corpore sive remotiori, sive propiori via recipiuntur. **9.3** Satis itaque habeo id explorasse, caussam hanc externam in contagio quodam consistere, cui rei argumento est 1:o violentia variolarum epidemica, nam ut *Schultzius* in Pathologia Speciali, §27, dicit, *illud certum est, variolas vix umquam sporadice grassari, sed simul plures hoc morbo corripi,* cui accedit *Lommius* qui in observationum medicinarum libro 2, p. 295, inquit, *Exanthemata haec sine pestis nota in populum, aeris vitio grassantur.* 2:o natura aegri, nam quamquam pancreatice valeas, sola tamen conversatione contaminaris, nisi ab iis olim sis correptus. 3:o modi variolas cum aliis communicandi, qui sunt: α conversatio, β insitio, γ emtio. **9.4** Atque hic tandem locum habet illud Avicennae: *Caussa* variolarum *est res adveniens extrincecus ebullire faciens occulta.* Illud vero posteris disquirendum relinquo, num contagium hoc, ex mente Nobilissimi *Linderstolpe*, sit alcalinum volatile aërem inficiens, infecturum mox illos, qui hoc morbo antea non occupati fuerunt[q]. De cetero heic non praetereunda sunt Celeberrimi *Schultzii* verba, quae haec sunt: *in genere certum est plerosque homines a contagione illum morbum (loquitur* autem de variolis*) suscipere, qui autem primi ab eo corripiuntur, in iis videtur omnino aëris quaedam specifica dispositio, ad hunc effectum provocandum valuisse*[r].

---

[p] *ejus Treatise on the small pox cap IX § 562.*
[q] *liber de venenis Cap 6 Thes 3.*
[r] *pathologiae specialis appendix de morbis infantum § 176.*

THE SECOND CHAPTER
On the possible method of preventing smallpox

§9.1 As we have already shown briefly, in the paragraphs above, from the very nature of smallpox, that this disease is to be counted among the inflammatory fevers, that it adequately is cured in accordance with the nature of these, and that the rating of them by *Boerhaave* is thus correct, I understand it to be my task also to further investigate the question, by what method the cure is to be brought about. Once again, I see that not only the aforementioned English censor, together with *Fischer*, is opposed to my opinions, but others as well, among these the foremost English physician, the famous *Mr. Mead*, who, for I do not know what reasons, condemns the opinions of those who support *Boerhaave*'s rating by their approval. Nonetheless, under the guidance of sound reason, and preceded by the authors to be named below, I wish to examine into, to what extent the method prescribed by Boerhaave would be sufficient to drive out the disease. **9.2** As he commands in the first place the elimination of inflammatory stimulus, perhaps somebody would ask, to begin with, what this stimulus is, and of what it consists. But, as nothing certain and well-founded could be said as regards the causes, I would postpone the answer. And from what successful treatments, if I may inquire, do the authors present their opinions on this matter? For me at least, it will be enough to put forward that, which, gathered from experience, long ago accurately was observed by the famous *Lobb*.[p] All this ends up with the stimulus being produced by a peculiar kind of fluid, which is spread by a contagion that spreads gradually through the air, and which is received in the infected body by some longer or shorter way. **9.3** Thus I think it is sufficient to have ascertained that this external cause consists of some kind of contagion, a conclusion for which the arguments are: 1st: the vehemently epidemic quality of smallpox, for, as *Schultz* says in *Pathologia specialis*, § 27: *this is sure, that smallpox almost never attacks separately, but several persons catch the disease at the same time*; of the same opinion is *Lommius*, who in *Observationes medicinales*, book 2, page 295, says: *This exanthematic disease, lacking the signs of the plague, goes around among the population because of some fault of the air*. 2nd: the nature of the suffering, for although you are healthy and strong as an athlete, you can be infected just by intercourse, if you have not been attacked before by the disease. 3rd: The ways to spread the smallpox to others, which are: α:intercourse, β:inoculation, γ:trade. **9.4** And here this well-known passage by Avicenna fits in: *The cause of* smallpox *is something that, coming from the outside, makes the hidden bubble up*. But the question, whether this contagion, as according to the Honourable *Linderstolpe*, is a volatile alkaline which infects the air, which will easily infect those, who have not before suffered from the disease,[q] I hand down to posterity to inquire into. As for the rest, the words of the famous *Schultz* should not be omitted here: *Generally it is sure that most human beings get this disease through infection* (he is talking about smallpox); *in those, however, who are the first to be infected, a certain disposition of the air seems to be able to bring this about* .[r]

---

[p] *His Treatise on the small pox, chapter IX, § 562.*

[q] *Liber de venenis, Chapter 6, thesis 3.*

[r] *Pathologia specialis, appendix de morbis infantum, § 176.*

§**10.1** Cum in eo jam sum, ut, in quo consistat stimulus inflammatorius, quem tollendum censet *Boerhavius*, explorem, illud quidem intelligitur, praeter caussam externam, ab effluviis variolosis contagii more provenientem, antequam plenam & absolutam stimuli inflammatorii notionem animo informes, aliud praeterea desiderari. Et, ut in hanc curam & cogitationem ulterius incumberem, experientia duce, effectum est. Ea vero in his praecipue cernitur: 1:o quotidie observamus non omnes aëri varioloso expositos morbum contrahere, 2:o multos, qui cum contaminatis diutius vixerunt, aegrius, alios, parum cum iis conversatos, citius inquinatos fuisse. Ex quo efficitur, praeter contagionem, etjam intestinum aliquod corpori inesse, quod stimulum creet. Probe vero cavendum ne opinionis errore in conjecturas §4 allatas adducar. **10.2** Itaque solam experientiam magistram sequar. Jam, uti parva materiae variolosae vis, sangvini permista, nunc in majorem, nunc in minorem molem accrescit, idque iis tantum accidit, qui morbo isto non sunt antea conflictati, necessaria consecutione fluit, humorum in corpore eum esse genium, qui materiam variolosam plus minus augeat. Illam vero illorum indolem quomodo consequi intelligentia poteris, nisi consensio quaedam humorum & contagii praestruatur? **10.3** Naturam illam sangvinis internam, sine alterius caussae adjumento, morbo producendo parem non esse, cum satis, ut opinor, sit exploratum: consequens est, ut utramque eam caussam ad stimuli notionem formandam constituamus. Prorsus itaque nostrum conjungimus judicium cum Celeberrimo *Lobb*, libro citato, eamque sententiam proxime ad veritatem accedere sentio, qua particulas variolosas, contagione adtractas, fluida corporis, proxime ad eam naturam accedentia, in suam plane indolem convertere putatur. De forma vero & figura particularum, non est, quod disquiram, cum eam mihi legem dixerim, ut quantum possim a conjecturis abstinere debeam. Sufficiat, me id ex dictis cogere potuisse, ea liquida, quae maximam cum contagione cognationem habent, facillime posse mutari, inque variolosi effluvii naturam abire, ex quo concipi recte potest diversitas morbi, ex eadem tamen contagione oriundi.

§**11.1** De eo jam disputandum est, quomodo miscendis cum sangvine particulis variolosis, sanguineque iis assimilando, sufficiens stimulus inflammatorius, morbo progenerando idoneus, produci possit. Hoc autem alia ratione illustrare non possum, quam si paria iterum fecero cum saepe laudato *Lobb*, & sic statuero: particulas fluidorum, quas modo nominavimus, alteratas & ex contagione coalescentes facili sanguinis cursui remoram injicere; nec posse per angustos vasorum meatus corporisque colatoria expelli.

110

§ **10.1** As I am now already investigating what the inflammatory stimulus which *Boerhaave* suggests should be eliminated consists of, it is at least clear that, above the external cause, originating in the manner of a contagion in a variolous outflow, something more is required before we could form an absolute idea of the inflammatory stimulus. And guided by experience I have further devoted myself to this matter, and to these thoughts. Mainly, these are the results: 1st: As we can see every day, not everyone who is exposed to this variolous air contracts the disease. 2nd: Many who have been living together with infected humans for a long time have not very easily been infected, while others who have spent little time with them have more quickly been so. Hence it follows, that above the contagion, there is also something internal in the body that creates the stimulus. I must, however, carefully avoid getting involved in the misconceptions put forth in the conjectures adduced in § 4. **10.2** I will therefore follow experience as my only master. Surely, as the small amount of variolous matter, when mixed with the blood, grows now into a bigger, now into a smaller lump, and as this only happens to those who have not been afflicted before by this disease, the conclusion necessarily follows, that there is, in the body, a special nature of the fluids, which to a larger or smaller extent adds to the variolous matter. But how is the nature of this possible to understand, unless we presume some correspondence between the fluids and the contagion? **10.3** This innate quality of the blood, without any support from external causes, is not able to produce the disease, as has, I believe, been sufficiently explained: consequently, let us agree upon both these origins in order to form an idea of the stimulus. Thus we can, in a word, join opinions with the famous *Lobb*, in the passage quoted above, and I believe that the opinion comes close to truth, according to which the variolous particles, attracted by infection, are thought to convert the bodily fluids, to which they are affined, entirely into their own nature. I have, however, no reason to investigate further into the shape of these particles, as I have drawn up as a rule to myself to avoid vague assumptions as far as possible. It would be enough that I, from what is said above, am able to prove that these liquids which have major affinity to the contagion very easily may change and be converted into variolous fluid, from which could be conceived a just notion of the varieties of this disease, which, however, arise from the same contagion.

§ **11.1** Now will be discussed how, through the mixture of the variolous particles with the blood and assimilating it more to those particles, enough of the inflammatory stimulus could be produced, capable of generating the disease. I cannot, however, explain this in any other way than by once again joining *Lobb*, whom I have often mentioned, and I will state this: The aforementioned particles of the fluids, altered and consolidated by the contagion, cause a hindrance to the free course of the blood; nor can they be expelled by passing through the narrow blood vessels or by the body's filtration.

11.2 Remanent itaque in sanguine, cum pluribus id genus conglobatae, quibus ad cor delatis pro ejus maxima irritabilitate[s] celerior illius vehementiorque sit contractio, unde non modo supervenientis ratio reddi potest febris, sed etjam obstructionis in superficie corporis minimisque vasis perceptae, ex magis magisque diminuta particularum continue accrescentium transeundi potestate explicandae. Experientia ulterius constat, ea, quae corpori inest materia, contagio assimilanda, sive per suppurationem destructa, sive, ab initio morbi, alia quacunque via expulsa, externum contagium quasi iners & morbo producendo impar esse.

11.3 Cum itaque nihil, quo cum conjungatur, habeat, per communes excretorias vias emanet necesse est, nullis excitatis variolarum symtomatibus. Et quae alia erit ratio, quare semel hoc morbo affecti, repetitis postea vicibus nullas fere ejus admonitiones sentiant, quamvis contaminatis diu multumque utantur. Neque quidem alias nutrices, & qui curam gerunt id genus aegrotorum, contagionis vim & incommoda effugerent, quum per vasa inhalantia & aperta pulmonum, magnam effluviorum copiam necessario imbibant, nisi particulae, nullo idoneo humore reperto, exire nequicquam cogerentur.

§12.1 Propero jam ad generalem illam indicationem, superius allatam, cui, qua ratione satisfiat, non difficile est existimare, postquam maxime naturalem ostendimus viam, qua possit stimulus inflammatorius intelligi. Observatum est, removendo *stimulo hocce sanari statum morbi praesentem, ulterioremque ejus progressum impediri.* Huic vero rationi persequendae, non nisi duplicem modum patere, ipse docet *Boerhavius*, alterum, qui in correctione per specifica versatur, alterum qui in methodo universali antiphlogistica. Quod ad illum attinet, quid fieri possit omnium primo dispiciendum est. **12.2** Hoc utpote ex analogia reliquorum morborum, qui cum inflammatione conjuncti sunt, intelligendum obiter tantum & tanquam in transitu, tangam: cum itaque in eo sum, ut ope specificorum stimulum inflammatorium vel auferam, vel corrigam, non alienum a proposito duxi, an sequentia mentem advertere **12.3** 1:o videndum est, an sit medicina quaedam, quae intra breve temporis spatium ita possit particulas variolosas, indolem & genium si spectes earum, mutare, ut corpori advenientes vim eam, quae in assimilandis sui generis humoribus cernitur, perdant & amittant: qua ratione nulla eruptio pustularum consequitur, particulis incassum abeuntibus. 2:o num qua dentur remedia, quae eo fluida corporis humani facile comparent. ut ex contagione adveniente permutari non possint.

---

[s] *confer Illustrissimis Halleri primae lineae physiologiae §§ 92 & 93.*

112

11.2 They thus remain in the blood, agglutinated to other particles of the same kind, and as they are transported to the heart, because of the great irritability of this organ[s] its contractions will be quicker and more vehement, from which an explanation can be given not only of the imminent fever, but also of the obstruction observable in the surface of the body and in the smallest blood vessels, an obstruction which is to be explained through the more and more increasing difficulty of the continuously growing particles to pass. From experience it is also clear that when this innate matter of the body, which can be assimilated to the contagion, has either been destroyed by suppuration, or expelled one way or the other at the beginning of the disease, then the external contagion is, so to speak, idle, and without any ability to produce the disease. **11.3** As the contagion thus has nothing to unite with, it has to leave through the ordinary secretory organs without bringing about any symptoms of smallpox. And what other reason could there be for why those who once have been afflicted by this disease, when they again are exposed to its force, almost never notice its impact, no matter how much time they spend together with infected humans or how often. Neither could wet-nurses and those who take care of this kind of patients escape the force and the disturbance of contagion, as they through the open and inhaling blood vessels of the lungs must inhale a large amount of contagious outlet, otherwise than if these particles, as no convenient fluid is found, are forced to leave the body without success.

§ **12.1** I now hastily move on to the general estimation mentioned above. It is by now easy to understand, how it can be supported, once the natural explanation of the inflammatory stimulus is put forth. It has been observed that by removing *this stimulus, the present state of disease is cured, and its further progress is stopped.* That there are two ways by which this method can be followed, *Boerhaave* himself tells us: one that consists in a specific cure for the symptoms, one that consists in a general anti-inflammatory method. Regarding the first alternative, first of all it should be investigated what can possibly be done. **12.2** As this could be understood from analogy with other diseases, connected with inflammation, I will merely touch it superficially and, as it were, in passing. Consequently, as I am about to, with all my strength, eliminate or cure the inflammatory stimulus by means of the specific cure, I have thought it appropriate to my task to direct my attention to the following:

12.3 1st: It must be investigated whether there is any medicine which in a short time could alter the variolous particles thus, with regard to their quality and nature, that they, upon invading the body, fail to obtain, and lose, the power to assimilate fluids of affinity to them that they have; in this way no eruption of pustules would follow, as the particles would leave without achieving anything. 2nd: It must be investigated whether there are any remedies that easily prepare the fluids of the body so completely, that these will not be able to change from the impact of the contagion.

---

[s] *Cf. the Famous Haller's Primae lineae physiologiae, §§ 92 and 93.*

12.4 Mirum vero nemini videatur, si versuram fecero a Celeberrimo *Lobb*, cujus librum citavi; nam cum certum sit, quoad valeant humeri, diligentissime hoc argumentum pertractare, fieri non potest, quin eum aliquando tramitem insistam, quem tanta eruditione spectatus apperiit medicus, non nihil tamen loci relicturus iis, quae experiendo sint cognita. Quod si jam id genus remedia obtineri possint, nihil impedit, quominus magni *Boerhavii* consilio sua constet utilitas: eaque specifica sint dicenda, quae singulari vi polleant, hujus morbi caussas dicta ratione mutandi, destruendi & removendi, haud secus ac cortex Peruvianus, ob easdem rationes, specificus audit, febres intermittentes si respicias.

§ **13.1** Quemadmodum stibii & antimonii adhibendi consilium dedit saepe laudatus *Boerhavius*[t] ut alteram rationem stimuli inflammatorii removendi commendatam faceret; ita in illud jam inquirendum est, num in haec quadrent, ea, quae § 12 quaesivimus. Notum est, antimonium nihil aliud esse, nisi corpus semimetallicum, quod parte regulina & sulphure constet. **13.2** Jam experientia patet, magnam ejus esse vim in reserandis obstructionibus emunctoriorum & diapnoë promovenda[u] item & in iis praeparatis, in quibus pars regulina sulphure non est destituta, insignem ejus esse omnibusque perspectam utilitatem, cum in vitiis lymphae emendandis, tum in venenis quibusdam expellendis. Hinc est, quod in lue venerea praestantissimus ejus sit usus: unde etiam Medici Batavi singularem ipsi efficaciam tribuunt, iis decoctorum formis addito, quae sangvini perpurgando destinantur.**13.3** Quae cum ita sint, in memoriam eorum si redierimus, quae modo requisivimus, quin ad variolas, ullo modo, cavendas recte referri possit antimonium, negari vix poterit; contagium enim, virtute ejus virus quodcunque debellante, destrui haud incommode videtur, quamobrem fieri nulla potest contagii sangvinisque assimilatio; quid quod vi stibii diapnöica particulae variolosae per corporis emunctoria ejiciantur? Cum vero, non sine multa opera, eam obtineamus antimonii penetrabilitatem, quam in hisce remediis praestrui vult *Boerhavius*, in eam curam magis incubuerunt medici, quomodo mercurium, alterum remedii genus, ad hoc consilium accomodatius, in suam traducerent utilitatem.

§ **14.1** Mercurii non solum in lympha attenuanda vitioque illius corrigendo, sed etiam in destruendo cujuscunque generis miasmate, singularem prorsus esse vim & efficaciam, multis periclitationibus stabilita experientia docet. Et quamquam sic dictus mercurius vivus, non nisi fortissimo quoque spiritu minerali acido, haud secus ad aurum, solvatur, non inde tamen efficitur, cum mitioribus quibusque corporis nostri humoribus nihil ab eo communicari posse, unde videmus quomodo vermes enecentur, epoto mane liquore, cui per noctem infusus fuerit mercurius vivus; quamobrem praeter vim, quae ipsi inest salivationem ciendi, non immerito aliam etjam ipsi assignamus humores vitiatos corrigendi facultatem.

---

[t] *aphorismi 1392.*
[u] *vide* Neumanni *Chemia, pagina mea 504, confer ibid p 1476.*

12.4 It should not, however, seem strange to anyone that I translate from the famous *Lobb*, whose book I have cited: for even if it is obvious that one cannot penetrate this discussion to the best of one's ability without sometimes treading the path which the respected physician has opened up through so much learning, though some space will be left for that, which is known by experience. Therefore, if this kind of remedy can be found, there will be no objection to the usefulness of the great *Boerhaave*'s advice. And those shall be named "the specific remedies" which have a special power to change, destroy, or remove the causes of this disease, in accordance with the method mentioned, in the same way as the cortex Peruvianus is called "specific" with respect to intermittent fevers.

§ **13.1** Exactly as the aforementioned *Boerhaave*[t] often gave prescriptions on how to use stibium and antimony in order to recommend another method to remove the inflammatory stimulus, it is now necessary to examine whether that which is inquired into in § 12 agrees with that method. It is known that antimony is nothing but a semi-metal matter, consisting of the regulus-part and sulphur. **13.2** It is already clear from experience that it has a great ability to relieve obstructions in the nostrils and to promote transpiration[u], and that also in the preparations, of which the regulus does not lack sulphur, its usefulness is remarkable and known to all, both in the correction of lymphatic diseases, and in the expulsion of certain poisons. This is why it is chiefly used in venereal diseases, whence also the physicians of the Netherlands ascribe to it a singular efficiency when added to those concoctions which are designed to purge the blood. **13.3** This being the case, if we recall what we just were inquiring, it is hardly possible to deny that antimony, in some way, could be used for avoiding smallpox. It seems that the contagion will be conveniently destroyed as the power fights down any poison and hence, there cannot be any assimilation of the contagion and the blood, not to mention the fact, that the variolous particles are blown out through the nose from the exhalation-promoting force of the stibium. But as this penetrating effect of antimony, which *Boerhaave* aims at in the case of these remedies, is not achieved without much effort, physicians are more at work with how mercury – another kind of remedy, and more suitable for this purpose – could be of use to them.

§ **14.1** That mercury possesses quite singular power not only to dilute the lymphatic fluid and to correct its defects, but also to destroy any kind of pollution, a well-founded experience teaches us from many experiments. And, even as the so called live mercury does not dissolve in anything but *spiritus mineralis acidus* just like gold, it does not follow that nothing of it could be transferred into the softer fluids of our bodies, whence we can see that worms are killed by drinking in the morning a fluid which has been left over night with live mercury added; therefore, in addition to the power to provoke salivation that it has, we could justly attribute to it another ability, viz. that to correct defect bodily fluids.

---

[t] *Aphorismi, 1392*
[u] *See* Neumann, *Chemia, p 504 in my copy, cf. ibid p 1476*

14.2 Mercurium dulcem si spectes, incomparabilem ejus esse usum, cum in impuritatibus eluendis, obstructionibusque inveteratis solvendis, tum maxime in miasmate venereo et scabioso in primis corrigendo & expellendo, nemo facile negaverit. Nihil vero aliud hic est, nisi mercurius vivus, forti spiritu salis solutus & sublimatus, cui iterum terendo, tantum mercurii vivi additur, ut ejus globuli cum spiculis mercurii sublimati prominentibus uniti, illa obtundant, quo mitius evadit mercuriale medicamentum. **14.3** Jam si ea repetamus, quae de mercurio praedicavimus, nihil obstat, quin eadem virtus, quam in aliud affert virus, item in supra nominato contagio varioloso exerceat[w]. Huic accedit, quod fontes salivales apperire valeat, dummodo id observes, transpiratione cohibita, ad hos ductus propellendum serum impurius esse. Cui geminum illud est, quod in variolis haud raro accidit, nisu quodam naturae, salivae excretionem progigni, quoniam, indiciis § 16 allatis, constat, inter humores gingivarum pedum manuumque, salivationem plurimum morbosae sordis, in purulentam alioqui corruptionem transiturae, salubriter exhaurire[x].

§ **15.1** Mirari ergo non convenit, cur, huic rei enodandae, suam operam dicaverit magnus *Boerhavius*, qui antimonio permiscendum mercurium eatenus censebat, quoad id efficeretur, ut illud quam optime cum humoribus communicari posset, hic vero ad cutem & exteriora corporis propelli[y]. Eodem etjam consilio Dominus *Lobb* egisse videtur, qui cum ab initio hujus rationis veritatem, tanquam chimaeram quandam in suspicionem adduxerit[z], deliberato tamen in eam venit opinionem, ut non tantum modum variolas praecavendi, sicut supra ostendimus, agnoverit, sed etjam aethiopem mineralem, tanquam optimum ad hunc morbum remedium praescripserit: quae curatio tam feliciter ipsi & ex sententia successit, ut ex quinque omnino hominibus, nondum variolis contaminatis, cum tamen aegrotis continue fere adstiterint, eorumque curam gesserint, quatuor immunes penitus evaserint, uno tantum leviter afflicto. **15.2** Immo, quod majus est, fuit quidem ex vicinia, qui, cum semel tantum propius ad aegrotos pervenisset, a remediis imparatus, illico contagionem attraxit & occubuit. Tota autem curatio Celeberrimi *Lobb* hisce momentis continebatur: Cum esset a contagione periculum, antequam indicia quaedam apparerent morbi, sumebantur pulveres, confecti, vel ex aethiopis mineralis drachmis duabus, florum sulphuris drachma una, in 8 partes divisi, qui propinabantur quavis vespera & mane, vel ex aethiops mineralis uncia semis, radicis enulae Campaniae drachmis duabus, myrrhae drachma una, camphorae scrupulo uno in 14 partes divisi, qui sumebantur bis de die, in mixtura quadam, ex aqua bryoniae composita, aut sola ad uncias binas data, cum syrupi quinque radicum aperientium unciis quatuor, syrupi baccarum sambuci unciis duobus, aut eadem hac aqua cum aqua cinnamomi fortis combinata, portione utriusque aequali ad unciam unam.

---

[w] *Recte itaque Neuman in Chemia pagina mea 509. Es ist,* inquit, *vor denen infallende variolis ein gutes reinigungs mittel und praeservativ.*

[x] *Confer Richteri citatum programma.*

[y] *Id quod videmus Boerhavium, bono cum sucessu, invenisse, ex libro, quem citat Richterus Germanico specie paradoxo, licet, eodem auctore in suo programmate observante,* pertaesus tot laborum & obtrectationum, noluerit in enodandis istis difficultatibus pergere.

[z] *Vide ejus librum citatum § 559.*

14.2 If you look at the calomel, it can hardly be denied that it is of unparalleled use to wash away impurities and to dissolve inveterate obstructions as well as, and above all, to correct and expel venereous and scabious miasm. But this is nothing else than live mercury dissolved and sublimated in strong hydrochloric acid, to which, by grinding, so much live mercury be added, that the drops of it, combined with the pungency of the mercury sublimate, will blunt that pungency, whereby the mercuric medicine becomes more mild. **14.3** If we now reconsider what we have said about mercury, there is no reason why it should not exercise the same power against the above mentioned variolous contagion as it does against other poisons[w]. In addition to this it has the ability to open up the sources of salivation, whereby it should be noted that as the transpiration is hindered, the impure serum has to be expelled that way. Similar to this is what often happens in smallpox, that salivation, from some effort of nature, is brought about, since it from the information in § 16 is clear, that among the fluids of the gingiva, the hands, and the feet, salivation exhausts the most of the pollution of sickness, which otherwise would break down into pus[x].

§ **15.1** There is therefore no need to wonder why the great *Boerhaave* devoted himself to investigating this question and suggested that mercury should be added to antimony in such quantity so that the best possible union of the latter with the fluids would be brought about, while the former would be driven towards the skin and exterior parts of the body[y]. Mr. *Lobb* seems to have acted in the same spirit; he, who first called this theory into question, as if it were a chimera[z], on second thought assumed the position of not only accepting the method described above to prevent smallpox, but also of prescribing *Æthiops mineralis* as the best remedy of it. This cure came out so successfully and in accordance with his ideas that out of all in all five persons, never before infected by smallpox, four turned out to be totally immune and one just leniently afflicted, even as they were in almost continuous contact with, and taking care of, patients. **15.2** Furthermore, which is more significant, there was a neighbour who had not prepared himself with this remedy, and who, though he was only in contact with the patients once, caught the infection and died. The cure was perfected by the famous *Lobb* according to this method: When infection was suspected, but before any symptoms of disease had shown, powders were taken, consisting either of two drachmae of *Æthiops mineralis* and one drachma of flowers of sulphur, which is divided into eight doses, of which one was taken every evening and morning, or of half an ounce of *Æthiops mineralis*, two drachmae of *radix enulae Campaniae*, one drachma of myrrh, and one scruple of camphor, which, divided into fourteen doses, was taken twice a day, in a mixture with either *aqua bryonia* only, in a dose of two ounces every time, with four ounces of *syrupus quinque radicum aperientium* and two ounces of *syrupus baccarum sambuci*, or else the same water combined with *aqua cinnamomi fortis* in equal parts, together one ounce.

---

[w] *Thus Neuman puts it correctly in Chemia, p 509 in my copy: "Es ist"* he says, *"vor denen infallende variolis ein gutes reinigungs mittel und praeservativ."*

[x] *Cf. the quoted program by Richter.*

[y] *Which we notice that Boerhaave successfully has discovered, according to a German book quoted by Richter as a paradox, even as the same author mentions in a program that* disgusted with all toils and envy, he did not want to proceed in unraveling these difficulties.

[z] *See his book, quoted above, § 559.*

15.3 Hisce autem sumtis biberent praeservaturi cerevisiam, cui herba rutae erat infusa. Fuere etiam alii, quibus vel solus aethiops mineralis ad unciam semis, coccinellae drachma una fucatus & in 8 partes aequales divisus praebebatur, sexta quavis hora, vini canariensis pauxillo immistus, quibus postea etiam dabatur vinum aqua temperatum: vel etjam saepius nominatur aethiopis scrupuli octo, cum pulveris e chelis cancrorum & coccinellae aequali portione ad scrupulos binos conjuncti, quibus factus pulvis, in 8 partes aequales divisus est, cumque supra dicto vehiculo propinatus. **15.4** Et quemadmodum auctor, praeter necessariam horum medicaminum cognitionem aeque heic, ac in reliquis, ubi adhibentur specifica, morbis, certam horum mensuram certo tempore sumendam censet, si ad consilia nostra opportuna erunt; ita sex horis drachmam minimum capi jubet, eamque medelam ab eo inde tempore, quo suspicionem contagionis concepimus, saepius continuari. Et haec summa fuit totius curationis a Celeberrimo *Lobb* praescriptae, quam eorum in gratiam inserui tractationi nostrae, qui libri ejus facultatem non habent.

§ **16.1** Sed missa jam facio testimonia aliorum, qui suis suffragiis usum mercurii insignem in cavendis variolis confirmant, ad unius Nobilissimi Domini *Praesidis* experientiam provocaturus. Hujus enim industria postquam factum est, ut varia variorum judicia hac de re accuratius exigerentur, nobisque quid de iis existimandum sit, innotesceret, eam ipsi sententiam placuisse animadvertimus, quae *Boerhavianam* rationem non improbat; & quemadmodum variolae, id quod in superioribus vicimus, non sine sangvinis vera inflammatione desinunt, non id tantum egit, ut mercurii ope contagium capite quasi deminueret, id quod ad stimulum inflammatorium removendum conducit, sed etjam, ut remedio quodam refrigerante phlogosin humorum jam ortam inhiberet & temperaret. **16.2** Cui rationi haud parum prospectum censet massa illa pilularum, quam ipse eum in modum composuit, ut loco basis Calomelano sumto, resina guajaci & aloës extractum aquosum sint excipientia, quibus camphoram tanquam caussam adjuvantem adstruxit. Eam vero ob caussam resina guajaci heic inprimis in censum venit, quod egregia ejus virtus, balsamica nempe, depurans & abstergens in affectibus scabiosis & catharralibus multum valeat, visque praeterea ejus leniter irritans omnia organa, cum secretoria, tum excretoria stimulet, quid quod camphorae virtute refrigerante & diapnoica ita corrigatur & adjuvetur reliquorum vis, ut quominus quae dicta sunt obtineantur, nemo dubitare posse videatur. **16.3** Haec autem ejus est methodus multiplici usu comprobata: Cum certo novimus vel vicinos, vel eos, qui in domo morantur cum variolis conflictari, aut cum a consortio eorum, qui cum variolosis conversantur, nos abstinere non possumus, jubet exempli gratia infantem primo lene laxans, ad purgandas primas vias, sumere, secundo suadet ad usum potus, solito largiorem quarto (*sic*) monet ut a liberiori aëre, quantum fieri potest coarceatur. quinto Praescribit pilulas praeservatorias, bis qualibet hebdomadum 4 vel 5 priorum, sumendas: exempli gratia vesperi diei lunae & martis. Deinde autem unicus tantum eorum usus, qualibet septimana, est necessarius. Forma pillularum est sequens:

15.3 After this has been taken, the person who is subject to this precautions should drink beer, with rue added. There have been others, as well, who have been given half an ounce of *Æthiops mineralis* alone, dyed with one drachma of cochineal and divided into eight equal doses, to be taken one every sixth hour, mixed with a little *vinum Canariense*; to these has also afterwards been given wine diluted with water. Or, more often, this is mentioned: eight scruples of *æthiops* combined with two scruples each of crayfish shell and cochineal, respectively, which powder thus manufactured is divided into eight equal parts, and taken with the above mentioned vehicle. **15.4** And just as the author prescribes, in addition to the necessary information about these medicines, that a certain dose of the medicine be taken at a certain time in this case in the same manner as in other diseases, where specific remedies are used, if it is to work according to our plans, he also states that as a minimum one drachma should be taken every sixth hour, and that this remedy should be taken more often from the moment when infection is suspected. This is the essential part of the cure prescribed by the famous *Lobb*, which I have inserted in my treatise as a service to those who do not have his book at hand.

§ **16.1** But now I will leave the testimonies of others, who with their support confirm the singular usefulness of mercury in preventing smallpox, in order to refer exclusively to the experience of the honourable *Praeses*. Since all kinds of ideas in this matter are sorted out more accurately as a result of his diligence and it becomes more clear to us what is to be thought about them, we have noticed that to him has been preferable an opinion that does not contradict the thoughts of *Boerhaave*. And as smallpox, as we have proved above, does not recede without a true inflammation of the blood, he has not only brought about, so to speak, that the contagion has been deprived, as it were, of its rights by the effect of mercury, which contributes to the removal of the inflammatory stimulus, but also that the inflammation of the fluids that has already started is restrained and tempered by some cooling remedy. **16.2** He is of the opinion that this matter is well provided for through the dough for these pills, which he himself has composed in such a way, that the basis should be made with calomel, and that *resina guajaci* and *aloës extractum aquosum* should be excipients, to which camphor is added as an adjuvant. But the reason for *resina guajaci* to be counted on here, especially, is that its splendid power, balsamic indeed, to cleanse and exsiccate is quite efficient in states of itch and in catarrhs, and also that its slightly irritating quality stimulates all organs, both secretory and excretory, and above that, as the force of the other substances is directed and assisted by the cooling and transpirational power of the camphor, no one could possibly doubt that what has been said is achieved. **16.3** This is his method, approved of by much use: When we know for sure that our neighbours or those who live in our house are suffering from smallpox, or when we cannot keep from intercourse with those who associate with smallpox-patients, he advises for instance 1st: that, for example, a child should take a mild laxative to purge the main ducts. 2nd: he recommends larger quantities of drink than the usual. 4th: (*sic*) he exhorts the protection, as far as possible, from open air. 5th: he prescribes prophylactic pills to be taken twice a week during the first four or five weeks, for example on monday and tuesday evenings. Thereafter it is only necessary to take the pills once a week. The formula of the pills is as follows:

16.4 Recipe   calomelanos rite praeparati, camphorae,
                   Extracti aloës aquosi ana grana tria;
                   Resinae guajaci grana quinque.
Misce, fac artis lege pilulae ponderis granorum 2, foliato argento obductae. Da.
Harum justa est portio, quae alvum infantis bis mane sequenti aperit. Viri autem
Nobilissimi experientia constat, fuisse infantes, qui 2 vel 3 menses, salutarem hujus
medicamenti vim experti, ne minimo quidem incommodi sensu, vel durante, vel finito
ejus usu, adfecti sunt.

§17.1 Postquam satis, ni fallor, exploratum est, quid de specificis, quibus caventur
variolae, Duce *Boerhavio,* sit existimandum, non abs re fuerit, in alia diversorum
auctorum remedia, huic fini accomodata, inquirere. Cum tamen & temporis & aliis
premar angustiis, satis habeo aliqua tantummodo medicorum super hac re cogitata
afferre. Quibus inprimis illa recensentur, quae de acidis quibusdam spiritibus
mineralibus, aqua quadam dilutis, circumferuntur. Haec vero ideo praesertim probata
videntur, quod materiam variolosam alcalinum aliquod esse voluerint, cui nostratem
Nobilissimum *Linderstolpium* accessisse antea innuimus. **17.2** Eorum vero remediorum
numero *phlegma victrioli, tinctura rosarum,* vel *florum papaveris erratici,* cum *spiritu victrioli
parata, & aqua* denique *picis navalis* habentur[a]. Quam praescriptionem, post
Sydenhamium, praeter medicos in Hassia celebres, secuti sunt *Dolaeus &Wadschmidius.*
Magnus vero *Hoffmannus* non dubiam tantum,sed & periculosam judicat[b]. Neque id
silentio transeundum putavi, quo Americani, non sine insigni utilitatis fructu utuntur,
ad variolarum atrociam minuendam. **17.3** Hoc erudito orbi primum innotuit, cura
MARLOWII, qui sic habet: *variolis optimum Medicamentum, fermentationem sangvinis nimis
vehementem cohibens, nec tamen facultatem expulsivam penitus ligans; Expectorationem promovet &
pulmones tutatur; caput & guttur, ne invadant variolae impedit. Marlovii observationes* Est autem
id *Ilex, Linnaei Materia Medica, 56,* cujus folia, in hunc usum infusa, inprimis,
gargarismatis instar adhibentur. Externe etjam, superioribus corporis partibus admota,
vehementiorem variolarum eruptionem cohibent. Alio nomine haec planta *Cassine,*
licet incommode, venit; quare cavendum ne, cum alia, id nominis, scilicet *Cassine libro
citato 153* commisceatur, cujus vis plane est diversa. Jam, cum in officinis nostris non
prostet herba nominata, haud exiguam a publico gratiam iniret, qui in nostro aquifolio,
Ilicis specie, experimentis factis, quaereret, numne hoc in locum alterius posset
surrogari.

§ 18.1 Sequeretur jam alterum indicationis, a *Boerhavio* propositae, momentum, quod
eo pertinet, ut methodus universalis antiphlogistica, in usus nostros traducatur.
Remediis hisce id innui dilucet, quod impedit, quominus liquida inflammata, in
angustiis vasorum haerentia, eadem vitali impetu destruant, viamque suppurationi
pandant. Quo refer ea genera, quae impacta solvant, obstructa referent, motumque a
tergo deminuant, ut venaesectiones, laxantia, diluentia, & quae sunt reliqua.

---

[a] *confer* Johannis Osterdyk *Schacht institutiones medicinae practicae, caput XIII.*
[b] *vide Hoffmani opera physica et medica.*

16.4 Take   of duly prepared calomel, camphor,
and *extractum aloës aquosum* three grains each,
and five grains of *resina guajaci.*

Mix to make, according to the rules, pills of the weight of two grains each, coated with silver foil. Administer.

The right dose of these is one that loosens the bowels of the child twice during the following morning. From the experiments of this honourable man it is clear, that there have been children who, benefiting from the salutary effects of this medicine for two or three months, have not felt any inconvenience from it, neither during the treatment nor afterwards.

§ 17.1 As it now, if I am not mistaken, has been well enough investigated into how the specific methods by which smallpox are prevented are to be judged, according to *Boerhaave*, it will not be irrelevant to inquire into other remedies designed for this purpose, recommended by various authors. As I am, however, afflicted with lack of time as well as of other things, I find it sufficient to put forth just a few thoughts by the physicians in this matter. Of those the opinions will mainly be surveyed that concern certain *acidis spiritibus mineralibus*, diluted by some kind of water. These seem to be approved of because the variolous matter is said to be an alkaline substance. I have previously mentioned that our compatriot *Linderstolpe* has assented to this view. **17.2** To this kind of remedies belong *phlegma vitrioli, tinctura rosarum* or *tinctura florum papaveris erratici* prepared with *spiritus victrioli* and finally *aqua picis navalis*[a]. This prescription has, after *Sydenham*, in addition to physicians known only in Hessia, *Dolaeus* and *Wadschmidius* followed. The great *Hoffmann*, however, considers it to be not only dubious, but also dangerous[b]. Neither have I thought it convenient to pass by in silence the method used by the Americans, with rather good results, to diminish the harshness of smallpox. **17.3** This method was first known to the world of scholars by mediation of MARLOW, who writes thus: *The best remedy of smallpox, which moderates the too strong fermentation of the blood without totally stopping the ability of excretion. It promotes coughing and protects the lungs, and stops the smallpox from invading the head and the throat. Marlow's observations.* This is the *ilex* described by *Linnæus* in *Materia Medica 56,* whose leaves are used in an infusion as a gargling fluid. Externally also, applicated to the upper parts of the body, it prevents a more violent eruption of pustules. This plant has also appeared under the name of *Cassine*, which however is quite inconvenient: one must take care not to confuse it with an other plant with the same name, i.e. *Cassine, 153 in the same book,* the effect of which is altogether different. Now, as this plant is not found in our pharmacies, he, who by experiment would examine whether our *aquifolium*, of the *ilex* species, possibly could replace it, would gain no small amount of gratitude from the people.

§ 18.1 Now for the other part of the policy, suggested by *Boerhaave*, which aims at transferring the general anti-inflammatory method to our benefit. It will become clear that the remedy referred to would be that which would prevent the inflamed liquids that are stuck in the narrow blood vessels from destroying those by their attacks, and from opening a way for the suppuration. To those remedies you could refer the kinds, that loosen compact matter, release the impeded, and from behind diminish the disturbances, like bloodletting, laxatives, diluents and what else similar.

---

[a] *Cf.* Johann osterdyk *Schacht: Institutiones medicinae practicae, ch XIII.*
[b] *See Hoffmann: opera physico-medica.*

18.2 Ad ista vero quod attinet, non quidem negarim antiphlogisticorum usum, magis ad morbi progressum mitigandum, quam ad eum penitus tollendum, conducere, quippe cum stimulus inflammatorius morbi continuandi radix, quantumvis facili humorum meatu, possit nihilo secius remanere. Nemo tamen ibit inficias, hanc methodum, cum usu specificorum, quae diximus, conjunctam, non utilem tantum, sed etjam necessariam esse. Et quid de usu venae sectionis sentiant auctores, cui volupe est scire, adeat saepe laudatum *Lobb*. Si alterum ejus usum, qui in eruptione & suppuratione penitus cavenda consistit, non consequaris, alterum tamen in eadem minuenda, accessionibusque mitigandis certe obtinebis. **18.3** Quod remedia laxantia attinet, eorum, cum opus sit, praestantiam in hoc morbo aeque immerito negabis, ac diluentium & antiphlogisticorum omnium. Ex recentioribus auctoribus *Dominem J. Freind* afferre sufficit, qui non solum de venae sectionis usu in variolis nos convincit in sua epistola, tres Hispaniae Reges adducendo, hac cura a morte liberatos, sed etjam de commodis laxantium felicem, in tertio quoque stadio morbi, adducit experientiam. Ea itaque, quae antea dixi, repeto, quod scilicet ejusmodi remediorum utilitatem, in principio morbi tantum abest ut refutare possimus, ut potius ex crebris, de usu eorum in progressu illius, observationibus non sine ratione concludere possimus eadem, cum reliquis conjuncta, quae in removendo stimulo inflammatorio conducunt, morbum satis feliciter praecavere posse.

§ **19.1** Cum vero nunc iis, quae jam dicta sunt, brevi sit ostensum, nullum esse dubium, quin possint variolae praeveniri, quaerat aliquis, quare non semper effectu id comprobent medici, tamque felicem praxin, recensitis remediis, quotidie exerceant? Respondemus, 1:o Quivis facile concedat prophylaxin iis nimis sero adhiberi, quibus morbus jam eas radices egit, ut caussae suum effectum in corpore exseruerint: nec enim in medicum, neque in medicamentum culpa redundet si fieri non potuerit, ut ea temporis oportunitate praescriptum sit remedium, quo maxime conveniat. 2:o Fit plerumque, quoniam plurium febrium signa in principio sunt communia, ut aut cum alio quocunque morbo confundantur variolae, aut levitate contagii epidemici, hoc vel illo tempore ingruentis, operae pretium non ducitur, de excludendo morbo curam adhibere, sed potius in id incumbunt aegroti, ut pro hac occasione omnia morbi stadia transeant: quid quod ea saepius ex pharmacopaeis & chirurgis praestruantur remedia, quae cum cura prophyllactica (*sic*) nullo pacto convenire possunt. 3:o Non adhuc experimentis satis est exploratum, quaenam ex rebus sic dictis non naturalibus mercurii, vel alius cujusdam effecta destruant, aut adjuvent, cum tamen notum sit, tutissima, nisi aequo regimine adhibeantur, pharmaca, suum fefellisse magistrum. **19.2** Ea itaque coronidis loco fateri necesse est, ut experientia, prima omnis medelae omniumque remediorum notitia acquiratur, ratione eorundem nexus, & Creatoris in iisdem nobis subministrandis summa sapientia & bonitas percipiatur, repetitis denique & assiduis experimentis acquisita cognitio augeatur, si omnium omnino verus & nobis quam maxime utilis obtineatur FINIS.

18.2 For that matter, I cannot deny that the use of antiinflammatory remedies contributes more to the mitigation of the disease's course than to the actual curing of it, because the inflammatory stimulus, being the root of continuous disease, however easy the flow of the fluids, nevertheless may remain. Noone will deny, however, that this method together with the more specific one that I have put forth is not only useful, but also necessary. And if anyone wants to know what the authors think about bloodletting, he might go to the often mentioned *Lobb*. If you will not have achieved one of its benefits, namely the one consisting in total avoidance of the outbreak of pocks and of suppuration, you will at least have the advantage of achieving the other, namely to minimize it, and to mitigate the fit of disease. **18.3** As for laxatives, to deny their great utility in this disease, when there is need for them, would be as unfair as to deny the use of all loosening and anti-inflammatory remedies. Of recent writers, it would be sufficient to refer to Mr. J. *Freind*, who not only in his letter gives proof of the benefit from bloodletting in smallpox – bringing evidence that three Spanish kings have been saved from death this way – but also puts forth convincing experimental evidence for the utility of laxation in the third and fourth stages of the disease. I will therefore repeat what I have said before: that it would be so far from me to refute the convenience of these remedies in the first stage of the disease, that, from many observations of its benefit in the more advanced stages, I am rather able, not without reason, to conclude that by the same remedies combined with others that contribute to the removal of inflammatory stimulus, this disease could be quite successfully prevented.

§ **19.1** As it now from what has been said has been succinctly shown that there is no doubt that the smallpox could be prevented, someone might ask, why the physicians do not always confirm this by practice, and why they do not regularly use such a successful method as the one consisting in the use of the abovementioned remedies. I will answer in this way: 1st: Anyone should admit that the prevention comes too late for those cases where the disease has already taken such roots that it brings about its effects in the body: for neither the physician nor the medicine should be blamed, if it is not possible to prescribe the most convenient remedy at the right time. 2nd: It often happens, since the symptoms of many fever diseases are common at first, either that smallpox is confused with some other disease, or that it, with regard to the fickle nature of the epidemic contagion that shows up from time to time does not seem worthwhile to take the trouble to keep the disease away, and that the patients rather go through all stages of the disease, not to mention that remedies often are composed by pharmacists and surgeons that in no way could fit in with the preventive treatment. 3rd: It has not yet been sufficiently explored which of the so-called non-natural things are destroyed or furthered by the effects of mercury or of some other element while it is well known that even the most reliable remedy, when not applied strictly in accordance with prescriptions, has let its master down. **19.2** As a concluding remark, it must be admitted that from experience is acquired the first notice of every cure and all remedies, that from reason is percieved their causal connexion and the wisdom and goodness of the Creator, who has handed them down to us, and finally, that the knowledge acquired is increased by repeated and continous experiments, if we keep the overall true, and for us most useful
END

Commentary, Martin

REGIARUM ACADEMIARUM … MEMBRO] The Royal Swedish Academy of Sciences (*Kungliga Vetenskapsakademin*) in Stockholm was founded in 1739 with the purpose of supporting research and scientific development in order to strengthen the Swedish economy; the *Academia Upsaliensis* mentioned must be the Royal Society of Sciences in Uppsala (*Kungliga Vetenskaps-Societeten i Uppsala*), which had been founded in 1710.

PRO GRADU DOCTORIS] The degree of MD was probably granted only once in Sweden before 1738, even if at least one more medical dissertation *pro gradu* from the 17th century does exist, viz. *De passione hypochondriaca*, defended by M. Detterberg under Rudbeck the Younger in 1697; according to Annerstedt, II:2, p 151, however, the doctoral degree was never conferred upon Detterberg.

During the following forty years, Swedish physicians generally took the degree abroad, most notably at Hardewijk, Holland, even if there was nothing to prevent a Swedish graduation except, perhaps, a lack of interested teachers of medicine.

Cf. "Biographical notes", footnote 22.

STIPENDIARIUS STIEGLERIANUS] The Stiegler scholarship was, according to Annerstedt (II:2, p 422sq), instituted in 1710 and amounted to 33 000 *daler silvermynt*; a just comparison to modern currency is difficult, but it might be noted that a mid-18th century farm hand earned ca. 1 ¾ *daler silvermynt* per week, while the price of a shirt was ca. 9 *daler silvermynt* (information obtained from the webpage *www.algonet.se/~hogman/slmynt.htm* as accessed in may, 2003).

IN AUDITORIO CAROLINO MAJORI] Even if a new main building (i.e. the "Gustavianum") for the University of Uppsala had been erected in 1622–25, the originally mediaeval *Academia Carolina* south of the cathedral continued to be in use until 1778, when it was finally pulled down.

CARL FREDRICH PIPER] (1700–70), Swedish count, official, influential politician and president of *Kammarkollegium* ('the Swedish Crown Lands Judiciary Board').

The Latin lapidary style had been used in Sweden since the early 17th century, in the beginning, however, seldom if ever written by native Swedes; according to Ridderstad, *Konsten att sätta punkt*, p 236, a breakthrough can be seen in 1662, in which year nine out of forty extant occasional prints contain Latin lapidary style.

In the 18th century, the popularity of the Latin lapidary style diminished, while the Swedish equivalent had become increasingly popular since late 17th century (the oldest extant example dates from 1675); from ca. 1745 the Swedish examples constitute a majority, even if Latin still was used in important official inscriptions.

The contents of the gratulatory "verse" are roughly as follows:

> The things which today support the reverence for the name "Piper" are no less the profound prudence, the impartiallity and the mildness of your mind than the honour which all Swedish men consent that you possess; these brilliant qualities have incited my hope that this work, through your protection, might gain the general acceptance that it could not achieve through my own efforts alone.

MAURITZ POSSE] (1712–87); probably the Mauritz Posse together with whom Nils Rosén made his European journey in 1728–30, a count who after serving in the French army had become a Swedish colonel; the contents of the poem are very much the same as those above.

1.2 *Nihil...valet*] *laus medicinae*; cf. e. g. a speech of Oosterdijk Schacht's, printed in his *Institutiones medicinae practicae*, 1747: *Ea scilicet Artis Medicae est indoles, ut si a perito tractetur, vix usu ipsi parem, superiorem certe inveniatis nullam* (p 322).

1.3 ἐξανθηματικούς] See ἐξανθηματικός, Greek word list, p 34.

accessiones] The translation of *accessio* may sometimes be rather uncertain in a medical context; the word can, according to different authors, have several slightly different meanings, both medical and non-medical (cf. TLL 284sqq; OLD p 19sq).

According to Langslow, p 196, the general meaning in Celsus is 'onset', as opposed to *recessio*; on the other hand, OLD, as well as providing the same translation s.v. *accessio* 2, also gives the translation 'a complication' s.v. *accessio* 4 d, with an example from Celsus 2.8.13: *dum febris ceteraeque accessiones huius morbi absint.*

In Cassius Felix 55, p 142 (447 AD), it is said: *accessiones quas Graeci episemasias vocant*, while Stephanus, s.v. ἐπισημασία, 1767 B-C explains ἐπισημασία as *ipsum Principium s. Insultus accessionis febris*.

In works which are more contemporary of the dissertations treated here, the word is explained as *deterius tempus in morbis intermittentibus* (Castelli 1713, s.v. *accessio*). Blancardus (1748), s.v. *paroxysmus*, provides the synonyms *periodus, exacerbatio* and *invasio*, but also his definition pertains to fluctuations *within* the course of a disease.

One possible way to sort this out is perhaps at first to consider *accessio* only in the general sense of 'an approaching' or 'a coming', then to consider, according to the context of each single occurrence, in what aspect the disease in question is involved; *morbi accessio* would then mean either 'the coming of a disease' or 'that, which comes to a disease'; we might further take into consideration that the *accessiones*, showing themselves as symptoms or signs, ἐπισημασίαι, probably could have been regarded by some physicians as originating from a latent disease, such as an intermittent fever, which then would give the sense of 'onset' or 'attack'; by other physicians the same symptoms might well be interpreted as manifestations of an other syndrom, i.e. 'a complication'; as might be seen from e.g **8.2** of Martin's text, physicians of the 18th century still had different views upon the nature of certain symptoms; in this case, *accessio* must be taken to mean 'complication' rather than 'attack' since it is contrasted against something that is *natura morbi dependens*.

In short, I believe that we should regard *accessio* in itself as being a polysemous technical term – if, indeed, a technical term at all – and that we must consequently interpret the word from its context in each particular case; in this paragraph, thus, as in **5.2** and **8.2**, I have regarded the meaning to be 'complication'; in **6.3** and **6.5**, I regard the sense to be 'attack', and in **7.3** and **18.2**, finally, the meaning might well be only that of 'manifestation' or 'symptom'.

2.1 *suppuratione*] See *Suppuratio*, Latin word list, p 49.

Variolae] See *Variola*, Latin word list, p 51.

2.2 *ejusque...adventum salutem hominum...oppugnare*] A military metaphor, see p 79sq.

2.3 *tenuitatis meae conscius*] See "Style: Modesty of the author", p 88.

pulcrum] An archaic spelling of *pulchrum*; even Cicero originally used this, as well as several other, unaspirated forms (cf. *Orator*, 160), which is mentioned by Noltenius, who nevertheless points out that the aspirated forms constitute a majority.

Candide Lector] See "Style: Interaction", p 84sq.

omnem movere...lapidem] This expression is found in Petri Gothus, s.v. *Lapis*, without further reference. It is however treated in Desiderius Erasmus' (1467–1536) *Adagia*, 1.4.30; according to Erasmus, the expression might have its origin in the following story: when the treasure-hunting Polycrates of Thebes at first could not find the gold buried by Xerxes' general Mardonius during the battle at Plataeae (479 BC), he consulted the oracle at Delphi, and recieved the answer: πάντα λίθον κίνει, by which method the treasure finally was found. The Greek expression is also found in Zenobios' (*fl.* during the reign of Hadrian, 117–138 BC) collection of proverbs, as nr. 5.63, where the same story about Polycrates is told; cf. also Euripides' (c. 485–406 BC) *Heraclidae*, 1002: πάντα κινῆσαι πέτρον, which is also used in a proverbial sense.

Further, Erasmus has a reference to Pliny the younger, Letter 1.20, where both the Greek and the Latin form of the expression occur.

Cf. Erasmus' *Adagiorum opus...ex postrema autoris recognitione* (1550), col 169.

3.1 *ab ovo*] Cf. Horace *Sat.* 1.3.6: *ab ovo usque ad mala*; *Ars p.* 147: *nec gemino bellum Troianum orditur ab ovo* (i.e, the egg of Leda, from which Helen of Troy was said to have been hatched together with Polydeukes/Pollux); Otto points out, s.v. *ovum*, p 261, that the latter example was in Horace's time *noch nicht sprichwörtlich*, but says further that it later has become *einer gangbaren und auch in weiterer Bedeutung gebrauchten Formel*; he has also a reference to the grammarian Atilius Fortunatianus (3rd–4th century), p 278 K: *altius et ab ovo mihi, quod aiunt, repetenda res est.*

3.2–3.3 This passage is, by and large, derived from Richard Mead's (1673–1754) *De variolis et morbillis liber* (1747), chapter 1, p 2sq; the corresponding passages in Mead read as follows:

MORBVM hunc novum esse, hoc est, antiquis medicis tam Graecis quam Romanis ignotum, extra dubium esse videtur. Frustra enim sunt, qui ἄνθρακας, ἐπινυκτίδας, *et consimilia in cute* ἐξανθήματα, *variolas nostras esse contendunt.* [– – –]

Ex Arabum igitur medicorum libris petenda est prima morbi hujus notitia. Horum facile princeps Rhazes circa annum aerae Christianae nongentesimum inclaruit. Ille in volumine ingenti, quod Continens inscribitur, ... Aaronem quendam tradit triginta libros De medicina scripsisse; in quibus signa variolarum, genera diversa, et curandi modum explicuit ... Hinc conjecit doctissimus Freindius in Aegypto fortasse prima exordia habuisse variolarum morbum. At paulo antiquiorem originem ejus reperit vir Arabice doctissimus, Johannes Jacobus Reiske, qui in veteri codice Arabico manuscripto bibliothecae Leidensis haec verba se legisse dicit: Hoc demum anno comparuerunt primum in terris Arabum variolae et morbilli. Annus autem ille erat post Christum natum DLXXII, quo natus est ipse Mahumedes.

3.2 *Werlhof*] Paul Gottlieb Werlhof (1699–1767), German physician.

calculum] *Calculus* for 'vote' is originally a legal term, pertaining to the use of a white or black pebble to indicate a vote for acquittal or condemnation, respectively; there are occurrences in ancient Latin also of a figurative sense, as e.g. in Pliny *Ep.* 1.2.5: *si modo tu fortasse errori nostro album calculum adieceris.*

Krebs-Schmalz I, p 226 says that *calculus* can *für sich allein nicht Beifall bedeuten, sondern nur mit dem Beiworte albus;* in Petri Gothus, s.v. *calculus,* the expression *Addere, Adjicere suum calculum* is however found, translated as Sw. *Samtyckia* (Eng. 'agree', 'consent').

ἀντράκας] Misprint for ἄνθρακας, Greek word list, p 31.

ἐτινυκτίδας] Misprint for ἐπινύκτιδας, Greek word list, p 34.

Rhazes] Abu Bakr Muhammad Ibn Zaharia al-Razi (860?–923), Persian physician, alchemist and medical writer; it is surprising that Martin's text reads *Araborum medicorum quidam* since Rhazes was well known as one of the most important mediators of ancient Greek medical knowledge – on which he however took an independent and critical view – to western Europe, much through *al-Hawi fi'l-tibb*, a posthumous edition of his notes and case studies, which were translated into Latin in 1279 as *Liber continens* (first printed ed. Brescia 1486).

The work hinted at here is *al-Judari wa al Hasabah*, known in western Europe as *De variolis et morbillis commentarius*, which, as we see, still was considered useful in the 18th century; a Latin translation was published in Richard Mead's *De variolis et morbillis liber*, and from the preface of Mead's book we might get some evidence as to the weight put upon getting the translation as correct as possible (cf. *De variolis et morbillis liber*, *praef*, p xii sqq).

Aaron] Cf. the second quotation from Mead, **3.2–3.3**, above.

Freindius] John Freind (1675–1728), English physician, philologist, and politician, who among other things published editions of Greek speeches and of Ovid; in 1722 Freind was elected an MP, only to be imprisoned in the Tower in 1723 for political reasons. During his imprisonment, Freind started working on *The history of physic from the time of Galen to the beginning of the 16. century*, which was published in 1725–26. Cf. **Bergius 10.30**

3.3 *Johannem Reiske*] Johann Jacob Reiske (1716–74) was originally intended on Arabian philology, but studied medicine as well; he achieved the degree of MD in 1746, and a professorship in Arabic in Leipzig in 1748; cf. the quotation from Mead, above, which is also quoted in Martin's footnote (a).

nec] *Nec* for *ne …quidem*; cf. Sz, § 241.B.b.

3.4 *Linderstolpe*] Johan Lindestolpe (1678–1724), prior to his ennoblement in 1719 Linder, Swedish physician, MD in Harderwijk 1706 and in Leiden 1707 (The Leiden dissertation was an earlier version of the *Liber de venenis* mentioned in footnote (b)). Lindestolpe published among other things a dissertation on syphilis, *De foeda lue venerea*, 1705 (Sw. ed. *Tanckar om then smittosame sjukdomen fransoser*, 1713), *Flora Wiksbergensis*, 1716; *Johan Linders Swenska Färge-Konst*, ('Johan Linder's Swedish Art of Dyeing') where methods for using Swedish vegetable dye were discussed, was published in 1720, and was to be of great economic importance.

Morbi ... luxu] This is a quotation from *Liber de venenis*, p 308sq.

Stenzelius] Christian Gottfried Stentzel (1698–1748), professor of medicine in Wittenberg, who was the editor of the 1739 edition of Lindestolpe's *Liber de venenis*.

Zacutum Lusitanum] Abraham Zacuto (1575–1642), Portuguese physician; the *Medicorum principorum historia* was published 1629–42 in twelve parts.

Hahnii scriptum] Johann Gottfried von Hahn (1694–1753), German physician; published *Variolarum antiquitates* in 1733.

(In footnote (c)) *SCHULTZ*] Johann Heinrich Schulz (1687–1744), German physician.

3.5 *rotunde dilucideque*] *Rotunde*, designating a "well rounded" phrase, is found in Cicero's *De fin.* 4.7: *ista ipsa, quae tu breviter: regem ... solum esse sapientem, a te ... apte ac rotunde; quippe; habes enim a rhetoribus*, while *dilucide*, meaning 'clearly' or 'distinctly' is found in his *De vat.* 37: *cum mea lex dilucide vetet*, and in e.g. Celsus 2.14.2: *Neque dubitari potest, quin latius quidem et dilucidius ... Asclepiades praeceperit ...*.

4.1 προκαταρτικοίς (*sic*) & προηγουμένοις] Originally philosophical terms, see "Language: Greek words", p 20.

4.2 *in eam putredinem abirent*] *Abeo* is used to express a transition from one state to another, a transformation, by e.g. Ovid *Met.* 1.236: *in villos abeunt vestes* and Pliny *NH* 3.70: *Stabiae oppidum ... quod nunc in villam abiit*, cf. TLL, s.v. *abeo*, 71.43; cf. also **5.1** and **10.3**, below.

4.3 *quo...assimilatur*] Although indicated by italics, this seems not to be an exact quote from any Latin edition of Rhazes. It does however much resemble the translation of Rhazes' book on smallpox and measles included in Richard Mead's *Opera medica*, Tome 1, p 89sqq, which reads: *Quapropter assimilatur sanguis infantium & puerorum musto, in quo nondum incepit fieri coctio perducens ad maturationem perfectam, & cui nec dum competit motio ad fervefactionem. Assimilatur vero sanguis juvenum musto, e quo fit effervescentia & erumpunt vapores, usque dum tranquillum & maturum sit vinum.* So where did Martin get his ablative? Probably just by miswriting *quo* for *cui*.

4.4 *Alexander Petronius Trajanus*] Alessandro Petronio (?–1585), Italian physician, physician-in-ordinary to the Pope Gregory XIII; his most important work was *De victu Romanorum et de sanitate tuenda libri V*, which was published in 1581.

Acta Breslaviensia] A publication, which I have not succeded in locating.

4.5 *Kircherus*] Athanasius Kircher (1601/2–80), German jesuit, educated in Paderborn and Cologne; taught Greek and mechanics in Mainz, from 1629 teacher of mathematics and Oriental languages at the jesuit college in Würzburg, where he also experimented with magnetism and published his *Magnesia* (1630).

In 1631 Kircher, fleeing from the victorious Protestant forces of Gustavus Adolphus, left Würzburg, and arrived the following year in Avignon, where he took up research upon astronomy and optics and published *Gnomonica Catoptrica* (1634) on the projection of sun dial scales by reflection; he also started investigating into the Egyptian hieroglyphs.

In 1635, Kircher was appointed mathematician to the court in Vienna, but arrived, after a shipwreck, in Rome, where he obtained a professorship in mathematics at the *Collegium Romanum*. Kircher was to spend the rest of his life in Rome, where he also became the major scientific "consultant" to the Vatican, which led to vast international contacts, e.g. with the Vatican delegates to the Ethiopian Coptic church; from a Coptic–Latin word list, Kircher tried to perfect his interpretation of the hieroglyphs, which eventually led to the publishing of *Oedipus Aegyptiacus* (1652–54), which, however, turned out to be a work full of misunderstandings and erroneous assumptions.

Upon his death in 1680, Kircher's collections were to form a museum, *Kircherianum*, containing *inter alia* archeological relics, works of art, mechanical inventions, and a collection of ancient and modern obelisks, among them one dedicated to Queen Christina of Sweden. The work hinted at in Martin's text might possibly be the *Scrutinium Physico-Medicum* (1658).

Hauptman] August Hauptman (1607–74?), German physician, who believed all diseases to be caused by different worms etc.

Langius] Probably Christian Lange (1619–62), German physiologist, anatomist, surgeon and pathologist, who held professorships in all these disciplines; his *Miscellanea medica curiosa: annexa disputatione de morbillis, quam prodromum esse voluit novae suae pathologiae animatae* …was posthumously published in 1666.

Rivinus] Augustus Q. Rivinus/Bachmann (1652–1723), German physiologist and botanist.

Lancisius] Giovanni Lancisi (1654–1720), Italian; physician-in-ordinary to the Popes Innocentus XI, Innocentus XII and Clemens XI.

Chesneau] Nicolas Chesneau/Quercetanus (1601?–?), Frenchman, whose *Observationum libri quinque...* were published in 1672.

4.6 *Lister*] Martin Lister (1638–1711), Englishman, best known as an entomologist.

Bergero] Johann Gottfried von Berger (1659–1756), German, published *Dissertatio de usu venaesectionis & clysterum in curatione variolarum* in 1711.

Hoffmanni] Friedrich Hoffmann (1660–1742), German physician, active in Halle.

Hoffmann believed every living organism to be formed out of "fibres", the movements of which prevented the body from decomposition; the foremost cause of those movements, thus of life, he believed however to be the "ether", which pervaded the entire Universe; respiration allowed the entrance into the body of this ether, which then was stored in the ventricles of the brain, from which location it was then spread via the spinal cord and nerves into the fibres, providing those with the right *tonus*; if the movements of the ether was disturbed, sickness was brought about; in his practice, Hoffmann however left most of the cure to Nature's own abilities, which perhaps is why he was considered a successful physician.

chyloso] See *chylosus*, Greek word list, p 33.

lymphatico] See *lymphaticus*, Greek word list, p 36.

medullae spinalis] See *medulla spinalis*, Latin word list, p 43.

4.7 *Merito …praeterimus alias aliorum opiniones*] See "Style: Metaphors", p 78.

meconii] See *meconium*, Greek word list, p 36.

(In footnote (d)) *Fhalstrom*] Johan Fahlström (?–1699), Swedish physician, educated at Uppsala, where he defended a dissertation *De flatibus* under P. Hoffwenius in 1681.

Fahlström achieved the degree of MD in Reims in 1685 by defending a dissertation *De variolis* – according to the title page under the presidency of God – whereupon he returned to a position as physician at the copper mine in Falun.

pulmentorum esu] According to Varro *L* 5.108, *pulmentum* in ancient Latin was something *quod edebant cum pulte, ab eo pulmentum,* later probably of more elaborate dishes, e.g. in Apuleius *Met.* 4.7: *cuncta suavi sapore percocta pulmenta praesto sunt.*

Here, however, it does probably mean the porridge itself, cf. Petri Gothus, who gives the translation *Gröot/moos* (Eng 'porridge/mash').

convellere] *Convello* in the figurative sense of 'overthrow', 'subvert', etc, is known e.g. from Cicero *Har.* 41: *T. Gracchus convellit statum civitatis,* and *Phil.* 2.83: *nolo plura, ne acta Dolabellae videar convellere* (OLD, s.v. *convello* 2 e).

(in footnote (e)) *Guido Patinus*] Guy Patin (1601–72), French physician and surgeon, one of the most prominent anti-Paracelsists, especially as regards the use of antimony; otherwise characterized in *Lexikon der hervorragenden Ärzte* as a *therapeutischer Sonderling,* which seems to agree well with this view of porridge.

aëre elastico] *Elasticus,* from Gr. ἐλατήρ, 'driver', of ἐλαύνω, 'to drive', occurs, probably for the first time, in Jean Pecquet's (1622–74) *Dissertatio anatomica* (1651) where *elastica vis* is the "impulsive force" which Torricelli had shown to cause those phaenomena which had previously been ascribed to Nature's *horror vacui.*

Elasticus later came to be used for the property of resuming "normal bulk or shape after having been contracted, dilated, or distorted by external force", which is the normal sense today. Cf. OED s.v. "elastic".

stasis] Greek word list, p 39.

oriretur] In classical Latin, the flexion of *orior* in imperfect subjunctive was normally made by the 3rd conjugation; cf. however A. J. Tiderus: *Grammatica Latina …,* 1688, where the only flexion indicated is the one present here, by the 4th conjugation.

4.8 *Dicant mihi…? Qua ratione…? & quis…vidit?*] Cf. "Style: Rhetorical questions", p 84.

4.9 *evaderet*] *Evado* for 'become' is known from Classical Latin, e.g. Cicero *Div.* 2.146: *si somnium verum evasit.* Krebs-Schmalz points out, however (I, p 480), that this sense is possible in Classical Latin only with the nuance of 'turn out as', etc.

130

In Neo-Latin, on the other hand, the sense of 'become', is extremely common; there are several occurrences also in this text, e.g. in **6.4**: *de die in diem flavior evadit*, **6.5**: *Majores quidem de die in diem evadunt*, **6.7**: *Salivatio autem parcior evadit*, **14.2**: *mitius evadit mercuriale medicamentum*; cf. also **Bergius**: **5.19**: *variolaeque adeo vel verrucosae, durae, pallentes &c. si effusio magna sit, evadant*, **5.27**: *Si vero variolae vacuae & rugosae evadunt*, and **Schröder**: **20**: *ne in idem semper decumbendo latus, gibber forte evadat*.

5–6 These two paragraphs are derived from Johannes Oosterdijk Schacht's (1704–55), *Institutiones Medicinae practicae* (1747), ch. 13, and from Thomas Sydenham's *Processus integri* (1695), pp 34–43; as a sample are provided the passages of Sydenham's and Schacht's texts which correspond to **Martin 6.1–2** (my italics in all three authors):

Sydenham p 34sq	Schacht p 39	Martin
In distinctis invadunt *rigor & horror, calor intensus, capitis & dorsi dolor* vehemens, *vomituritio, in adultis ingens in sudores propensio* (& hinc minimè confluxuras esse licet conjicere) *dolor sub scrobiculo cordis* si manu prematur, *stupor & somnolentia*, nonnunquam & *insultus epileptici* (in infantibus praesertim) quibus si, dentitione peracta corripiantur, in procinctu esse variolas possis praedicere, ita ut si fortè insultum epilepticum sub vesperam patiantur, sequenti Aurorâ in conspectum se daturae sunt variolae.	In primo stadio haec sunt Phaenomena: *vagus horror. rigor. calor intensior. dolor capitis, dorsi:* nausea: *vomituritio:* anxietas: *dolor acutus circa praecordia:* dolores colici, nephritici, Pleuritici: *ingens in sudores propensio*, potissimum *in adultis:* splendor oculorum, lacrimatio: rarius tussis & sternutatio: febris continua acuta: saepe deliria: interdum narium & mensium fluxus: in adultis alvus strictior: in infantibus aliquoties diarrhoea: tum & *stupor, somnolentia: convulsiones Epilepticae:* Sanguis tenuis, floridus, dissolutus, acer: Eruptio papularum inchoata.	In primo stadio haec exstant indicia, qua distinctas. Post meridiem plerumque incidunt, tumque adest *rigor & horror vagus, calor intensus* & vertiginosa turbatio, nausea & *vomituritio, dolor circa praecordia*, inprimis si manu premantur, *dolores capitis & dorsi* tensorii & leviter punctorii, accedunt colici, nephritici, pleuritici; *propensio in sudores*, praesertim *in adultis*, oculorum splendor, lacrimatio; Interdum sternutatio, tussis, oppletio pectoris, febris, continuata saepe deliria, haud raro narium & mensium fluxus, *stupor & somnolentia*, Alvus stricta in adultis, in infantibus saepius diarrhoea. Non numquam in iisdem *insultus epileptici*, quibus si corripiuntur dentitione peracta, in procinctu variolas esse, possis praedicere, sub his quoque non raro eruptio fieri solet.

Even if the fact that the three passages are descriptions of the same disease would necessarily lead to correspondences between the texts, we might note instances, where almost exactly the same expression occurs in all authors, most notably *in adultis ingens in sudores propensio/ingens in sudores propensio, potissimum in adultis/propensio in sudores, praesertim in adultis*; since Sydenham's posthumous importance was tremendous, and this particular book of his was to be used well into the 19th century, it does not seem to be too far-fetched an assumption that Schacht had also studied it; we should not, however, regard these correspondencies as mere plagiarism; for one thing, Sydenham was above all famous for his accurate observations of symptoms; why then bother to make a list entirely of one's own instead of just adding any complementary information available? As we see, Schacht does in fact provide some additions of his own in accordance with contemporary medical theories, inasmuch as he mentions the assumed quality of the blood during the process, while Martin provides a somewhat more elaborated description of the symptoms.

5.1–5.2 This entire paragraph is a good example of the predilection for systematic categorisation at this time; one might consider the *Nouvelles classes de maladies* (1731–34) by Boissier de Sauvages (see **Bergius 1.7**), Petrus Artedi's (1705–35) posthumous *Ichthyologia* (1738; edited by Linnaeus), and of course Linnaeus' own *Systema Naturae* (1735). Cf. my commentary to **Bergius 1.7**, *species* and **7.6**, *e regno animali*.

5.1 *Ut …propius …veniam*] A metaphor of movement, see p 78sq.

dividendi rationem] *Divisio* in the sense of a 'categorisation' or 'classification' is known from e.g. Cicero *Fin.* 2: *cupiditates non Epicuri divisione finiebat*, and Quintilian *Inst.* 11.1.2: *divisione hac utimur, ut ab eo, quod deceat, utilitatem separemus.*

Cf. also OED, s.v. "division", 6: "Of Divisions, one is a distribution of the Genus into Species, and of the whole into parts … Another is of a word into divers significations, when the same may be taken several ways" (1656).

spuriae] These "false smallpox" are perhaps the chicken pox?

rarius in pus abeunt] Cf. **4.2** and **10.3**.

pus] Latin word list, p 45.

5.2 *curatius*] There are no occurrences of the adverb *curate* in the positive to be found in Classical Latin, but the comparative is used by Tacitus: *negotii initium … curatius disseram* (*Ann.* 2.27), and by Pliny the younger: *hortatus es ut epistulas, si quas paulo curatius scripsissem, colligerem* (*Ep.* 1.1), in about the same sense as here.

contagii] See *Contagio and contagium*, Latin word list, p 40.

inflammationis] See *Inflammatio and inflammatiuncula*, Latin word list, p 42.

prolapsus] here not used in the ordinary medical sense of 'prolapse', but rather as meaning 'collapse'; cf OLD s. v. *prolabor* 5.b.

6.1 *qua*] *Qua* in the sense of 'as regards' is not found in Ancient Latin, but, being a useful construction, it is often used in factual Neo-Latin texts (however, as it seems, not in texts written by those authors who are particularly skilled stylists, such as the *professor Skytteanus* Johan Ihre); the examples provided below are mainly taken from as yet unpublished material by Professor Hans Helander.

There are occurrences in a few dissertations, e.g. *Sponsalia plantarum* (pr. Linnaeus, resp. Wahlbom) 1746: *semina ... tam qua figuram, quam magnitudinem, eandem tamen plantam proferant* (in *Amoenitates academicae*, I, p 379) and *De dentitione difficili* (pr. Aurivillius, resp. Halenius) 1757: *ego ... morbum istum praesenti dissertatiuncula qua indolem ... describere in animum induxi.* (p 5); further in e.g. Swedenborg: *Quod mundus per easdem series subsistat, per quas existit; quodque qua subsistentiam, et qua existentiam perpetuo primum suum respiciat* (*Principia* 2.2), and in the *Nova Literaria Maris Balthici & Septentrionis*: *utilitatem venationis exponit, qua animum, qua corpus ...* (1706, p 251)

vertiginosa] See *Vertigo* and *Vertiginosus*, Latin word list, p 52.

nausea] Greek word list, p 37.

vomituritio] Latin word list, p 53.

praecordia] Latin word list, p 45.

dolores tensorii] *Dolor tensorius* is probably synonymous with the *dolor tensivus* in **6.4**, below; the formation of adjectives on *-orius* is very common in the Neo-Latin period; Hoven (p 424sq) lists almost 120 such forms. Cf. also *punctorii* below, and *Excretorius*, *Inflammatorius* and *Secretorius* in my Latin word list.

Even if several different kinds of pain are listed in contemporary sources, such as Zedler, it does not seem as though there existed, at the time, any general and univocal system for a detailed classification of pains; in the dissertation *De doloribus* (1765), defended by E. O. Rydbäck under the presidency of S. Aurivillius, one distinction proposed, however, is that between *dolores obtusi* and *dolores acuti*, while any more detailed categorisation is avoided, apparently since the perception of pain is highly individual and often not possible to adequately communicate: *Dolores ... alii alios queruntur ... immo tales, quibus nomina non inveniuntur* (Ry, p 3); *Sensum ... alterius alter non percipit.* (id. p 4).

(As a matter of fact – and quite an embarrassing one, too – this opinion has not yet obtained a footing with everybody involved in medical care.)

punctorii] *Dolor punctorius* is found in Zedler s.v. *Dolor*, and explained as *Wenn es wie mit Steck-Nadeln sticht.*

colici] See *Colicus*, Greek word list, p 33.

nephritici] See *Nephriticus*, Greek word list, p 37.

pleuritici] See *Pleuriticus*, Greek word list, p 38.

tussis] Latin word list, p 50.

deliria] See *Delirium*, Latin word list, p 41.

stupor] Latin word list, p 48.

diarrhoea] Greek word list, p 34.

6.2 *insultus epileptici*] For *insultus*, see Latin word list, p 43, for *epileptici*, see *Epilepsia*, Greek word list, p 34; cf. also *Colicus, Nephriticus,* and *Pleuriticus.*

in procinctu variolas esse possis praedicere] Another military metaphor, see p 79sq.

6.3 *pustulae*] See *Pustula*, Latin word list, p 46.

prodeuntes] A military metaphor, see p 79sq.

acicularum] *Acicula* or *acucula*, a 'pin' or 'needle', is, acc. to TLL, s.v. *acucula*, a Late Latin word; it is perhaps found, then spelled *acicla*, in *Mulomedicina Chironis*, 102 (Buecheler), even if the preferred reading seems to be *aciola.*

6.4 *vesiculas*] See *Vesicula*, Latin word list, p 53.

ab insultu] Another military metaphor, see p 79sq.

doloreque tensivo] *Dolor tensivus* is found in Zedler, where it is translated as *dehnender Schmertz*, cf. *dolores tensorii*, above.
Adjectives and adverbs on *-ivus* and *-ive*, respectively, are another common feature of the Neo-Latin language; cf. *indolis corrosivae* in **6.9**; Hoven (p 416) has ca. thirty-five forms of the kind.

de die in diem] This phrase, here used by the author three times in less than two pages, is also to be found in Oosterdijk Schacht's chapter on smallpox.
The phrase is by Noltenius regarded as having a somewhat unjust reputation for being a Hebraism. It is to be found in the Vulgate, e.g. *Ps* 60.9: *Ut reddam vota mea de die in diem*; 2 *Petr.* 2.8: *habitans apud eos, qui de die in diem animam iustam iniquis operibus cruciabant*, but Noltenius argues that there is also one occurrence in Pliny's *NH* 8.1, which however is not the case in modern edd.
In Krebs-Schmalz I, p 357, the phrase is regarded as a Late Latin vulgarism for *ex die in diem*, which is found in Cato, *pro L. Autronio*, frag (ed. Jordan, p 63): *iussisti adesse in diem ex die*, and in Cicero *ep. ad Brut* I.1: *in diem ex die dilata sunt.*
One might note, however, that both these phrases as used in extant older occurrences indicate a duration (cf. the Vatican Psalms version of 1947, where the phrase has been changed to *omni die*), whereas the point in Schacht/Martin rather seems to be the change from day to day, as is also suggested by the comparative: *de die in diem flavior evadit; majores … de die in diem evadunt*, or by the verb itself: *de die in diem augeri … videtur.*

vesica] Latin word list, p 53.

phrenitis] Greek word list, p 37.

coma] Greek word list, p 33.

petechiae] Latin word list, p 45.

haemorrhagia] Greek word list, p 35.

6.6 *palphebrae*] See *palphebra*, Latin word list, p 44.

rosarum Damascenarum aemulum] According to Johan Gottschalk Wallerius'
PRAELECTIONES PHARMACEUTICAE ad normam Pharmacopeae Londinensis …MDCCLIV
(UUB ms D 251), p. 164, these are ordinary red roses: *Rosae rubrae vulgares Damascenae
appellantur*, according to Zedler, 32, col 836sq, however, a *Rosa damascena* can be either
(1) a pink rose, *die blaßrothe Zuckerrose*, or (2) the white *Muscat- oder Damascerrose*.
   Today, *Rosae damascenae* seems to denote a group of hybrid roses of several
colours, ranging from white to dark red; with all probability, however, the colour
indicated by Wallerius is that, which is relevant in this text, since *color floridus* would
not be a very likely way to describe a pale or white nuance.

6.7 (footnote (g)) *Lommius*] Joost van Lom (c. 1500–63/64), physician in Brussels,
physician-in-ordinary to Philip II.

6.8 *emetiuntur*] *Emetior* for 'pass through', 'complete', etc, seems to be known in ancient
Latin only in connexion with human beings and, as regards actual distances, celestial
bodies; there are occurrences of the verb used in a temporal sense in e.g. Valerius
Maximus, 8.13: *Masinissa … hunc modum excessit, regni spatium LX annis emensus*, and
Tacitus *Hist.* 1.49: *hunc exitum habuit Servius Galba, tribus et septuaginta annis quinque
principes emensus*. Cf. TLL s.v. *emetior*, 481 sq.

viscera nobiliora] See *Viscera*, Latin word list, p 53.

per metastasin] See *Metastasis*, Greek word list, p 36.

desquamantur] The plural indicates that the subject here is not *cutis*, but rather *crustae*.

tubercula] See *Tuberculum*, Latin word list, p 50.

6.9 *…vergant …abscedant …flavescunt …confluxerint …proripiunt*] This sentence, which
otherwise is a direct quotation from *Processus integri*, p 38, differs from its source
inasmuch as Sydenham has the indicative forms *vergunt* and *abscedunt*, respectively; as is
pointed out by Östlund, p 40, and Helander (95), p 25sq, there was an uncertainty
regarding mood in this kind of *quod*-clauses, which could explain this difference.

indolis corrosivae] The adjective *corrosivus* is not known from ancient Latin; cf. *doloreque
tensivo*, above.

ptyalismus] Greek word list, p 38.

7.1 *invaserunt*] For military metaphors, see p 79sq.

fluxus] Latin word list, p 41.

7.2 *globulorum sanguinis*] See *Globulus sanguinis ruber*, Latin word list, p 42.

vasorum] See *Vasa*, Latin word list, p 51.

Boerhavii] Herman Boerhaave (1668–1738), Dutch physician, professor of medicine, botany and chemistry at Leiden; probably the most famous physician of the 18ᵗʰ century.

Boerhaave, the son of the apparently unusually well-educated Rev. Jacobus Boerhaave, studied Latin, Greek and history at home under the supervision of his father until he in 1682 was sent to the grammar school in Leiden, where he also took up university studies in 1685, primarily in philosophy – which also included natural science – and classics, with the intention of eventually becoming a clergyman; he did, however, also study mathematics.

After achieving his degree in philosophy in 1690, Boerhaave continued his education by studying theology while supporting himself through the teaching of mathematics and by undertaking the cataloguing of recent additions to the university library.

Following the advice of the secretary Jan Van den Berg, Boerhaave decided to take up medicine along with his theological studies; without attending any medical lecture in Leiden, but rather by studying the Greek and Latin authors chronologically, from Hippocrates to Sydenham, with the addition of studies also in chemistry and botany, he completed his medical education, and achieved the degree of MD at Hardewijk in 1693.

Instead of re-establishing himself as a student of theology, Boerhaave set out on a medical career while continuing his studies in chemistry until he was appointed lecturer in medicine at the University of Leiden in 1701; his predilection for Hippocrates in combination with his knowledge of chemistry, mathematics and natural science led him to establish a medical theory of his own, the main point of which was the need for natural science to be included in medicine as well as the careful observation of each single patient; while he was critical of the iatrochemical idea, that all diseases were due to fluctuations of the balance between *acidum* and *alkali*, he also recognised the importance of chemistry to the physician.

For the benefit of his students, Boerhaave published his *Institutiones medicae* in 1708, and in 1709 his *Aphorismi de cognoscendis et curandis morbis*. In 1709, he was also appointed *professor medicinae et botanices*, which in effect was much more a chair in botany than a chair in medicine; it was not until 1714 that Boerhaave could take up the teaching of clinical medicine, which above all would make him famous.

In 1718, Boerhaave was appointed professor also of chemistry, and thus lectured on three subjects until 1729, when he resigned from the professorships of chemistry and botany for health reasons; he did, however, continue his medical lecturing until just before his death.

Boerhaave was, much like Nils Rosén, not famous for any major scientific discovery, but rather for being a successful and observant practitioner; above all, his Hippocratic view of medicine lead to the regarding of the patient as an individual.

Among Boerhaave's most famous disciples were Albrecht von Haller, Gerard van Swieten and Julien Offray de la Mettrie. Cf. Lindeboom: *Herman Boerhaave The Man and his Work*.

resolutio] today, "resolution" in a medical technical sense is "the subsidence of a pathological state" (Dorland), which is probably the case in this text also.

gangraenam] See *Gangraena*, Greek word list, p 35.

8.1 *solis luce clarius est*] The comparison with daylight to indicate obviousness is a feature, which is known also from ancient Latin; Otto (p 203, s.v. *lux*) has examples e.g. from Cicero, such as *Cat.* 1.3.6: *Luce sunt clariora nobis tua consilia omnia, Tusc.* 1.37.90: *quod est luce clarius*, and *De divin.* 1.3.6: *solis luce ... clarius*.

qua via maxime conveniat morbo occurrere] Another military metaphor, see p 79sq.

8.2 *in hac virium mearum tenuitate*] Cf. "Style: Modesty of the author", p 88; cf also **2.3**.

dicam scribere] *Dica*, Gr δίκη, is in Latin a legal term denoting a lawsuit etc, whereas the Greek word could have several meanings. Cf. Plautus *Aul.* 759: *tibi scribam dicam*; *Poen.* 800: *subscribam homini dicam*, TLL, 957.37ff.

Censor Anglus] Unfortunately, I have not been able to obtain any information on this journal (or writer).

crisis] Greek word list, p 33.

8.3 *Richter*] A physician whose identity I have not been able to establish.

Id ...afferam me intelligentia consequi non posse] Cf. **10.2**.

8.4 *Fischerus*] Daniel Fischer (1695–1745), Hungarian physician.

9.1 *indicationi ...comprobant*] comprobo should, classically, have an acc.

9.2 *Et quo ...autores?*] Cf. "Style: Rhetorical questions", p 84.

Lobb] Theophilus Lobb (1678–1763), Englishman; the *Treatise on the small pox* of footnote (p) was published in 1731.

me respondendo sustinere vellem] Cf. Cicero *Luc* (*Academica 2*). 104: *cum se a respondendo ... sustineat.*

Quae ... eo recedunt] *Recedo* in this sense does not seem to be known from Classical Latin.

contagione serpente] See *Contagio and contagium*, Latin word list, p 40.

9.3 *sporadice*] This adverb, originally from Gr. noun σπορά, 'sowing', adj. σποραδικός, 'scattered' (while the Greek adv. seems normally to be σποράδην), is not found in ancient or mediaeval Latin.

Quamquam ...valeas] *Quamquam* in Classical Latin normally occurs with the indicative, but could, as in Sallust *Iug.* 3.2: *quamquam et possis et delicta corrigas*, and in this case, be found with a potential subjunctive; in general, the construction with the subjunctive becomes more usual towards the end of the Classical period – even if it is not relevant for this case, one might note one example in Celsus 1 *pr.* 47 – and in Tacitus and Pliny the younger it is the preferred construction; cf. K-St, § 221.5; Sz, § 325 with further references.

pancreatice] This is an amusing mistake, which is quite understandable in a physician intent on questions belonging to his profession; *pancreatice* has nothing to do with the pancreas, but is rather a misprint for adv. *pancratice* (from Gr. *παγχρατικως*), 'like a combatant in the *pancratium* (i.e. a combination of boxing and wrestling)', a word which is found in Plautus *Bac.* 248: *benene usque valuit? –pancratice atque athletice.*

insitio] Normally, *insitio* in ancient Latin is a technical term from agriculture, meaning 'grafting', as in Cato *Agr.* 41.2: *altera insitio est: si vitis vitem continget, utriusque vitem teneram praeacuito, oblique inter sese ... conligato;* Columella 5.11.1: *tria genera ... insitionum antiqui tradiderunt, unum, quo resecta et fissa arbor ... surculos accipit ... tertium, quo ipsas gemmas cum exiguo cortice in partem sui delibratam recipit, quam vocant agricolae emplastrationem, vel ut quidam, inoculationem.*

From the descriptions in Cato and Columella, it is easily understood why *insitio* and *inoculatio* both have been used to denote the smallpox inoculation; not only is it, both in agricultural and medical usage, an act of deliberately making one thing "grow" upon another, but the actual techniques do also very much resemble each other, as might be seen from eye-witness reports, most notably a letter (april, 1717) by Lady Mary Wortley Montagu (1689–1762), the wife of the English ambassador in Constantinople, who had came in contact with the Turkish method:

> The small pox ... is here entirely harmless, by the invention of ingrafting, which is the term they give it ... they make parties for this purpose, and when they are met ... the old woman comes with a nut-shell full of the matter of the best sort of small pox and asks what vein you please to have opened. She immediately rips open that ... with a large needle ... and puts into the vein as much matter as can lie upon the head of her needle, and after that, binds up the little wound ...

This letter is perhaps the most famous early description, by a European, of the smallpox inoculation, but it was not the first; in the *Philosophical transactions*, vol. 339, there is a summary by John Woodward (cf. **Bergius 3.5**) of a letter on the matter from one Emanuel Timonius, MD, dated in Constantinople, December, 1713, where the same method is described; according to Woodward's summary, the method, which has "metaphorically, the name of Insition or Inoculation", has been introduced among the Turks by "Circassians, Georgians, and other Asiaticks ... for about the space of forty Years"; in vol. 347 of the same periodical there is another letter on the *Nova & tuta Variolas excitandi per Transplantationem Methodus, nuper inventa & in usum tracta*, by Jacobus Pylarinus, MD, who, according to the letter, had recently been the Venetian consul in Smyrna.

In this letter, the *nuper inventa methodus* is actually said to have had its origin in Thessalia, whence it had spread to Constantinople and for a few years been used by common people, however not by physicians and the upper classes until the outbreak of a smallpox epidemic in 1701; as for terminology, Pylarinus says that *hujusmodi ...Variolarum excitatio fit per Metaphorice sic dictam Insitionem sive Transplantationem*; since the first occurrence of Eng. "insition" in this sense is the passage from Timonius/Woodward quoted above (cf. OED, s.v. *insition* 1), the Latin *insitio* in the same sense is probably also coined at this time.

In this context, something might also be said about the development of smallpox inoculation in Sweden; according to A.O. Lindfors' *Minnesord öfver Nils Rosén von Rosenstein*, p 13, the physician-in-ordinary to the Swedish king, Karl XII, dr Samuel Skragge, had obtained the information communicated by the above-mentioned

Timonius in Bender, Turkey, where the king was staying at the time; inoculation was, however, apparently not put to practical use in Sweden until 1754, when J.J. Haartman (cf. **Bergius 8.30**) inoculated a daughter of professor J. Leche in Åbo and S. Aurivillius performed one inoculation in Uppsala.

The success, however, seems to have been limited; according to J.A. Murray's *Historia insitionis variolarum in Svecia* …, only four inoculations were performed until 1756 (p 58), when David Schultz (later von Schulzenheim), who had been studying inoculation in London, published his book *Berättelse om koppors ympande* (Eng. "Report on the inoculation of smallpox"); according to Lindroth (p 459) this book, together with Rosén's calendar articles, was an important reason for inoculation's increasing popularity during the 1760s; in 1769, even the successor to the throne, crown prince Gustav, was inoculated under the supervision of Nils Rosén, apparently by David Schultz.

Inoculation was to be used to some extent throughout the 18th century, but in 1801 Eberhard Munck af Rosenschöld (who, by the way, was related to Nils Rosén, inasmuch as the family descended from the daughter of Eberhard Rosén (Rosenblad)) performed the first *vaccination* according to the method described by Edward Jenner, and in 1816, new legislation made vaccination compulsory for all Swedish children under the age of two.

emtio] That smallpox were actually bought, as a kind of variolisation, seems evident from Rosén's *Underrättelser om barnsjukdomar*, p 97: [*Kopporna fortplantas*] … *4:o Genom kjöpande, som länge warit brukeligt i Sachsen, uti Öster- och Wäster-Göthland …Barnet* [*föres*] *til en som har goda Koppor, och begärer at få köpa 5 eller 7. Penningarna … läggas … på en mogen söndergången Koppa, så att Wahr fastnar wid dem. Dessa Penningar läggas sedan på Benen på Barnet, och bindas fast, då någon del av Wahret drager sig in … hwaraf det sedan får Koppor.* ("[The Pox are propagated] … (4) Through purchase, which has since long been customary in Saxony, in the provinces of Östergötland and Västergötland … The Child [is taken] to one who has good Pox, and asks to buy five or seven. The Coins … are placed on a mature bursted Pock, so that Pus sticks to them. These Coins are then placed on the Legs of the Child, and tied there, by which some part of the Pus is drawn in … whence it then attracts the Pox.")

9.4 *Avicennae*] Abn al Hosain ibn Abdallah ibn Sina (980–1037), Islamic philosopher and physician, who, according to his autobiography, was fully educated in all sciences of his time at the age of sixteen.

Avicenna served several Persian potentates and was a productive author, not only on medical subjects, but also on philosophy, astronomy and mathematics, among other things; his most famous medical work, and one of the most influential medical books of all times, is *Al-Qanun fi-l-tibb*, in Europe known as *Canon*, which was translated into Latin already in the 12th century, and was to become the major textbook in European medical education well towards the late 16th century; it was printed in several editions from 1470 on.

alcalinum volatile] A term from chemistry; however, as it seems, not a very exact one.

According to Zedler, s.v. *Alcalinum*, this term could be used about any of the *erdigte und irdische Cörper* that either contains an alkaline salt or has some property in common with such a salt; s.v. *Alkali* the alkaline salt is defined as any salt with a taste that is *urinös und laugenhafftig*, there is further a distinction made between volatile alkaline salts, such as *sal volatile cornu cervi* (i.e. ammonium carbonate), and fixed alkaline salts, e.g. *sal tartari* (pottassium carbonate).

The conclusion of this would be that *alcalinum volatile* is, roughly, 'some unspecified volatile substance with alkaline qualities'.

qui hoc morbo ... non occupati fuerunt] Another military metaphor; see p. 79sq.

10.1 *inquinatos*] Classically, *inquinatus* does not mean 'infected' in a literal sense, as it appears to do here.

10.2 *quomodo consequi intelligentia poteris, nisi ... praestruatur?*] cf. **8.3.**

10.3 *cogere*] Here in the sense of 'prove', known from e.g. Cicero *Leg.* 2.33: *ex quibus id, quod volumus, efficitur et cogitur*, cf. TLL, s.v. *cogo*, 1532.13sqq.

abire] Cf. **4.2,** above

11.1 *si paria ... fecero cum ... Lobb*] The expression *paria facio* in its original sense indicates the squaring of accounts, both literally, as e.g. in Columella 1.8.13: *negotiatio curam vilici avocat nec umquam patietur eum cum rationibus domini paria facere*, and figuratively, as in Pliny *NH* 2.202: *nascuntur ... alio modo terrae ... velut paria secum faciente natura*; here, however, the sense is clearly more of 'join', etc.

colatoria] The adj. *colatorius* is found in the compound *colatoria ossa*, denoting the bones of the nostrils, in the 1607 ed. of Castelli's *Lexicon medicum*, where the reason for the name is said to be the cavernous structure of these bones; in Zedler, VI, 642 – where it is said to be *ein zwar nicht recht gebräuchlich Wort* – *colatorius* denotes an organ, which disposes of superfluous matter; as an example is given the kidney; in the same sense, the word is found in C, while B only has the noun *colatorium*, Germ. *Durchschlag*, meaning 'a strainer'.

The English form "colatory" is, acc. to OED, also known in a medical sense: "The holes of the eyes and the collatores of the nosethrylles" (R. Copland, *Guydon's Quest. Cyrurg*, 1541); "Two holes, whyche ar called Colatories or Strayners of the nastrelles" (Traheron, *Vigo's Chirurg.* I.iii.4, 1543); "The Liver ... is a Colatory of the Blood" (*Brit. Apollo* II. *Quarterly* No. 1, 1710). For the 16th century examples; cf. the entry in Castelli 1607, above.

We might also note that the noun *transcolatio* is found in the dissertation *De functionibus corporis humani primariis*, 1695 (pr. O. Rudbeck, Jr, resp. J. Dalin), where it is used about the absorption of nutritive substances from food in the digestive tract.

11.2 (footnote (s)) *Halleri*] Albrecht von Haller (1708–77), Swiss anatomist, physiologist and botanist, studied under Boerhaave in Leiden, and subsequently in London, Paris and Basel. Professor in Göttingen for seventeen years.

Haller upheld a vast correspondence with several colleagues all over Europe, among them Nils Rosén, who also used Haller's *Primae lineae physiologiae* (1747) as a basis for his lectures; cf. also "Biographical notes: Nils Rosén", p 13.

11.3 *vasa inhalantia & aperta pulmonum*] In all probability, *vasa inhalantia* does not denote any particular part of the respiratory apparatus, but indicate only that the blood vessels of the lungs are thought to "inhale" the air (and the contagion). Cf. *Vasa*, Latin word list, p 51.

12.1 *Propero jam*] A metaphor of movement, see "Style: Metaphors", p 78.

antiphlogistica] See "Drug categories", p 56.

stimulum inflammatorium ... corrigam] The sense of *corrigo* here is clearly closer to 'change' or 'alter' in a more thorough way than the usual sense of 'correct' would indicate; this also seems to be a possible interpretation in some cases pertaining to medical matters in ancient Latin, e.g. in Pliny *NH* 22, 88: *Erasistratus ... monstrat ... oris graveolentiam corrigi.*

12.4 *quoad valeant humeri*] Cf. Horace *Ars p.* 39sq: *versate diu, quid ferre recusent, quid valeant humeri.*

Eum ...tramitem insistam] This is another metaphor of movement, see "Style: Metaphors", p 78.

cortex Peruvianus] See *Cortex chinae*, Pharmacological word list, p 63.

13.1 *stibii & antimonii*] See *Antimonium*, Pharmacological word list, p 60.

corpus semimetallicum] At this time the metal antimony was not known; Zedler lists e.g. only six metals altogether, viz. gold, silver, copper, iron, lead and tin; on antimony, or rather stibnite, he says, however, that it is a substance *so einem Metalle gar nahe kommt*, which might be roughly the same as a *corpus semimetallicum.*

parte regulina & sulphure] Pars *regulina* is probably synonymous to *regulus*, i.e. what in this case is the metal which today is known as antimony, cf. *Antimonium*, Pharmacological word list, p 60; since stibnite does in fact consist of antimony and sulphur, Martin's statement is basically correct.

13.2 *emunctoriorum*] Emunctoria (from *emungo*, to 'wipe or blow the nose') is a collective term for the excretory organs and ducts (cf. *colatoria*, above); the word *emunctorium* is otherwise known also from the Vulgate, however in the sense of 'snuffers': *Emunctoria quoque et ubi quae emuncta sunt extinguantur, fiant de auro purissimo* (*Exod.* 25:38). Both senses of course pertain to the getting rid of superfluous matter of some kind.

diapnoë] Greek word list, p 34.

(in footnote (u)) *Neumanni Chemia*] Caspar Neumann (1683–1737), German pharmacist and professor of chemistry in Berlin.

lue venerea] See *Lues venerea*, Latin word list, p 43.

13.3 *virtute ...virus quodcunque debellante*] A military metaphor, see p 79sq.

mercurium] See *Mercurius vivus*, Pharmacological word list, p 67.

14.1 *miasmate*] See *Miasma*, Greek word list, p 36.

spiritu minerali acido] A chemical term of somewhat uncertain meaning; according to L&G II, p 50, *spiritus mineralis* was coined by Friedrich Hoffmann to denote carbonic acid, which could not possibly be the sense here.

Since the dissolution of gold is mentioned in the context, we must rather assume that what is intended is the *aqua regis* or *acidum chloro-nitrosum* – which was the only substance used to dissolve gold – even if it does not seem very likely for an author in this period to use any other term than *aqua regis* for this mixture.

14.2 *mercurium dulcem*] See *Mercurius dulcis*, Pharmacological word list, p 67.

scabioso] See *Scabies* and *scabiosus*, Latin word list, p 47.

spiritu salis] See *Spiritus salis*, Pharmacological word list, p 73.

sublimatus] From *sublimo*, 'elevate' or 'raise', used in Classical Latin both literally and figuratively.

In Latham, *Revised Medieval Word-list*, s.v. *sublimatio*, the word is translated as 'sublimation/vaporization' and said to be a term from alchemy, known from 1144, however without any indication of the source; it is also found, in a similar sense, in Petrus de Crescentiis (c. 1300), *de Agricultura* 1.8: *sublimatio quidem et distillatio aquas rectificant malas* (duCange s.v. *sublimare*).

In chemical usage, the term denotes more specifically the equivalent to destillation as regards those solid inorganic substances, which, when heated, vaporize without previously adopting a liquid state of aggregation; thus a meaning, which agrees well with both the literal (the vapors rising) and the figurative (the end result being a purified, "elevated" substance) sense in Classical Latin.

terendo] Indicates the method of pulverizing a substance by grating.

ejus globuli cum spiculis … uniti, illa obtundant, quo mitius evadit … medicamentum]
For once, this is not a metaphor, but rather another good example of the iatromechanical way of thinking, inasmuch as the added mercury is believed to mechanically blunt the sublimate.

14.3 *eadem virtus*] *Virtus* for a particularly prominent property of something, as opposed to the normal sense of 'the qualities typical of a true man', is known from ancient Latin, e.g. from Vitruvius 8.2.1: *quae ex imbribus aqua colligitur, salubriores habet virtutes* (OLD, s.v. *virtus* 6), where the sense seems to be very close to the medical usage for 'drug effect'; this sense is also frequently found in Mediaeval Latin, e.g. in Gregorius Holmiensis' *Miracula defixionis Domini*, p. 10: *oculus ille sanus et integer cum … visiva virtute ad locum suum naturalem rediit* (GMS, s.v. *virtus* 2).

In Linnaeus' *Materia medica*, however, the word used for 'drug effect' is not *virtus*, but rather *vis*. Cf. also **16.2** *ejus virtus, balsamica nempe*, below.

15.1 *tanquam chimaeram quandam*] Chimaera, from Greek χίμαιρα, 'goat' is in ancient Latin a monster, mentioned e.g. in Cicero *Nat. Deorum* 2.5: *Quis enim Hippocentaurum fuisse aut Chimaeram putat…?* and in Lucretius, 5.905, where also a description is provided: *prima leo, postrema draco, media ipsa, Chimaera.*

As used here, however, as in modern usage, the only surviving feature of the original *chimaera* is its actual non-existence.

aethiopem mineralem] See *Aethiops mineralis*, Pharmacological word list, p 59.

15.2 *drachmis duabus*] See "Weight units", p 55.

floris sulphuris] See *Flos sulphuris*, Pharmacological word list, p 66.

propinabantur] *Propino* in the medical technical sense of 'offering to drink as a remedy' is known from Pliny *NH*, e.g. 21.145: *splenicis propinant ex aceto*, 25.169: *ischiadicis drachmam cum oxymelite ab ambulatione propinavere*. Cf **Bergius 8.8**.

quavis vespera & mane] *Quivis* for *unusquisque* is a quite common feature in Neo-Latin; cf. Erikson: *En undersökning av Anders Spoles Sphaerica et usus globorum, 1694* (1974), p 26.
   The usage is otherwise known also from Medieval Latin, e.g. the *Chartae Traiectanae*, (i.e. the records of the diocese of Utrecht) 1845 p 107.29 from the year 1273: *si me sine filio mori contingerit ... frater meus mihi succedet in eisdem bonis, quivis successive post obitum alterius* (*Lexicon latinitatis Nederlandicae medii aevi*, s.v. *quivis*). Cf. **Bergius 10.8**

uncia semis] See "Weight units", p 55.

radicis enulae Campaniae] See *Radix enulae Campaniae*, Pharmacological word list, p 70.

myrrhae] See *Myrrha*, Pharmacological word list, p 68.

camphorae] See *Camphora*, Pharmacological word list, p 62.

scrupulo uno] See "Weight units", p 55.

aqua bryoniae] Pharmacological word list, p 61.

syrupi baccarum sambuci] See *Syrupus baccarum sambuci*, Pharmacological word list, p 73.

aqua cinnamomi fortis] See *Aqua cinnamomi*, Pharmacological word list, p 61.

15.3 *praeservaturi*] *Praeservare* is by Krebs-Schmalz, II, p 331, regarded as "sehr *Sp.L.*", and only used in the sense of 'consider beforehand' etc; cf. Caelius Aurelianus *Acut* 3, 8, 90: *naturam vel aetates ac vitae consuetudinem ... praeservare*. In this case, the future participle seems to be substantivated and used in an absolute sense of 'those who want to be provident'.

herba rutae] Pharmacological word list, p 66.

coccinellae] See *Coccinella*, Pharmacological word list, p 63.

pulveris e chelis cancrorum & coccinella] See *Pulvis e chelis cancrorum & coccinella*, Pharmacological word list, p 69.

vehiculo] *Vehiculum* in Classical Latin usually denotes a means of transportation such as a ship or, normally, a wagon; the more specific medical sense of a medically inactive excipient, as in this case, is still the normal meaning in medical usage; the English form "vehicle" is known from early 17th century, and OED, s.v. "vehicle" I.1 lists several examples of this sense, e.g: "Let all your Vehicles for your Medicines ... be soft and pleasing to your Patients." (1612); "Let him have of the same pill in a convenient vehicle, of four grains" (1658); "I seldom give less than half a spoonful, ... diluted with a sufficient measure of a temperate Vehicle."(1689); "Mineral Chalybeat Waters ... are the most agreeable and beneficial Vehicle for such Medicines."(1733).

16.1 *ad ... experientiam provocaturus*] An intransitive *provoco* in the sense of 'appeal' is known e.g. from Cicero *Phil.* 1.21: *damnati ad populum provocent*; in a transferred sense from Apuleius *Apologia* 84: *ad litteras Pudentillae provocastis*, cf. OLD, s.v. *provoco* 7.

Nobilissimi Domini Praesidis experientiam] Sometimes this kind of reference has been taken as an indication that the *respondens* has written his dissertation himself.

As is shown by Östlund, p 16, however, the mentioning of the *praeses* in 3rd person does not mean that he cannot be the author of the dissertation; in Östlund's case, extant drafts by Ihre's hand clearly indicated him as the author of e.g. *De runarum patria et origine*, 1770 (resp. J.G. Stenberg); nevertheless, the *Nobilissimus Dominus Praeses* is mentioned in §VI of this dissertation.

id quod in superioribus vicimus] This construction represents *Vinco* with acc. c. inf, which is used in the sense of 'carry a point', etc, already in early Latin, e.g. in Plautus *Am.* 433: *vincon argumentis te non esse Sosiam?*, but also in the Classical period, e.g. by Cicero: *Peripatetici ... haec ipsa ... a se peti vincerent oportere* (*De orat.* 1.43).

ut ... capite quasi deminueret] *Capite deminuere* for 'deprive of civil rights' is known from e.g. Cicero *Top.* 29: *qui capite non sunt deminuti* and Livy 22.60.15: *deminuti capite ... servi Carthaginiensium facti*.

phlogosin] See *Phlogosis*, Greek word list, p 37.

16.2 *Calomelano*] See *Calomelanum*, Pharmacological word list, p 62.

resina guajaci] Pharmacological word list, p 71.

aloës extractum] See *Extractum aloes*, Pharmacological word list, p 66.

excipientia] Cf. **15.3** *vehiculo* above.

ejus virtus, balsamica nempe] See *Balsamica*, "Drug categories", p 56; cf. **14.3** *eadem virtus*, above.

depurans & abstergens] See *Depurantia* and *Abstergentia*, "Drug categories", pp 57 and 55, respectively.

catharralibus] Misprint for *catarrhalibus*, see *Catarrhalis*, Greek word list, p 32.

secretoria] See *Secretorius*, Latin word list, p 48.

144

excretoria] See *Excretorius*, Latin word list, p 41.

16.3 *conflictari*] Another military metaphor, see p 79sq.

laxans] See *Laxantia*, "Drug categories", p 58.

pilulas praeservatorias] Cf. **15.3** *praeservaturi*, above.

16.4 *Recipe …Da*] This is a genuine prescription, as will appear from the *invocatio* (the imperative *recipe*, sometimes written as a ℞, which, acc. to Bendz, *Latin för medicinare*, 1950, p 339, originally was the ♃-sign, indicating the invocation of Jupiter, later of God), from the *praescriptio*, with the amounts of each substance involved being indicated, and from the *subscriptio* (the imperatives *misce* and *fac*) regarding method of preparation; cf. Dorland, s.v. *prescription*.

grana tria] See "Weight units", p 55.

foliato argento obductae] According to Lindgren & Gentz, II, p 230, the practice of coating pills with a thin silver foil might trace its origin back to an old alchemistic and astrological belief, that silver, which was believed to be connected to the moon, had an especially salutary effect on the heart.

17.1 *Cum… & temporis & aliis premar angustiis*] See "Style: Modesty of the author", p 88.

17.2 *phlegma victrioli*] Pharmacological word list, p 69.

tinctura rosarum] Pharmacological word list, p 75.

florum papaveris erratici] See *Syrupus floris papaveris rhoeadis*, Pharmacological word list, p 73.

spiritu victrioli] See *Spiritus victrioli*, Pharmacological word list, p 73.

aqua picis navalis] Pharmacological word list, p 61.

Sydenhamium] Thomas Sydenham (1624–89), English physician, who apparently was particularly intended on the observation of actual symptoms, as opposed to the theoretical speculations of the contemporary medical science; because of this, but perhaps also because of his serving as a captain in Cromwell's army, Sydenham never held a professorship, but published medical works of considerable importance, such as *Observationes medicae* (1676), where e.g. Scarlet fever is first described as a particular disease. Cf. **Bergius 2.1**

Praeter medicos in Hassia celebres] Since both Dolaeus and Waldschmiedt would be included in the category *medici in Hassia celebres*, this probably hints at a bunch of physicians known *only* in Hesse.

Dolaeus] Johann Dolaeus (1651–1707), German physician, *archiater* of Hesse-Kassel.

Wadschmidius] Wilhelm H. Waldschmiedt (1669–1731), German physician, imperial army-surgeon in Hesse, professor of anatomy, botany, and physics in Kiel.

Hoffmannus] Cf. **4.6** *Hoffmanni*, above

17.3 *Marlowii*] This is apparently an American physician, whom I, however, have not been able to identify.

gargarismatis] See *Gargarisma*, "Drug categories", p 58.

Cassine] Pharmacological word list, p 62.

aquifolio] Probably *Ilex aquifolium*, the holly; cf. André: *Lexique des termes de botanique en latin*, p 37; Pliny *NH* 16.19: *in provinciis aquifolia sunt ilices*, 16.73: *Montes amant ... aquifolia.*

18.1 *motumque a tergo deminuant*] The phrase *a tergo*, in the sense of 'from behind', is known from ancient Latin, e.g. Cicero *Mil.* 29: *ut a tergo Milonem adorirentur*, and Livy 25.26.1: *ne qua ab tergo vis hostium ... suos turbaret*; the underlying thought here might be that the action of the remedy consists in preventing suppuration (i.e. efflorescence of pustules) by interfering, not at the surface of the body, but rather from within the body, which then would be *a tergo* from the struggling inflamed liquids' point of view.

venaesectiones] See *Venaesectio*, Latin word list, p 52.

diluentia] See "Drug categories", p 57.

18.2 *cui volupe est scire*] *Volupe*, generally spelled *volup*, an adv. meaning 'pleasurably', is an archaic word, known mainly from eighteen occurrences in Plautus, e.g. in *Men.* 677: *Scio, ut tibi ex me sit volup*. Cf. **Bergius 10.20.**

18.3 *in sua epistola*] I.e. *De purgantibus in secunda variolarum confluentium febri adhibendis epistola*, written by Freind to Richard Mead in 1719.

hac cura] *Cura* in the medical sense of 'cure' or 'treatment' is found already in Cato *Agr.* 157.10: *cito sanum facies hac cura*, but also in Pliny *NH* 7.58: *si quando medicina et cura vicere.*

19.1 *praxin*] See "Language", footnote 46, p 19.

prophylaxin] See *Prophylaxis*, Greek word list, p 38.

morbus ... radices egit] *Agere* for 'put forth' or 'send out' roots etc. is known from ancient Latin, certainly regarding plants, etc, but also in a metaphorical sense, as e.g. in Cicero *De off.* 2.43: *vera gloria radices agit*; there are, however, no extant ancient Latin occurrences of the phrase being used about a disease.

chirurgis] See *Chirurgus*, Greek word list, p 32.

The conflict hinted at here, between physicians and surgeons, who were craftsmen with no compulsory university education, was to be important later on in Roland Martin's career: after studying and practising anatomy and surgery in Paris, he was

appointed professor of these disciplines in Stockholm in 1756, a professorship which
to great extent had been created to prevent the surgeons, most notably Acrel, from
lecturing on the subject; Acrel had in fact been given a professorship in 1755. After a
few years, Martin was however elected a member of the Surgical society, much to the
annoyance of e.g. Linnaeus, only to be brought back to the *Collegium medicum* in 1766;
he did however continue with his lecturing to surgeons, which probably were essential
in bringing surgery closer to medicine.

sex rebus sic dictis non naturalibus] These things are (1) air, (2) food and drink, (3) motion
and rest, (4) sleep and wake, (5) excretions and retentions, and (6) emotions.

As all of these are essential to normal life, they have of course been treated very
early in medical writing, even if the idea of a more comprehensive term seems to
originate from Galen, in his "introduction" to medicine, τέχνη ἰατρική.

This work was translated into Latin probably as early as the 6th century (Ottosson,
p 23), and used in the education of physicians throughout the Middle Ages.

The term used for these essential things in the τέχνη ἰατρική is τινα ἐξ ἀνάγκης
(23.6); Galen lists, however, only air, food and drink, and wake and sleep.

Early Latin translations of Galen seem to have used *res necessariae*, which indeed is
more readily intelligible than *res non naturales*, which has nothing to do with 'unnatural',
but denote necessary things which do not depend upon the innate nature of human
beings, but which can contribute to health or sickness; the exact phrase *res non naturales*
was apparently first used in the *Isagoge Johannitii*, an introduction to Galen's work,
possibly written by Hunayn ibn Ishaq (800–873), where they were not, however,
divided into the aforementioned six parts (Ottosson, p 25sq).

As regards the notion of *res non naturales* in 18th-century medicine, one might also
consider Linnaeus' *Dietetik* (p 25), where chapter 3, *Principia diaetetica*, starts with the
list *1. Aër. 2. Somnus et Vigiliae. 3. Qvies et Motus. 4. Ingesta. 5. Excreta et Retenta. 6. Sensus
Externi et Animi pathemata*, which, as we see, comprises all the things mentioned above,
albeit not in the same order; one might also note that the editor of *Dietetik*, A.O.
Lindfors, apparently has not understood the specific sense of *non naturales* in this
context; he uses the term *res naturales*, but says in footnote (1): *Ofta men felaktigt kallade
non naturales* (Often, but erroneously, called *non naturales*).

19.2 *coronidis loco*] *Coronis*, Greek κορωνίς, is a colophon; the word is used in ancient
Latin by Martial: *si nimius videor seraque coronide longus | esse liber* (10.1.1sq)

De variolis curandis, resp. Petrus Jonas Bergius,
text and translation

DEO DUCE
DISSERTATIO MEDICA
DE

VARIOLIS
CURANDIS

QUAM
CONSENSU EXPERIENTISSIMAE FACULTATIS MEDICAE
IN REGIA ACADEMIA UPSALIENSI
PRAESIDE

VIRO NOBILISSIMO & EXPERIENTISSIMO
DOMINO DOCTORE NICOLAO
ROSÉN
SACRAE REGIAE MAJESTATIS ARCHIATRO, MEDICINAE ET ANATOMIAE
PROFESSORE REGIO & ORDINARIO. REGIARUM ACADEMIARUM SCIENTIARUM
STOCKHOLMENSIS & UPSALIENSIS MEMBRO
PRO GRADU DOCTORIS
PUBLICO ERUDITORUM EXAMINI SUBJICIET
STIPENDIARIUS REGIUS
PETRUS JONAS BERGIUS
SMOLANDUS
IN AUDITORIO CAROLINO MAJORI DIE XII JUNII
ANNI MDCCLIV
HORIS ANTE & POST MERIDIEM SOLITIS

———

UPSALIAE, Excudit LAURENTIUS M. HÖIJER, Regiae Academiae typographus

THE CURING
OF SMALLPOX

WHICH,

WITH THE PERMISSION OF THE MOST EXPERIENCED FACULTY OF MEDICINE
AT THE ROYAL UNIVERSITY OF UPSALA

UNDER THE PRESIDENCY OF

THE MOST HONOURABLE AND EXPERIENCED

DOCTOR NILS
ROSÉN

PHYSICIAN IN ORDINARY TO THEIR ROYAL MAJESTIES, PROFESSOR REGIUS ET
ORDINARIUS OF MEDICINE AND ANATOMY. MEMBER OF THE ROYAL SOCIETIES OF
SCIENCES IN STOCKHOLM AND UPPSALA,
THE STIPENDIARIUS REGIUS

PETRUS JONAS BERGIUS

FROM SMÅLAND

WILL PUT FORTH TO BE EXAMINED IN PUBLIC BY LEARNED MEN
FOR THE DOCTORAL DEGREE,
IN THE MAJOR CAROLINE AUDITORIUM, ON JUNE, THE 12TH
1754
AT THE USUAL TIME AM AND PM

―――

Printed in *UPSALA* by LAURENTIUS M. HÖIJER, Typographer to the Royal University

§ **1.1** Variola febris exanthematica est, cum inflammatiunculis cutaneis, suppurantibus, siccescentibus, cicatrices plerumque relinquentibus. Memoria dictos tenenti characteres, variolas, a ceteris febrium exanthematicarum generibus, facile erit distinguere. **1.2** Bubones & anthraces Pestis comiter, distinctissimum constituunt genus. **1.3** Miliariae papulae elevatae, rotundae, durae, confertae, furfurascentes, satis a variolis differunt. **1.4** Pariter ab iisdem non multo cum negotio licet discernere, ex maculis parum elevatis, parvis, rubris, aequalibus, furfurascentibus, Rubeolam SAUVAGES; **1.5** ex maculis inaequalibus, latioribus haud elevatis, prurientibus, fugacibus, furfurascentibus, Uredinem; **1.6** ex maculis parvis, morsus instar Pulicum, non prurientibus, colore maxime variantibus, non furfurascentibus, Petechias; **1.7** ex ampullis solitariis, diaphanis cum basi inflammata Bullosam SAUVAGES; **1.8** denique & Erysipelas, ex inflammatione leviore, vix elevata, sed latissima coloris rosei, qui, pressa cute, evanescit, mox, cessante pressione, rediturus; quod, aeque ac cetera enumerata genera, a variolis maxime diversum est.

§ **2.1** *Species,* si velis, hae esse possunt: Variolae *Interstinctae* SYDENHAMUS pagina mea 161. **2.2** Variolae *Cohaerentes* MORTON *Pyretologia de variolis p. 38.* **2.3** Variolae *Confluentes* SYDENHAMUS p. 165. **2.4** Variolae *anomalae nigrae* SYDENHAMUS pp. 250, 294. **2.5** Variolae *durae ovales* WERLHOF de Variolis & Anthracibus, p 11. **2.6** Variolae *Complicatae,* e.gr. cum petechiis J.G. Hahn *de Variolarum ratione p. 50 et sequentes.* cum miliaria *Acta medica Berolinensia, dec. 1 vol. 2 p 18 seqq.* cum morbillis G. HARRIS *observationes 7, pagina mea 15.* cum Haemorrhagiis ut Haemoptoë MORTON *libro citato 142, 183.* **2.7** Variolae *Crystallinae* SCHENCK *observationes liber 6, observatio 112, Richard* MEAD *de Variolis & morbillis p 17.* **2.8** Variolae *cum pustulis sangvine plenis* HILDANUS *centuria 6, observatio 77,* R. MEAD, *libro citato, p 18.* **2.9** variolae *Chronicae,* de quibus J. H. SCHULZ, *acta Physico-medica Academiae Naturae Curiosorum, volumen 1 p 533.* licet dubio non careat vera illarum existentia. **2.10** Allatas vero species propius considerare, instituti non sinit ratio, neque historiam dare variolarum, aut cursum illarum describere: in qua re Medicinam & facientibus & discentibus abunde satisfecerunt SYDENHAMUS, ac post illum bene multi. Nonnullas tantum observationes practicas, imprimis circa variolas Confluentes, exponere, constitutum nobis est.

§ **3.1** *Caussam* tamen variolarum paucis attingere liceat. Quin valde sit abstrusa, variisque illius ab Auctoribus tentatae explicationes laborent tricis inficias iverit nemo. **3.2** Etenim quot fere in eam inquisiverunt Medici, tot sunt varietates sententiarum; quas allegare omnes, quum nimis longum foret, paucas tantummodo libare sufficiat. **3.3** Sanguinis menstrui reliquias in fetu caussam variolarum statuebant olim *Arabes,* dein LIDDELIUS *libri 3 de febribus caput 8.* WILLIS *de febribus caput 15.* FORESTUS &c.

In the Name of Jesus

§**1.1** *Smallpox is an exanthematic fever, with small inflammations in the skin, which suppurate, dry up and often leave scars.* Keeping these characteristics in mind, it is easy to distinguish smallpox from the other exanthematic fevers. **1.2** The boils and carbuncles associated with *the plague* form their own distinct kind. **1.3** The raised, rounded, hard, closely spaced, desquamating pimples of *miliaria* are quite different from the smallpox. **1.4** Likewise it is possible, without difficulty, to distinguish from smallpox the following diseases: *rubeola* (acc. to SAUVAGES), from its just slightly raised, small, red, even, desquamating spots; **1.5** *uredo* by its uneven, wider, but less elevated, itchy, diffuse and desquamating spots; **1.6** *petechiae* by its small spots, like flea-bites, that do not itch, that have varied colour, but do not desquamate; **1.7** *Bullosa* (acc. to SAUVAGES) by its distinct blisters, transparent, with inflamed base, **1.8** and finally *erysipelas* from the milder, hardly elevated but very wide inflammation of a rosy colour which, when the skin is pressed vanishes, but as the pressure is released reappears. This illness, as the other ones mentioned, is much different from the smallpox.

§**2.1** These different *species*, if you like the word, can appear: *discrete* smallpox: SYDENHAM, in my copy page 161; **2.2** *Coherent* smallpox: MORTON: *Pyretologia de variolis p. 38*; **2.3** *Confluent* smallpox: Sydenham, p. 165; **2.4** *Abnormal, black* smallpox: SYDENHAM, p. 250, 294; **2.5** *Hard, oval* smallpox: WERLHOF, De variolis & anthracibus p. 11; **2.6** *Complicated* smallpox, for example by petechiae: J. G. HAHN, *De variolarum ratione p. 50 and following,* by miliaria: *Acta medica Berolinensia dec. 1. vol. 2 p. 18 and following,* with measles: G. HARRIS *Observationes 7, in my copy p.15*; with bleedings, such as hæmoptoë, MORTON, *the aforementioned book, 142, 183*; **2.7** *Crystalline* smallpox: SCHENCK, *Observationes, book 6, observatio 112, Richard* MEAD, *De variolis & morbillis, p.17*; **2.8** smallpox *with bloodfilled pustules:* HILDANUS *centuria 6, observatio 77,* R. MEAD, *the aforementioned book, p.18*; **2.9** *Chronical* smallpox, which are mentioned by J. H. SCHULTZ in *Acta Physico-medica Academiae Naturae Curiosorum vol. 1, p. 533,* even if their very existence is doubtful. **2.10** My scheme does not offer the opportunity to deal more closely with the species mentioned here, neither to give an accurate description of smallpox, nor to describe their course: in this respect SYDENHAM has fully satisfied both the practitioners and students of medicine, and after him many others quite well. My aim is to put forth just a few practical observations, mainly dealing with confluent smallpox.

§**3.1** Here might shortly be dealt with the *cause* of smallpox. No one will deny that this cause is well concealed, and that the attempts at explanation by various authors suffer from confusion. **3.2** But even as the opinions are almost as many as the number of physicians who have been investigating into the matter, it may be enough, since it would be too tedious to enter all of them, to merely touch just a few. **3.3** The *Arabs* once stated that residue of menstrual blood in the fetus was the cause, and after them LIDDEL, in *libri 3 De febribus, caput 8,* and WILLIS, in *De febribus, caput 15* FOREST, and others.

3.4 Morbum haereditarium esse variolas crediderunt GENTILIS *de* FULGINEO, MERCURIALIS &c. **3.5** Acidum ex reliquiis lactis nutrivi corruptis exortum accusavit SYLVIUS *de morbis infantum caput 9* & ETMÜLLER *Opera omnia pagina mea 67*; idemque, sed a biliosa & putrida lympha proveniens WOODWARD *De morborum statu & variolis p 71*. **3.6** Salia denique fixa particulis sulphureis maritata SIDOBRIUS. **3.7** A venenata bestiola variolas esse putavit M. LISTER *e variolis pagina mea 5 et sequentes*.
3.8 Sideribus aliquam inesse vim variolosam materiem in motum vocandi, variolasque provocandi, arrisit N. CHESNEAU *observationum libri 4 p 478*. **3.9** Nuperrime in liquore renum succenturiatorum caussam quaesivit *Ph*. VIOLANTE *de variolis et morbillis p 21*.
3.10 Et pariter ex recentissimis est J. G. HAHN libro citato p. 78, qui variolas actum esse statuit, evolutionis corporis, quo vasa sangvinea arteriosa, motuum vitalium virtute, e cute efflorescunt; pustulas variolarum cum plantarum gemmis & floribus, illarumque crustas cum fructuum perianthiis comparans. **3.11** Harum vero opinionum plurimas ad levia prorsus figmenta, ceteras ad incertas conjecturas, referre non dubitaverim, quidquid in quibusdam insit ingeniosi, & in argumentis auctorum ad hypotheses veri specie induendas docti & eruditi. Nec fateri quenquam pudeat, caussam contagiosi hujus morbi, ut aliorum quamplurimorum, adhuc latere. **3.12** Si qua vero sententia ceteris praeferenda, probalitate se commendat illa, quae contagium, ut cujuscunque generis, ita & variolosum animalculis constare affirmat; in satis quidem obscura re caussam quaerens, cui tamen tantum & lucis & verisimilitudinis lucratur, praeter alia, scabiei theoria, ut optandum sit, diligentiori fidaque observatione quid ipsi insit veri certique perquiratur.

§ **4.1** *Subjecta* quae variolis corripiuntur maximam partem sunt infantes, pueri & adolescentes; sed aetate quoque provectiores illas invadere haud rari casus probant. Morbo hoc semel convalescentibus, reliquum vitae ab ejus incursu immune agere, fere ab omnibus statuitur; interim tamen exempla memorantur, licet rarissima, hominum bis afflictorum; quale est mulieris, septies variolis infectae, & nihilo tamen minus aetatis annorum 118 illis exstinctae, quod refert BORELLI *observationum 10 centuria 3*.

§ **5.1** Certam in morbis *prognosin* tradere maxima medici laus est, plurimumque ad felicem praxin famaeque amplitudinem confert. Ultra limites vero excurremus, si singula conquireremus prognostica signa, in morbo, de quo agimus, notanda; quare vagis omissis, constantiora saltem recensere animus est.
    5.2 *Stadium 1* Si quem variolae adoriuntur, dum morbus aliquis gravis alius generis epidemicus est, verendum, ne illis hic semet associet, vide HUXHAM *essai sur les Fievres p 168*. **5.3** Postquam variolae diutius aliquo in loco grassatae sunt, ceteris paribus, naturam induunt illae, quam sub initio, mitiorem; quod & in Minorca ubi pessima epidemia erat variolarum, obtinuisse observavit *George* CLEGHORN *observations on the epidemical diseases in Minorca, p. 275*. **5.4** *Stupor* magnus variolas bonas non praesagit. *Hydroas* SAUVAGES satis copiose interdum, simul variolis erumpentes, tam in pueris quam adultioribus, sed absque graviori aegrotum discrimine, vidimus.

3.4 GENTILIS *de* FULGINEO, MERCURIALIS, and others, believed the smallpox to be an hereditary disease. **3.5** SYLVIUS accuses, in *De morbis infantum, caput 9* an acid, originating from residue of bad milk from the nurse, as does ETMÜLLER in *Opera omnia, page 67 in my copy* and WOODWARD, in *De morborum statu & variolis page 71*, even if the latter believes the acid to originate from lymphatic fluid, polluted with bile, and rotting. **3.6** SIDOBRIUS, then, believes in *salia fixa* combined with particles of sulphur. **3.7** M. LISTER thinks, in *De variolis, in my copy page 5 and following*, that the smallpox come from some poisonous animal. **3.8** That there is some power in the stars, which can set the variolous matter in motion and cause smallpox to appear is a pleasant theory to N. CHESNEAU in *Observationum libri 4, page 478*. **3.9** Recently *Ph.* VIOLANTE has been searching the causes in the fluids of the adrenal glands, in his *De variolis et morbillis, page 21*. **3.10** Also belonging to the more recent is J. G. HAHN in the aforementioned book, page 78, who states that smallpox are the result of some bodily process, whereby the arteries from vital power spring up from the skin; he compares the pustules of smallpox to buds and flowers of plants, the crusts to the perianths of the fruits. **3.11** Of these opinions I will not hesitate to regard some as pure fabrications, the rest as uncertain assumptions, no matter how ingenious some of them are, or how wise and learned the arguments, by which the author wants to cover his hypothesis under the semblance of truth. No one should be ashamed to admit that the cause of this disease, as of many others, is still concealed. **3.12** If any opinion is to be preferred to the others, however, the one that stands out by its probability is the one stating that the contagion of the variolous kind, like any other kind, consists of small animals. This theory, certainly searching for the cause in a quite obscure matter, benefits so much, regarding both general enlightenment and particular likeness, from the theory of scabies, above all, that it would be desirable that it were diligently investigated into what is true and certain about it.

§ **4.1** The *victims* of smallpox are mostly children, youngsters and younger adults, but not so few cases show, that the disease also afflicts older people. It is almost universally stated that, once having recovered from this disease, one spends the rest of life immune to its impact; at times, however, it is reported, though very seldom, that someone has been infected twice. One such case is that of a woman, who was infected by smallpox seven times, but nevertheless died from it at the age of 118 years, according to BORELLI, in *Observationes 10, centuria 3*.

§ **5.1** To be able to put forth a certain *prognose* is most commendable to the physician, and contributes much to a profitable practice and a good reputation. It would be beyond the limits to collect every single prognostic sign possible to note in the disease with which we are dealing; consequently, the idea is to go through the more reliable, with the omission of the more vague.

5.2 *Stage 1.* If smallpox is imminent during an epidemic of some other grave disease, there will be the risk of that disease associating the smallpox with itself, see HUXHAM: *Essai sur les fievres page 168*. **5.3** When smallpox have been prevalent for some time in a certain place, they will, under otherwise similar conditions, assume a more lenient character, which was observed to have happened in Minorca, where there was a serious epidemic, by *George* CLEGHORN, in *Observations on the epidemical diseases in Minorca, page 275*. **5.4** A grave *confusion* does not portent benignant smallpox. *Hydroa*, according to SAUVAGES, from time to time quite abundant, breaking out at the same time as the smallpox, have been seen among children as well as among adults, but without any great danger to the patient.

5.5 *Insultus epileptici* (Eclampsia SAUVAGES) infantes corripientes vix ominis mali sunt, vehementissimos si exceperis; significant enim variolas in procinctu esse ad erumpendum. **5.6** *Deglutiendi difficultas* stadio 1. annexa, malum vix praesagit; in Stadio vero 2. attentionem meretur majorem, at stadio 3. periculosa, inprimis si inflammatoria sit. **5.7** *Delirium* leve, huic stadio superveniens, vix Medicum terreat, eruptionem enim brevi insecuturam antecedit. **5.8** *Haemorrhagia* narium, si moderata, bona, nisi febris status nimis depressus sit. **5.9** Variolae *tarde*, hoc est 4. die erumpentes, symptomate omni quod eruptionem alias remorari valet exule, semper meliores sunt *cito* erumpentibus. Ratio in promptu est illis, qui exanthemata variolosa critica putant; hoc enim posito, sequitur quo tardior crisis fuerit, eo meliorem fore & comminutionem particularum peccantium; **5.10** si vero animalculis debeatur stimulus febrim excitans, quaerenda est tum in illorum structura, tum in modo quo corpus ingressa vitales functiones laedere valent, qui vero non magis quam ipsa animalcula, adhuc nobis cognita. **5.11** *Debilitas* sine caussa manifesta, in hoc stadio non adeo pertimescenda, quippe quae miasma variolosum orificium ventriculi, quod Cardiam vocant, lacessivisse indicat, unde idem effectus, debilitas scilicet, sequitur, ac cum ciborum cruditates illud ventriculi orificium aggrediuntur; **5.12** quae omnia irritationi plexus nervosi, ibi degentis & a pari Nervorum octavo potissimum orti, quod cum reliquo fere corpore communicat, adscribenda. **5.13** *Pulsus* circa finem stadii hujus solito fortior, signum, ceteris paribus, dat variolas intra horarum paucas erupturas; quod etiam HAHN *libro citato p. 23* in aegro suo 5:to observasse constat. **5.14** De cetero, *si aegri vires tantae sint, ut 4. Morbi tempora sustinere valeant, felix; at si a febris & symptomatum magnitudine ita obruantur, ut vix ad flatum usque sufficere possint, infelix erit eventus,* ut verbis utar DIEMERBROEKI *de variolis, pagina mea 276.*

5.15 *Stadium 2.* Variolae semet non *elevantes*, sed depressae, durae, pallentes, non optimae censendae sunt; docent enim versus peripheriam corporis turbatam esse circulationem, vide BOERHAVII *aphorismi § 1398.* **5.16** Quo plures in *capite* erumpunt, eo ob cerebri viciniam periculosiores. **5.17** *Haemorrhagiae*, sive e naribus, sive alio ex loco prodeuntes, periculosae sunt; hinc fluxum mensium suspectum censuerunt Scriptores, nisi in stadio 1, & periodi tempore fluant; hincque mictum cruentum pro certo signo mortis habuit SYDENHAMUS. **5.18** Ratio patet, significat enim sanguinem vel adeo dissolutum esse, ut vasis contineri nequeat, vel circulum sanguinis adeo esse vehementem, ut aut vasa rumpantur, aut dilatatis extremitatibus arteriarum, sanguis exeat. **5.19** Quicquid horum existat, prono quasi fluit alveolo, in primo horum casuum fieri quod nequit, quin maculae non bonae notae, malignitatem morbi prodentes, erumpant; in binis reliquis, necesse est, circulatio ambitum versus imminuatur, variolaeque adeo vel verrucosae, durae, pallentes &c. si effusio magna sit, evadant, vel retrocessionis illarum in propinquo adsint caussae.

5.5 *Epileptic fits* (according to SAUVAGES: Eclampsy) that afflict children are hardly a bad sign, with the exception of the most vehement ones; they show that the pustules are about to erupt. **5.6** *Difficulty in swallowing* during the first stage hardly portends a malignant case; in the second stage, however, it deserves major attention. But in the third stage it is dangerous, especially when of an inflammatory quality. **5.7** Slight *delirium* appearing in this stage should hardly frighten the physician, as it precedes the eruption briefly to follow. **5.8** *Bleeding* from the nose is good if it is moderate, as long as the state of fever is not kept down too much. **5.9** Smallpox that break out *late*, i. e. on the fourth day, when there is no symptom present of anything that could otherwise retard the outbreak, are always more benignant than those which break out *earlier*. The reason for this is obvious to those who consider the variolous rash to be critical: from this assumption follows that the later this crisis would arise, the better would also the reduction of the faulty particles be. **5.10** But if the stimulus that brings about fever is caused by some small animals, then the structure of those is to be examined, as is also the manner by which they, having arrived in the body, are able to damage the vital functions, a matter which really is not known to any greater extent than are the animals themselves. **5.11** *Debility* without any obvious reason should not give reason to very much alarm in this stage, since it only shows that the variolous miasma has irritated the orifice of the stomach, which is called cardia, whence this effect, the debility, follows as when undigested food assembles at this orifice. **5.12** All this could be attributed to the irritation of the nerve plexus on this location, which comes mainly from the eighth nerve couple, which communicates with almost the whole rest of the body. **5.13** A *pulse* stronger than usually at the end of this stage signifies, if there are no other changes, that the pustules are about to erupt in a few hours, which also HAHN *in the aforementioned book, page 23*, clearly has observed in his fifth case. **5.14** For the rest, *if the strength of the patient is such, that it could sustain the four phases of the disease, the event will be lucky; but if his strength is to such extent broken by the vehemence of fever and symptoms that it is hardly sufficient to sustain his breath, then the end will be unhappy*, to cite DIEMERBROEK'S *de variolis, in my copy p. 276*.

 5.15 *Stage 2*: Pocks that are not *raised*, but depressed, hard, and pale, should not be considered the best, for they show that the circulation about the outskirts of the body is disturbed, see BOERHAVE, *Aphorismi, § 1398*. **5.16** The more of them that burst out on the *head*, the more dangerous it is, because of the nearness to the brain. **5.17** *Bleeding* from the nose or from some other part alike is dangerous; hence the writers consider menstrual flow to be suspect, if it does not occur in stage 1 and in its due time; hence SYDENHAM regarded blood in the urine as a certain portent of death. **5.18** The reason is obvious: the bleeding shows, namely, either that the blood is disintegrated to such extent, that it cannot be kept inside the blood vessels, or that the blood circulation is so vehement, that either the vessels burst, or the blood gets out through the dilated outer parts of the arteries. **5.19** Whatever happens out of those things, the blood flows in a violent current, and in the first case, nothing else could be the result, than that spots, a bad sign, forerunning the outbreak of malignant disease, burst out; in the two other cases the circulation towards the peripheral parts is necessarily diminished, and the pustules are either wart-like, hard, pale, etc. if the outlet of blood is widely spread, or else there is a recess of pustules closest to the place of the outlet.

5.20 Idem etiam de *Diarrhoea* valet. Variolae enim diarrhoeae per totum morbi cursum junctae, horrendisque symptomatibus indies aggravatae, ut difficultate respirandi, inquietudine & jactitationibus manuum pedumque, febri fere vehementissima, insultibus epilepticis: extensione scilicet brachiorum spasmodica, retortione oculorum, stridore dentium, quem interrumpebat hiatus oris, conjunctus cum motitatione capitis momentanea; debilitate maxima, palpebris flaccidis, excretis per alvum nigris, plus simplici vice a nobis observatae sunt. **5.21** *Vomitus & Dolores Lumborum* vel scrobiculi cordis, si adhuc continuent, indicant majore adhuc numero variolas erupturas. **5.22** Si pustulae subito *retrocedant* pulsu duro, dolore faucium, micturitione, urina aquea, inquietudine, anxietate, rubedine oculorum &c. pessimum est; delirium enim non longe abesse indicatur. **5.23** Si pulsus in carpis languidus, carotides autem & temporales vehementer pulsent, itidem pessimum est; significat enim liberum sanguinis per pulmones non esse transitum, unde peripneumonia, deliriis stipata horrendis, facile enasci potest. **5.24** Si potulenta ori ingesta per nasum redeant, malum indicans est; oesophagum enim rearis esse inflammatum; sin vero sorbitionem liquidorum subito sequantur vomitus gravissimi, ventriculum ipsum inflammatum esse certocertius scimus. **5.25** Si pustulis innascantur puncta nigra, vel si papulae nigro, viridi, violaceo, plumbeo, sangvineove coloratae evadunt, raro periculum effugiunt aegroti.

5.26 *Stadium 3.* Pustularum bases & interstitia si inflammata, apices vero, quibus sensim punctum rubrum, non aliter ac in pustulis scabiei suppuratis, ideoque *maturationis* dicendum, innascatur, fastigiati sint, variolis rite suppurantibus, optimum est. **5.27** Si vero variolae vacuae & rugosae evadunt, febrisque cum putredine vix toleranda in magnum excrescat gradum, non boni ominis est, praesertim si accedat delirium, somnolentia, pleuritis, vel alia febris inflammatoria; significatur enim pus e pustulis in massam sangvineam absorberi, atque ad loca infecta dudum pulsum esse. **5.28** Si pustularum *sanies* salsum praebeat saporem praesagium triste adest, pro certo enim signo mortis a quibusdam habetur. **5.29** Si sputa sistantur nondum debita facta evacuatione, malum est. Si tumorem faciei retrocedentem, manuum & pedum non sequatur, nec copiosus compenset ptyalismus, pessimum jure censetur. **5.30** In variolis malignis non contemnendi sunt abscessus passim in corpore provenientes; constat enim ex observationibus, haud raro maxime salutares illos exstitisse, si maturantibus ad suppurationem redacti & postea aperti fuerint.

5.31 *Stadium 4.* Si variolae placide exsiccentur, optimum est; sin vero exsiccationi febris cum inflammationibus vel alia sinistra signa se adjungant, malum est. **5.32** Dum *Miliaria* eadem tempore, ac variolae, epidemica fuit, debilitatem periodicam post meridiem, per horas nonnullas durantem, quamvis ne minima quidem conspicerentur eruptionis miliariae vestigia, interdum observavimus; illam tamen periculosam non fuisse debilitatem simul didicimus.

5.20 The same thing is true about *diarrhoea* as well. I have more than once observed smallpox being joined by diarrhoea throughout its entire course, and day by day aggravated by horrible symptoms, like respiratory distress, anguish, and jerks of hands and feet, mostly violent fever, epileptic fits, spasmodic stretchings – of the arms, that is – rolling of the eyes, grinding of teeth, which wide opening of the mouth interrupted, together with sudden movements of the head; major faintness, flaccid eyelids, black excretion from the bowels. **5.21** *Vomiting and pain in the back* or in the pit of the stomach, if still present, indicate that an even larger number of pustules are about to burst out. **5.22** If the pustules suddenly *recede*, accompanied by hard pulse, pain in the throat, micturition, waterclear urine, agitation, anguish, reddening of the eyes, etc., that is very bad, as it indicates that delirium is imminent. **5.23** If the pulse is faint in the wrists, but the carotids and the temples beat vehemently, this is also very bad, as it indicates that the blood does not have free passage through the lungs, whence pneumonia accompanied by dreadful fits of delirium easily can follow. **5.24** If drink, when poured into the mouth, comes out through the nose, that is a bad sign, as you can count upon the oesophagus being inflamed; but if abundant vomiting suddenly follows from swallowing of liquid, then we know for sure that the stomach itself is inflamed. **5.25** If black dots arise in the pustules, or if they turn black, green, violet, livid or blood coloured, the patients rarely escape the danger alive.

5.26 *Stage 3.* If the base and middle part of the pustules are inflamed, but the peaks, where little by little a red point, just like in suppurating pustules of scabies, and therefore to be called *the point of maturation*, arises, are pointed, and the pustules are duly suppurating, that is very good. **5.27** But if the pustules become empty and wrinkled, and the fever increases to a very high level together with a hardly tolerable stench, that is not a good sign, especially if delirium, somnolence and pleurisy are added, or some other inflammatory fever, as this shows that pus from the pustules has been absorbed by the blood, and is already driven to the infected parts. **5.28** If the *ichorous matter* of the pustules has a salty taste, this is a sinister portent, as it by some is regarded as a certain sign of death. **5.29** If there are no longer any expectoration while due evacuation not yet has been brought about, that is bad. If swelling of hands and feet does not follow, as the swelling of the face recedes, or it is not compensated for by increasing salivation, this is rightly considered to be very bad. **5.30** In malignant smallpox, abscesses in various parts of the body should not be despised, as it is perfectly clear from experience, that these quite often have shown to be salutary to great extent if they, when maturing, suppurate and are then opened.

5.31 *Stage 4.* If the pustules quietly dry up, that is the best; but if fever with inflammations or other serious symptoms join the exsiccation, this is bad. **5.32** When an epidemic of *Miliaria* has been about at the same time as the smallpox I have at times observed a temporary feebleness in the afternoon, lasting for several hours, even if no trace whatsoever of any outbreak of miliaria has been seen; at the same time, though, I have learned that this feebleness is not dangerous.

§ **6.1** En itaque *curam variolarum*, absoluta prognosi, paucis tradendam momentis! Juberet quidem ordinis ratio methodum praemitti praeservatoriam, nisi hac in re otium nobis fecisset Dominus Doctor Roland MARTIN per integram dissertationem *de variolis praecavendis, Upsaliae 1751.* **6.2** Heic tamen intactum linquere noluimus, Norlandiam & inprimis Westrobotniam inhabitantes, per longum temporis spatium amuleto, quod Moscho conficiunt, & collo suspendunt, insigni cum fructu usos fuisse. Ex propria, quod dictis addamus, experientia, nihil quidem habemus; certo tamen scimus, experimentum hocce per totam Epidemiam variolarum upsaliensem 1753 ita feliciter cessisse, ut integrae domui, moscho usae, penitus pepercerint variolae.

§ **7.1** *Regimen* variolas curaturo maxime necessarium & observatu dignum est, cum illo magnam partem felix ipsius curae sucessus innitatur. Accedit, quod primum medico negotium incumbit, regimen accuratum adstantibus praedicere, antequam ad pharmaceutica praescribenda manum admoveat. **7.2** *Temperies* itaque caloris in cubili, ubi decumbit aeger, probe observanda est, ne aut modum excedat, aut deficiat ita, ut frigida nimis sit aura. Medium tenere praestat. Dissimulandum tamen non est, cum febris interdum exaestuet, regimen frigidiusculum in primo stadio praestare calido; cum vero interdum (quod rarius) febris ad diem usque 8. justo mitior pergat, vide HUXHAM *libro citato, p 163,* non possum non regimen paulo calidius commendare, lectumque maxime necessarium, a primo invasionis momento, dicere. **7.3** Aër semper servandus est purus, praecipue binis posterioribus stadiis, nam quantum ad felicem eventum valeat puritatem aëris observasse, incredibile dictu; variolas enim, dum suppurant & arescunt, putridum vaporem exhalare, eumque pulmonibus exceptum, noxam afferre, quis non videt? **7.4** Cubile itaque altis parietibus eligendum, quos velamenta probe tegant, ut frigidam excludant auram, aegro magnopere nocituram. **7.5** Pavimento quotidie injiciantur sarmenta abietina vel juniperina concisa, quae stadio 4:to aceto, vel vino quodam acido irrigari queunt. **7.6** *Diaeta* aegro sancte servanda; vitanda sunt omnia, quae e regno animali desumuntur, & facile alcalescunt, ut carnes, juscula carnium, lardum, ova &c. quatenus humores magis acres reddunt; eligenda autem e contrario plurima e regno vegetabili acescentia leniterque gelatinosa, ut lac recens, decocta ex Avena, Pruneolis, Oryza, Festuca, Sagu &c. **7.7** Potui esse possunt serum lactis, cerevisia tenuis, infusum Theae, decoctum Coffeae, ubi stimulantibus eget natura &c. **7.8** Liquores spirituosi magnopere aegro interdicendi, autoptae loquimur, cum extremum efflare spiritum, illorum ergo, coactos fuisse miseros, cum horrore saepius cognoverimus, (confer FORESTI *libri 6, observatio 41*); Spirituosorum tamen prudentem usum non ideo volumus exclusum.

§ **8.1** His praemissis ad Remedia filum tractationis nos ducit. Ut autem distinctius tota succedat tractatio, stadia sequi singula, quaeque in unoquoque maxime scitu necessaria tradere lubet.

§ **6.1** And now, behold the *cure for smallpox* being transmitted in a few moments, as the prognosis now has been dealt with! The principle of order would indeed demand that the methods of prevention be dealt with first, were it not that Doctor Roland MARTIN has relieved me of this through a whole dissertation on the subject: *De variolis praecavendis*, Uppsala, 1751. **6.2** I will not, however, ignore that the inhabitants of Norrland, and especially of Västerbotten since long have been using an amulet made out of musk, and worn around the neck, with good results. I have no experience of my own to be added in this matter, but I do know for sure that this has been tried successfully during the epidemic of smallpox in Uppsala, 1753, as the smallpox then entirely spared a house where all the inhabitants used musk.

§ **7.1** *Guidelines* are utterly necessary and noteworthy to anyone who is about to cure smallpox, since the sucess of the cure supports itself to great extent upon these. Besides, the first duty that rests upon the physician is to dictate the right guidelines to the persons taking care of the patient, before he passes on to prescribing medicines. **7.2** The *temperature* of the patients room must be carefully observed, so that it neither exceeds the normal, nor gets below it, so that the air gets too cold. It is best to keep to the middle. It should not be concealed, however, that as the fever sometimes burns more vehemently, in the first stage a somewhat cooler temperature is to be preferred to a warm; but when, at times, (which is unusual) a fever, less vehement than normal, persists till the eighth day (see HUXHAM, *the book cited above, p. 163*), I cannot neglect to prescribe a somewhat higher temperature, and commend the bed as necessary from the beginning of the illness. **7.3** Clean air is to be kept always, especially in the two later stages, for it is incredible, how much it contributes to a fortunate outcome to have kept the purity of the air; who would not realise that the pocks as they suppurate and dry up excrete rotting vapours, which, if they are received by the lungs, bring about damage? **7.4** A bedroom with high walls should then be chosen, covered by tapestry to exclude the cold air, which is very harmful to the patient. **7.5** The floor should every day be strewn with chopped twigs of spruce or juniper, which in the fourth stage may be moistened with vinegar or some sour wine. **7.6** A *diet* is to be kept rigorously by the patient: everything that is taken from the animal kingdom should be avoided, as should anything that easily becomes alkaline, like meat, broth, lard, eggs, etc, with regard to what extent they make the bodily fluids more sharp; one should on the contrary chose the most from the vegetable kingdom, which will become acid, and which is somewhat gelatinous, like fresh milk, decoctions of oat, plums, rice, wild oats, sago, etc. **7.7** To drink could be used whey, small beer, infusion of tea, decoction of coffee when nature needs stimulation, etc. **7.8** Strong liquor should be strictly forbidden. I say this from my own experience, since I have often seen, to my horror, wretched humans being compelled to pull their last breath because of it. (cf. FOREST: *book 6, observation 41*). A more prudent use of alcohol I would not therefore ban, however.

§ **8.1** As this now has been said, the outline of this treatise leads us to the remedies. To make the whole treatise come out more clear, I will deal with the stages separately and put forth from each of them what is most necessary to know.

8.2 STADIUM I. Si ea Medico contingat felicitas, ut sub ipsius morbi initio ad aegrotum accersitus fuerit, ante omnia scrupulosius inquirat, utrum evacuantibus, an corrigentibus morbo occurrendum; scrupulosius inquam, cum in hocce stadio fundamenta jaciantur subsecuturi exitus morbi. **8.3** Itaque genio morbi probe examinato, si Medicus dolores artuum, dorsi, lumborum & scrobiculi cordis vehementes esse; si cephalalgiam adeo vehementem, ut ad delirandum aeger pronus videatur; si oppressiones pectoris, spirandique difficultatem praevalidam; si pulsum durum, fortem; si calorem magnum; si in flore aetatis aegrum constitutum; si diaetam aegri praegressam lautam, animalem, vinosam fuisse; si febres inflammatorias epidemicas esse, quarum naturam variolas facile suscepturas merito suspicari possit; si haemoptysin vel mictum cruentum, aliamve haemorrhagiam periculosam praesentem, cognoverit, vena statim amplo vulnere secanda est. **8.4** Plures tamen esse, qui statuunt Venaesectionem in variolis minime exercendam esse, idque plurimis demonstrare rationibus adnituntur, nos non fugit, *vide Andreas* HOFFART *de variolis Vratislavis grassentibus p 39, Lucas* TOZZI, *commentarii in aphorismis Hippocratis liber 1, aphorismus 3, J.* WOODWARD *libro citato p. 95.* Qui vero de Venaesectionis genuino usu convictus esse cupit, evolvat *Dissertationem* J.G. a BERGER *de usu Venaesectionis et Clysterum in variolarum curatione,* alios ut taceam. **8.5** Phlebotomia efficitur, ut globuli sanguinis rubri, omnium ponderosissimi, minuantur; minuta autem ratione globulorum rubrorum, minuitur etiam attritus & impetus; minutis hisce, tollitur calor, consequenter febris vehementia remittitur. **8.6** Sed ut scopo huic magis adhuc fiat satis, non inconsultum arbitramur, refrigerantia adjungere medicamina. In usum itaque vocandi sunt Pulveres e Nitro purissimo crystallino, vel sale Ammoniaco, ubi metus est diarrhoeae, Morsuli Citri; syrupi Acidi ut Cerasorum Nigrorum, Acetositatis citri, Ruborum Idaeorum, Mororum &c. Si vero febris urget, clysma, more *Sydenhamiano,* proxime post sanguinis missionem injici juvat. **8.7** Haec omnia autem cum grano salis sumenda volumus, nam accidit non raro, ut variolae in statu depresso sint, scilicet ut febris lenta, pulsus debilis, celer sed vacillans; habitus corporis pallidus & languidus; urina cruda; aeger sine calore & siti, continua tamen gravedine capitis, nausea & conatibus vomendi, afflictus fit; variolae tardissime erumpant, (7 aut 8 die) & sessiles, pallidae, depressae, ichore claro & male digesto plenae sint, *vide* HUXHAM *libro citato, p 162* CLEGHORN *libro citato p 273.* **8.8** In hoc casu tantum abest ut Venaesectio & refrigerantia celebranda, ut potius excitantia, febrimque augentia praescribenda sint. Hanc itaque ob caussam, *vesicatoria* brachiis vel suris applicantur, serum lactis cum vino Rhenano paratum largiter adhibetur, interponendo aquam Alexiteriam simplicem Londinensem, Contrayervam, Serpentariam Virginianam, in infusione floris Sambuci propinandas. Nec ipsam Chinchinam omittendam putamus; adhibuit enim illam stadio primo, atque maturationem & bonum pus inde accelerari, observavit MONRO in *the Medical essays, volume 10, article 10.*

8.2 STAGE I. If the physician has the advantage of having been sent for during the very outset of the disease, he should above all carefully examine whether the disease should be fought with evacuant or correcting methods; carefully, I say, as the subsequent outcome of the disease is dependant on the basis laid in this stage. **8.3** So, when the kind of disease has been duly examined, if the physician finds out that the pains in the joints of the body, the back, the loins, and the pit of the stomach are violent; that the headache is so strong that the patient seems almost delirious; that the pressure upon the chest is strong; that there is great difficulty in pulling breath; that the pulse is hard and strong; that the temperature is high; that the patient is in the prime of life; that his diet, before disease, has been luxurious, rich in meat and wine; that there is reason to suspect some epidemic inflammatory fever, the quality of which the smallpox are likely to adopt; that there is spitting of blood, blood in the urine, or some other acute dangerous bleeding, then a vein should immediately be opened, by a wide cut. **8.4** It does not escape us that there are many who state that bloodletting should not at all be undertaken in smallpox, and who make every effort to show this by several methods of reasoning, see *Andreas* HOFFART: *De variolis Vratislavis grassantibus*, p. 39; *Luca* TOZZI: *Commentarii in aphorismos Hippocratis, book I, aphorism 3*; J. WOODWARD, the book cited above, p. 95. But he, who wants to be sure of the real usefulness of bloodletting may read J.G. von BERGER'S dissertation *De usu venaesectionis & clysterum in variolis curandis* not to mention others. **8.5** By phlebotomy is obtained that the number of red blood corpuscles, the heaviest kind of all, is reduced, but as the share of red corpuscles is diminished, the strain and vehemence is also reduced; as those are reduced, the heat is removed, and consequently the vehemence of the fever is subdued. **8.6** But in order to reach the aim all the better, I think it would be well-advised to add refrigerating medicine. Thus should be employed *pulveres e Nitro purissimo crystallisato* or *pulveres e sale Ammoniaco* or, when there is a risk of diarrhoea, *Morsuli Citri, syrupi acidi*, like *syrupus Cerasorum nigrorum, syrupus Acetositatis citri, syrupus Rubaeorum Idaeorum, syrupus Mororum*, etc. But if fever attacks, a clysm, according to *Sydenham's* method given right after the bloodletting, will help. **8.7** I would however want all this to be taken with a pinch of salt, as it quite often happens that the smallpox is in a state of depression, which means that the fever is tardy, the pulse is weak, quick but wavering; the state of the body is pale and lifeless; the urine is unconcocted; the patient does not feel heat or thirst, but is afflicted by continuous heaviness in the head, nausea and impulses to vomit; the pustules break out very late, (on the seventh or eighth day), and are low, pale, and depressed, full of clear ichor, which is not dissolved, see HUXHAM, *the book cited, p. 162*; CLEGHORN, *the book cited, p. 273*. **8.8** In such cases bloodletting and refrigerants are so far from being useful that preparations that are stimulating and raise the fever should rather be prescribed. For this reason, therefore, *vesicatories* are placed on the arms or calves, whey prepared with Rhine wine is used extensively, alternatingly *aqua Alexiteria simplex Londinensis, Contrayerva, Serpentaria Virginiana*, to be given with *infusio floris sambuci*. Neither do I recommend that *Chinchina* be omitted; MONRO made use of it in the first stage and has observed that the maturation and the good pus thereby was hastened, in *the Medical essays, volume 10, article 10*.

8.9 *Emetica* in variolis fere ab omnibus Auctoribus laudantur. Variolosus morbus contagiosus est (§ III) & miasmate suo ex uno in alterum propagatur. **8.10** Miasma per poros cutis corpus ingredi posse inoculatione variolarum evinci videtur; attamen experientia quotidie edocet, omnium primo ventriculum, viasque primas ex illo turbari, quod e nausea, vomitu, satis liquet: unde frequentem esse hanc inficiendi rationem, quae per os primasque vias peragitur, simul apparet. **8.11** Inde satis elucet emetica maximo esse usui in variolis, nec unquam, nisi contraindicantia adsint, ut inflammatio ventriculi &c. omittenda, quatenus reliquias ex alimentis, cruditates, deglutitum miasma evacuant, atque exorta ex illis concussione corporis, sudorem eliciunt. **8.12** Emeticorum necessitatem ex posteriori quoque evincunt historiae medicae. Unicum haud exigui ponderis, si fides ipsi habenda, exemplum afferamus ex WOODWARDO *libro citato p 69*, scilicet apparuere 4. die in facie, pectore & brachiis tubercula denso agmine. **8.13** Propinabatur eadem vespera emeticum, adeo exoptato cum effectu, ut postero die cuncta evanuerint symptomata, atque tubercula disparuerint singula. **8.14** Subjectis tamen plethoricis emeticum, sonticas ob caussas, ne propinetur, auctores sumus, nisi primum secta fuerit vena; namque cerebri vel aliarum partium nobilium vasa, sub vehementi, quam vomitus in corpore excitat, concussione facile rumpi posse, ultro patet. **8.15** Emeticum esse potest instar omnium radix Ipecacuanhae recens pulverisata sive in pulveribus a Drachmae β ad scrupulos II sive alia sub forma, e.g. Vinum Ipecacuanhae Londinense, Drachmae X &c. **8.16** At vero haud raro accidit, ut emetica penitus aversetur aeger, frustraque tale exhibere conatur medicus; quo in casu, statim cogitare de praescribenda catharsi debet.

8.17 *Laxantia* sane, in variolis propinata, non tanti sunt periculi ac perhibet supra allatus Woodward, *loco citato*; prudenter enim praescripta, nec diarrhoeam excitant, neque alias mali moris secum trahunt sequelas; contra vero summopere indicantur, ubi emetico locus non est, vel ubi obstipatio alvi in initio morbi aliquantum temporis duravit; nam sagax Medicus jure suspicari potest, si alvi exoneratio in hoc stadio non procedat, fore, ut scybala, loco calido, aërisque pleno retenta, putrescant, adeoque stadiis sequentibus diarrhoeam excitant symptomaticam, vel fomitis instar particulas acres sanguini immisceant, febrimque adeo perpetuo alant pabulo. **8.18** Cathartica maxime idonea, e Tamarindis, e.g. Decoctio Tamarindi cum senna; Cassia, Salibus catharticis, Senna, Mercurio dulce, ceterisque his cognatis parantur. In illis vero casibus, ubi emetica in usum vocantur, vel Laxantia illis combinari queunt, vel injici debent Clysmata.

8.19 Sed hisce omnibus copiose interponenda sunt *Diluentia*, in variolis & praecipue stadio hocce primo, adeo necessaria, ut merito dici possit: *bibendum vel moriendum est* HUXHAM *libro citato p 206*. Nam si diluentia non copiose ingurgitentur, maximo cum detrimento, in stadiis ultimis, experientur miseri aegri, tantam muci copiam fauces propemodum occludere, ut neque deglutire, neque spiritum trahere valeant.

8.9 *Emetics* in smallpox are praised by almost all authors. The smallpox disease is contagious (§ III) and is spread by its own miasma from one person to another. **8.10** That miasma is able to intrude into the body through the pores of the skin seems to be proved by inoculation of smallpox; nevertheless, experience tells us every day that first of all the stomach and the main ducts are disturbed by it, which is quite clear from the nausea and vomiting: at the same time it shows that the way of infection which goes through the mouth and main ducts is very common. **8.11** From this it is quite clear that emetics are of maximum use in smallpox, and never should be omitted, except for in case of contraindications, like inflammation of the stomach, etc, as they evacuate residues of food, undigested pieces, swallowed miasma and, by the concussion of the body brought about, evoke sweat. **8.12** The medical case descriptions also convince us of the need for emetics, with arguments from experience. I shall relate just one example, of considerable weight if it is reliable, from WOODWARD, *the above-cited book, p. 69*, namely, that on the fourth day appeared, in the face, the chest, and the arms, tubercles in close formation. **8.13** The same evening, an emetic was given, to such an excellent effect, that on the following day, all symptoms had disappeared and the specific tubercles were gone. **8.14** For plethoric patients, however, I recommend for good reasons that emetics should not be given, if bloodletting is not carried out first; for it goes without saying, that blood vessels in the brain or in some other vital part easily could burst from the violent concussion which the vomiting brings about in the body. **8.15** As an all-round emetic could be used recently powderised Ipecacuanha root, whether in dose-powders of half a drachm to two scruples each, or in some other form, for example ten drachms of *vinum ipecacuanhae Londinense* etc. **8.16** But it does happen quite often, that the patient totally rejects emetics, and that the physician tries in vain to offer such remedies; in such cases, he should at once consider prescribing a purging.

8.17 *Laxatives* are in fact not as dangerous when given in smallpox as the above-mentioned WOODWARD maintains in his book, *cited above*, as they, discerningly prescribed, neither provoke diarrhoea, nor bring about any other bad consequences; on the contrary, they should be strongly recommended, when there is no room for emetics, or when constipation in the initial stage of disease lasts somewhat longer; for the sagacious physician would rightly suspect that if the emptying of the bowels does not come about in this stage, the excrement will putrify, held back in this warm place, full of air, and even symptomatically bring about diarrhoea in the following stages, or mix sharp particles into the blood, like kindling-wood, and thus give permanent fuel to the fever. **8.18** The most suitable cathartic remedy is prepared from Tamarinds, e. g. *decoctio Tamarindi* with *senna, Cassia, Sales cathartici, Senna, Mercurius dulcis*, and other related substances. In those cases, however, where emetics are used, either laxatives could be combined with them, or clysters should be given.

8.19 But in all this large amounts of *diluents* should be included, which in smallpox, and especially in this first stage, are so essential, that it rightly could be said: *it comes down to drinking or dying*, HUXHAM, *the book cited, p. 206*. For if diluents are not taken in large quantities, the poor patients will, to their great detriment, experience, in the final stage, that their throats are almost choked up by so much mucus that they can neither swallow, nor pull their breath.

8.20 Ratio in promtu est; novimus enim sanguinem vena emissum, perseverante aliquantisper malo, maxime spissum, & corio obducti inflammatorio BOERHAAVE *aphorismi § 1384.* hinc patet illum partibus tenuioribus maxime spoliatum esse, quod partim salivationi, in confluentibus primoribus diebus se prodenti; partim propensioni adultorum ad sudandum, quam etiam in infantibus saepius observavimus; partim quoque secessioni liquidorum ad pus in pustulis formandum debetur.

8.21 Sed plurima mala ex sanguine adeo spisso redundatura, quis non videt? Ut stagnationem in vasis minoribus, unde pleuritis, peripneumonia, phrenesis, cetera ut taceamus. **8.22** Ex dictis patere crediderim necessitatem diluentium in variolis; sed ut rite debito fungantur officio, cum saponaceis mixta propinentur, alio enim in casu cum sanguine non miscentur, nec effectum optatum praestant. Admiscendum itaque censemus Mel; oxymel; syrupi Acetosae, Berberis, Cerasorum nigrorum, Ribium, Ruborum idaeorum, Mororum &c.

   8.23 Sed hisce non acquiescat Medicus, debet enim quoad ejus fieri potest, partes nobiliores corporis externas a variolis immunes servare & symptomatibus maturo occurrere auxilio. **8.24** *Oculis* itaque omnium primum consulendum; hunc ergo in finem lintea Camphora perfricentur, palpebris imponantur, bisque terve de die mutentur. *Laryngi* externe applicare solemus Theriacam Andromachi Camphora mixtam, eamque semper cum effectu. **8.25** Faciem a variolis conservare res est valde expetita, sed non adeo facilis effectu dare, Topica externa commendant, ut Balsamum Embryonale J.H. SCHULZ *Pathologia specialis p 140.* De lacte cum Croco & de aqua Cinnamomi narrat *Isbrand van* DIEMERBROEK *libro citato p 298, observationibus 12 & 13.* **8.26** Quidquid tamen sit, externa haecce commendare non ausimus, usque dum experientia ad oculum monstraverit nihil subesse periculi; nam semper suspicari svevimus, ne topica, eruptionem pustularum impediendo, derivationi miasmatis in cerebrum faveant, nisi fomentis aut epispasticis, pedibus applicatis, combinentur. **8.27** De *Fomentis & Balneis* pedum fidem faciunt Auctores; sic HUXHAM, *libro citato p 174* dicit se pluribus annis cum successu usurpasse balnea pedum in aqua calida simplici, vel lacte mixta. SYLVIUS & ADOLPHI successum vix negant, quamvis debilitates pedum & alia mala illis succedanea clamitent; confer FISCHER, *Relatio de variolis annorum 1740. 41 et 42 durante grassatione pestilentiae verae in Hungaria, epidemice grassantibus p. 93.* **8.28** Fomenta tamen innoxie usurpari posse, ex plena didicimus praxi. Fotus itaque e speciebus emollientibus nunquam omittendos esse putamus, quia re ipsa aliquid contribuunt ad materiam variolosam e facie revellendam. Id tamen dissimulandum non est, sinapismis longe debiliores illos esse. **8.29** *Sinapismi* enim, plantis pedum applicati, derivationem variolarum ad partes inferiores mirifice efficiunt, quatenus suo stimulo affluxum humorum huc vertunt. **8.30** Prolixi in hisce enarrandis non erimus; casum solummodo a *Celeberrimo Medicinae Licentiato* J. HAARTMAN observatum & communicatum afferre contenti. Vocatus erat ad aegrotum secundo morbi die, quo statim sinapismum plantis pedum applicabat. Nihilo tamen minus in facie die morbi 3. variolae erumpebant fere millenae. Fortissimum loco praedicto subito admovebat sinapismum, quem tollere adstantibus interdictum, priusquam vesiculas excitasset. Quo facto ipsas pustulas faciem reliquisse, ingentem vero earum copiam pedes occupasse videbat.

8.20 The reason is obvious: we know that blood let out from the veins, as the evil remains for some time, is very thick, and is covered by an inflammatory coating, BOERHAVE, *Aphorismi,* § 1384, hence it is obvious that *it is deprived of its thinner parts,* which is due partly to the salivation that appears during the first days in confluent smallpox, partly to the tendency, among adults, to sweat, which I have often observed among children as well; partly also to the transition of fluids to form pus in the pustules. **8.21** But who would not realize that much evil will result in abundance from a blood that is this thick? As, for instance, stopping in the minor vessels, whence pleurisy, pneumonia and frenzy, to say nothing of the rest. **8.22** I should think that the need for diluents in smallpox is obvious from what has been said, but to make them fulfil their duty, they should be given with saponaceous substances, as they otherwise do not mix with the blood, and do not have the wanted effect. Thus I think that *Mel, oxymel, syrupus Acetosae, syrupus Berberis, syrupus Cerasorum nigrorum, syrupus Ribium, syrupus Ruborum idaeorum, syrupus Mororum* etc. should be added.

8.23 But the physician must not be satisfied with this, as he to the greatest possible extent should protect the most noble outer parts of the body against the pocks and promptly stand up against the symptoms. **8.24** Thus, the *eyes* should be taken care of first of all; for this purpose cloths should be rubbed with camphor and applied to the eyelids; they should be replaced two or three times a day. To the *larynx* I usually apply *Theriaca Andromachi* mixed with camphor, which has always turned out to be effective. **8.25** To protect the face from smallpox is largely desirable, but not very easy to achieve. They recommend locally efficient external remedieses, like *Balsamum Embryonale* J.H. SCHULTZ, *Pathologia specialis,* p. 140. *Isbrand* van DIEMERBROEK mentions *lac cum croco* and *aqua cinnamomi* in the *book cited above, p. 298, observations 12 and 13.* **8.26** I would not dare to commend those external remedies, whatever they are, however, until experience has shown, before my own eyes, that they do not involve any risks; for I always suspect that *topica* by impeding the eruption of pustules promote the transference of miasma to the brain, if they are not combined with poultices or extractive substances, applied to the feet. **8.27** *Poultices* and *baths* for the feet are well attested by the authors: thus HUXHAM says *in the book cited above, p. 174,* that he for several years has been making use of foot baths consisting of hot water only, or mixed with milk. SYLVIUS and ADOLPHI hardly refute the good results, even if they claim weakness of the feet and other bad consequences of the method, cf. FISCHER: *Relatio de variolis annorum 1740. 41 et 42 durante grassatione pestilentiae verae in Hungaria, epidemice grassantibus,* p. 93. **8.28** Poultices could however be made use of without damage, as I have learned from extensive practice. Consequently I think that a warming bandage of *species emollientes* should never be omitted, as it in itself contributes to the pulling away of variolous matter from the face. It should not be concealed, however, that they are far less powerful than mustard poultices. **8.29** The *mustard poultices,* when applied to the soles of the feet, bring about, in an extraordinary way, a transfer of pocks to the lower parts of the body, as the flow of humours is directed this way by their influence. **8.30** I will not talk extensively about this; it will be enough to put forth only one case, observed and described by the famous *Licentiatus* of Medicine J. HAARTMAN. He was sent for to the patient on the second day of disease, when he immediately applied mustard poultices to the soles. Nevertheless about a thousand pocks burst out in the face on the third day. He then at once applied a very strong mustard poultice to the aforementioned place, which he prohibited those tending the patient from removing before it had brought about blisters. As this had been made, he saw that the pustules had left the face, but that a great number of them had occupied the feet.

8.31 Sequuntur jam *Symptomata* stadii hujus, quibus occurrendum. *Difficultatem deglutiendi* optime profligavimus Gargarismate ab infuso Herbae Menthae crispae, Salviae, cum pauxillo Camphorae composito. **8.32** *Haemorrhagia narium* si copiosa & ultra modum sit, moderanda aqua Vitrioli caerulea Londinensi turundarum ope naribus admota; vel pulvere ex Alumine crystallino & Vitriolo Martis, in nares attracto. **8.33** *Dolores Lumbi & scrobiculi cordis* mitigantur Herba Menthae crispae vino leniter cocta & applicata. *Vomitus* nunquam contemnendus est; casum vidimus, ubi ita praevaluit, ut nec cibum, neque medicamenta retinere potuerit aeger. Mitigatur externe applicato regioni ventriculi cataplasmate cum Herba Menthae crispae & Croco, vino leniter coctis; interne vero hausta mixtura salina *Riverii*, quae ita omnium optime concinnari videtur: Recipe Salis Absinthii vere alcalinis Drachmam I, Succi Citri Unciam β, aut quantum satis ad saturationem, Aquae stillatae menthae crispae Uncias III, Syrupi Menthae crispae quantum satis ad gratum saporem. Miscetur. **8.34** *Eclampsia* infantibus & pueris frequens, semper feliciter cessit Moscho a granis III ad VIII, pro ratione aetatis propinato, qui omnibus aliis expellentibus hoc in casu praeferendus, quatenus materiam variolosam fortiter expellit, vique sua antispasmodica spasmos tollit.

§**9.1** STADIUM II. Stadium hoc quum ingressus est aeger, ambitum petiit miasma variolosum & sanguinem deseruit. In variolis itaque benignis remittuntur febris & symptomata, non vero item in confluentibus. In benignis medicamento nihil opus est, diluentibus solum utatur aeger, cum natura sibi sufficiat ipsa. In confluentibus febris durat & symptomata, ut stupor, vomitus & dolores, non raro adhuc urgent. **9.2** Febrem semper normae & regulae instar sequamur, quae si vehemens sit, Venaesectione & refrigerantibus minuenda. Si pustulae tarde erumpunt, expellentia ut Moschus, flores Sulphuris, Ulmaria, flores Sambuci, Camphora, propinanda sunt. **9.3** *Diarrhoea* mature curanda est, cum elevationi pustularum obsit; praestat itaque adhibere Decocta alba Londinensia Rhabarbarina; quae vero si nihil valeant, ad Opiatas, e.g. Diascordium Fracastorii, &c. confugiendum. **9.4** Si *Somnolentia, stupor & delirium vagum* praesto sint, indicatur plus miasmatis corpori inesse & cerebrum petiisse; vesicatoria ideo statim nuchae, & sinapismi plantis pedum, eum in finem applicandi, ut materiam peccantem mobilem reddant, atque ad inferiora revellant. **9.5** *Sputa* confluentibus laborantium, hocce in stadio plerumque manare incipiunt, unde attento nunc consideranda oculo. In benignis raro, nisi in ultimis stadiis, & parce, fluunt. In confluentium initio tenuia & pellucida, omnique conjuncta cum facilitate fluunt; versus diem autem 10 aut 11 magis spissa & mucosa evadunt, nec sine screatu, molimine molesto & suffocationis metu expelluntur. **9.6** Diluentia itaque saponaceis mixta, copiose, per totum, quo fluunt tempus, hauriantur; frigus cane angueque pejus vitetur; lac tepidum ore detineatur, quamprimum spissescunt; & si nimis fiant tenacia, siphone injiciantur Gargarismata, cum pauxillo spiritu Salis mixta, quae irritando fluxum humorum revocant. **9.7** Infantibus non semper exspectanda sunt, cum Natura lenem diarrhoeam horum loco substituat, quae, si vehemens, moderanda, non vero sistenda. Biennibus tamen ptyalismum fluxisse, vidit FISCHERUS, *libro citato p 99*, quod certe insolens est.

8.31 Now follows, how the *symptoms* of this stage are to be dealt with. *Difficulty in swallowing* is best overcome with a gargling fluid consisting of *infusio herbae menthae crispae, Salviae,* with a little camphor added. **8.32** *Nose bleeding,* if profuse and immoderate, could be subdued by *aqua Vitrioli caerulea Londinensis* applied to the nostrils with a pad of lint; or by *pulvis ex Alumine crystallino & Vitriolo martis* drawn into the nostrils. **8.33** *Pains in the back and in the pit of the stomach* are mitigated by mint, lightly boiled in wine and applied. *Vomiting* should never be neglected; I have seen a case, where it was so vehement, that the patient could keep neither food, nor medicine. It is mitigated by external application, on the stomach, by a plaster of mint and crocus, lightly boiled in wine; internally however by drinking *mixtura salina Riveri,* which seems to be best prepared as follows: take one drachm of *Sal Absinthi vere alcalinus;* half an ounce of lemon juice, or a sufficient amount for saturation; three ounces of *Aqua stillatitia menthae crispae;* a sufficient amount of *Syrupus Menthae crispae* to give a pleasant taste; To be mixed. **8.34** *Eclampsy* which is common among infants and children always yield to musk, of which from three to eight grains are given, according to age, which in this case should be preferred to all other expellants, as it forcefully expels the variolous matter, and by its antispasmodic power takes away the spasms.

§ **9.1** STAGE II. As the patient has entered this stage, the miasma has moved on to the periphery, which is afflicted by pocks, and left the blood. Therefore, the fever and symptoms recede in benign smallpox, but not so in confluent. In the benign, there is no need for medicine, the patient should only use some diluant, as nature will help itself. In confluent pocks, the fever remains and symptoms like unconsciousness, vomiting, and pains quite often still oppress the patient. **9.2** I always keep a record of the fever as a rule and guide; if it is vehement, it should be subdued by bloodletting and refrigerants. If the pustules erupt tardily, expellants, like musk, flowers of sulphur, *Ulmaria, flores Sambuci* or camphor should be given. **9.3** Diarrhoea should rapidly be cured, as it hinders the elevation of pustules; it is thus best to take to *Decoctum album Londinense Rhabarbarinum;* if this should fail, however, one should resort to opiates, for example *Diascordium Fracastorii* etc. **9.4** If *somnolence, unconsciousness,* and *a vague delirium* are present, it indicates that more miasma is in the body and has invaded the brain; therefore vesicatories should immediately be applied to the back of the neck, and mustard poultices to the soles, to the purpose to mobilize the faulty matter, and pull it towards the lower parts. **9.5** *Saliva* begins, among those suffering from confluent smallpox, often to flow in this stage, wherefore it should be closely observed. In benign pocks it seldom runs, except for in the final stages, and then sparsely. In the beginning of confluent smallpox, it is thin and clear, and runs, on the whole, easily; but towards the tenth or eleventh day it becomes thicker and more mucous, and cannot be expelled without hawking, tiresome efforts, and risk of choking. **9.6** Diluants, mixed with saponaceous substances, should therefore be taken in large quantities during the whole period of salivation, cold, worse than dogs and snakes, should be avoided; tepid milk should be kept in the mouth as soon as the saliva starts to thicken, and if it gets too sticky, a gargling fluid, mixed with a little *spiritus salis* should be given by a siphon, which by irritation will restore the flow of humours. **9.7** Among children, this is not always to be expected, since nature provides a mild diarrhoea as a substitute, which, if it is vehement, should be moderated, but not stopped. FISCHER, *in the cited book, p. 99,* has however seen salivation in children at the age of two, which indeed is unusual.

§10.1 STADIUM III. Variolis plene eruptis in generationem puris omnes intendit natura vires. Pustulae itaque inflammantur; hinc dolore, rubore & calore afficiuntur; nervi cutis irritantur, unde febris oritur (confer van SVIETEN, *commentarii in Boerhavii aphorismos, § 382, vol 1 p 649*) quae ideo *Secundaria* audit, & vera est inflammatoria. **10.2** Resolutio nulla heic speranda, adeoque placida promovenda suppuratio, & gangraena omni studio avertenda. Utrumque obtinetur febrim moderando: depressam evehendo; nimis evectam deprimendo. **10.3** Si vis naturae deficiat, & febris nimis depressa sit, ut impulsus liquidi, a tergo urgentis, vasa inflammata separare, & cum liquidis effusis in liquamen vertere nequeat; bonum pus minime generari posse constat; vis ergo vitae augenda remediis est, quae circulationem intendunt & versus peripheriam derivant. **10.4** Huc spectat serum lactis vinosum, Crocus, Myrrha, Contrayerva, Chinchina; verbo: omnia, quae robur solidorum augent, ut reactio vasorum in fluida efficacior evadat. **10.5** *Chinchinam* non propria solum, sed plurimorum Illustrium Auctorum experientia edocti, commendamus. Contigit nobis in praxi videre aegrotum 4. Annorum, cui variolae erumpebant die 2 ab invasione; **10.6** diarrhoea levi, per tres sedes quotidie laborabat; febris urgebat, & integros ejulando dies consumebat aeger. Pulveres nitrosos porrigebamus, quos, qua de caussa ignotum, neglectos postmodum conspiciebamus. Facies die 4 intumescens, valde tumida apparebat. Anxietates turbulentae eadem nocte cum tumoris incremento valide ingruebant. Pustulae maxime confluentes, depressae & pallidae erant. Febris indies quasi increscebat cum pulsu citato, minime autem forti vel duro. **10.7** Consultum itaque visum Corticem Chinae propinare ad Scrupulos IV quotidie, idque tam bonis auspiciis factum, ut pulsus sedatior incederet; inquietudines diurnae placide levarentur; variolae colorem favi reciperent, & punctum maturationis spem nobis faceret, morbum deinde periculi expertem fore. **10.8** Anodyna quavis vespera sumebantur. Tumor feliciter ad inferiora migravit. Sed quid ad propriam experientiam provocemus? Cum praeclaras observationes de insigni Chinchinae utilitate in 3 & 4 stadiis abunde orbi erudito communicaverit *Richard* MORTON. **10.9** Erupuere, ut habet, variolae die 3 juveni robusto. Die 6 confluentes erant, cum maturescere inciperent; ea nocte sociam se jungebat febris secundaria, cum deliquiis, ferocia, vigiliis, quas anodynis mitigabat, non autem tollebat. **10.10** Propinata insuper Chinchina tanto effectu, ut nec postea deliraret aeger, nec febris ante diem 11, eo autem cum urinae quadam difficultate, rediret; quae tamen mingendi molestia, aeque ac febris ipsa, cortice profligabatur. *Vide Pyretologia p158, historiam 23; confer historiis 24, 22, 25, 28, 8.* **10.11** Hisce observatis scribit *libro citato* p. 101. *Ubi autem febris sub initium maturationis suborta exacerbationibus & remissionibus periodice recurrentibus* συνεχέως *typum servaverit, apprime convenit durante remissione Corticis Peruviani doses saepius exhibere, unde 2 aut 3 dierum spatio, febre prorsus exulante, variolae citissime more benignarum maturantur.*

§. **10.1** STAGE III. As the pocks are completely erupted, nature directs all its forces to generating pus. The pustules therefore are inflamed; hence pain, redness, and heat are brought about; the nerves of the skin are irritated, whence fever arises, (cf. v. SVIETEN: *Commentarii in Boerhavii aphorismos,* § 382, vol I, p. 649) which therefore is called *secondary* and truly is inflammatory. **10.2** There is no hope for resolution here, and therefore a gentle suppuration should be promoted, and gangrenes averted, with all strength. Both these things are accomplished by moderation of the fever: by raising the low, and lowering the too high. **10.3** If nature's power should fall short, and the fever is too low, so that the pressure of the fluids, urging from behind, cannot severe the inflamed vessels and direct itself towards the liquids together with the suffused fluids, then it is clear that the good pus could not be generated at all; thus the power of life has to be augmented by remedies, which strengthen the circulation and direct it towards the periphery. **10.4** To this end serve *serum lactis vinosum,* saffron, myrrh, *contrayerva, chinchina,* in one word, all that increase the strength of the solid matters, so that the reaction of the vessels to the fluids becomes more effective. **10.5** I commend *Chinchina* guided not only by my own experience, but also by that of several famous authors. I have had the opportunity to see in my practice a patient, four years of age, in whom the pocks burst out on the second day after the infection: **10.6** he suffered from light diarrhoea, with three evacuations a day: the fever tormented him, and the patient spent the whole days moaning. I offered *Pulveres nitrosi,* which, I learned afterwards, had not been taken, for what reasons I do not know. The face, starting to swell on the fourth day, looked very swollen. Violent anguish attacked the same night, with an increase of the tumour. The pustules were maximally confluent, depressed, and pale. The fever grew higher, almost day by day, with quick pulse, which was not at all, however, strong or hard. **10.7** Hence it seemed convenient to offer China bark at 4 scruples a day; this was done with the good result that the pulse was calmed down; the daily anxiety was mitigated; the pocks adopted the colour of a honeycomb, and the maturation point gave reason for hope that the disease henceforth would not be dangerous. **10.8** Every evening analgesics were taken. The swelling moved safely towards the lower parts. But why should I appeal to my own experience, when *Richard* MORTON has extensively communicated to the learned world his eminent observations on the splendid use for *Chinchina* in the third and fourth stages? **10.9** On the third day erupted, according to him, pocks on a strong young man. On the sixth day they were confluent, as they began to mature; the same night a secondary fever appeared in addition, with fainting, rage, sleeplessness, which he mitigated with analgesics, but did not remove. **10.10** Chinchina was also offered, with the result that neither was the patient delirious thereafter, nor did the fever reappear until the eleventh day, then, however, together with a certain difficulty in passing water; this urination problem, however, and the fever itself, was expelled by this bark, see *Pyretologia p. 158, historia 23: cf. historiae 24, 22, 25, 26 and 8.* **10.11** On these observations he writes in *the work quoted, p.101: But when a fever, occurring about the beginning of maturation, has preserved its character through periodically and continuously recurring exacerbations and remissions, above all it is convenient to give doses of cortex Peruvianus frequently during the remission, whence, in two or three days, as the fever is expelled, the pocks quickly mature in the same manner as the benign.*

10.12 Ex dictis patet eandem esse curam, si variolae semet *elevare* nolint. Sed si haec minus arrideret, utendum est sero lactis cum vino Rhenano parato, cui adjungenda sunt expellentia. **10.13** Quanto cum successu lacte, in hoc casu, interne usi sint aegri, praesertim expellentibus adjectis, pulcrae testantur apud scriptores historiae, vide: D. FISCHERI *Observationes de usu lactis dulcis interno in variolis, propria experientia notatae, p. 127,* HAHNI *librum citatum 59.* **10.14** Vaporem lactis tepidi externe adhibuit *Illustris* Dominus PRAESES, eo cum effectu, ut intra horae spatium semet elevaverint pustulae; cautela vero summa hic opus est, ut probe arceatur frigus, ne retrocessioni pustularum occasio detur.

10.15 Si pustulae *retrocedant,* res certe altioris est indaginis, & mortis praenuncia, nisi feliciter iterum expelli possint. Scimus equidem nonnullos esse, qui retrocessionem negant, vide VIOLANTE, *librum citatum, p. 68.* Sed hypothesios amore abrepti non rationali nixi praxi videtur. **10.16** Caussa retrocessionis in genere duplex, externa vel interna est. Ad priorem pertinet frigus, vel alia retropellentia temere adhibita; ad posteriorem vero omnia, quae aequilibrium & resistentiam solidorum atque fluidorum tollunt. **10.17** Hinc in variolis Contiguis vel Confluentibus exstirpata nimis febre, retrocessioni caussa subministratur; hinc fortiores evacuationes, ut diarrhoea, haemorrhagiae &c. retrocessionem faciunt. **10.18** Sequelae variae infaustae sunt, nempe delirium, lethargus, oppressiones pectoris, anxietates, inquietudines, peripneumonia, febris. Curatur, in priori casu, expellentibus, vesicatoriis vel sinapismis. In posteriori vero casu cardiacis, ut sero lactis vinoso, vel vino ipso Hispanico, cum expellentibus & epispasticis, pro re nata, interpositis.

10.19 *Oculi* plerumque tumore faciei clauduntur, quod tamen nihil mali portendit, modo, tumore extremitates inferiores petente, aperiantur. **10.20** Nihilo tamen minus si oculos servare volupe fuerit apertos, linctu optime procedit; si vero hoc nihil efficiatur, convenit linteolum quoddam in lac calidum cum Croco ebullito, immittere, atque humiditate expressa, palpebris admovere. **10.21** J. Z. PLATNERUS *institutiones Chirurgiae, p. 172,* statuit oculos optime custodiri si palpebrae conglutinentur, & diductionem palpebrarum, arte factam, non approbat. Ipsi largiri possumus, fotus emollientes, vel nimiam indulgentiam emollientium periculi plenam esse. **10.22** Quicquid sit, praxi didicimus, palpebris, post diem 11 morbi, ad tempus clausis, nec convenienti modo unquam apertis, id accidisse, ut diductis tandem iisdem, membrana totum oculum texerit, in aegrotorum maximum damnum; quod DIEMERBROEK *libro citato, historia 16. p. 300.* etiam observavit. **10.23** Quid? quod aegrotum biennem, die morbi circiter 16, variolosis symptomatibus adeo exhaustum, ut palpebrae pendulae essent, & purulenta forte materia conglutinatae vidimus. Parentes de restitutione prorsus desperantes, religioni duxerunt palpebras dimovere, unde die circiter 21, palpebris diductis, ambo oculi quasi suppurati apparuerunt.

10.12 From what has been said, it is obvious that the cure is the same, if the pocks do not want to rise. But if this is not satisfactory, whey prepared with Rhine wine, to which expellants are added, should be used. **10.13** With how great success patients have used milk internally in these cases, especially added with expellants, is excellently attested in the authors of case descriptions, see D. FISCHER: *observationes de usu lactis in variolis, p.127*; HAHN: *the work quoted, p. 59*. **10.14** The *famous* PRAESES has made use, externally, of the vapours of tepid milk, with the result that the pustules elevated within an hour; here is the utmost caution necessary, to protect well against the cold, not to bring about a recession of the pustules. **10.15** If the pustules *recede*, it is definitely a matter for deeper investigation, and a forerunner of death, if they cannot once again be safely brought out. For my part, I know that there are many who deny this regression, see VIOLANTE: *the work quoted, p.68*. But they seem to be lead astray by love of their hypotheses, not supported by rational practice. **10.16** The reason for this regression is, generally speaking, twofold, external or internal. To the former is to be referred cold, or other checking means, employed without due care; to the latter, though, all that remove the balance and resistance of the solid and fluid parts. **10.17** Hence, when the fever is too profoundly rooted out in contiguous or confluent pocks, a reason for regression is provided; hence the more vehement evacuations, like diarrhoea, bleedings, etc. bring about a regression. **10.18** There are various unfortunate results, to be more exact delirium, lethargy, obstruction of the chest, fits of anguish, unrest, pneumonia, fever. In the former case expellants, vesicatories or mustard poultices should be effected. In the latter case, though, cordials, like whey with wine, or Spanish wine only, alternatingly with expellents and antispasmodics, according to the circumstances.

10.19 *The eyes* are often closed from the swelling of the face, which however does not portend anything bad, as long as they are opened when the swelling moves towards the lower extremities. **10.20** Nevertheless, if one wants to keep the eyes open, one would succeed best by an electuary, but if nothing is accomplished this way, it is useful to soak a linen towel in hot milk with boiled saffron, wring out the moisture, and apply it to the eyelids. **10.21** J.Z. PLATNERUS states in *institutiones Chirurgiae, p. 172*, that the eyes are best protected if the eyelids are stuck together, and does not approve of separating the eyelids by artificial means. I can myself admit that softening fomentations, or an excessive use of softeners, is dangerous. **10.22** Anyway, from my practice I have learned that when the eyelids after the eleventh day of sickness are closed, and have never been opened by any convenient method, it has happened, that when they finally are separated, a membrane has covered the eyes completely, to major detriment for the patient; something that DIEMERBROEK *the quoted work, historia 16, p.300*, has also observed. **10.23** What more? That I have seen a two year old patient, who, on about the sixteenth day was so exhausted by the smallpox' symptoms that his eyelids were hanging down, and strongly stuck together by purulent matter. The parents, who despaired of a recovery, had strong misgivings towards opening the eyelids, whence, as the eyelids were opened, on about the twenty-first day, both eyes showed to have suppurated.

10.24 Si vero febris nimis evecta sit, cum pulsu duro inflammatorio, non est quod de China propinanda cogitemus; auget enim phlogosin sanguinis, & plurima mala secum trahit. E contrario Venaesectiones largae, Clysmata, Nitrosa, Julapia acidula, in usum vocanda sunt. **10.25** Si vero febris mediocris sit, atque natura satis vigoris habeat ad suppurationem placidam promovendam, supervacanea sunt omnia medicamenta, solaque diluentia & paregorica versus noctes, omne punctum absolvunt.

10.26 *Febris Secundaria* nunc consideranda. Incipit in Confluentibus die plerumque 6; in benignis vero non ante diem 8. animadvertitur. Amphimerinam quodammodo refert exacerbationibus suis nocturnis; eo autem differt quod exacerbationes nocturnae diebus criticis incidentes longe sint vehementiores. **10.27** Dies Critici sunt 8. 11. 14. 17. 20 &c. Quavis itaque nocte per quemcumque horum dierum altius evehitur febris, &, si dicere liceat, eodem modo ac Quotidiana composita cum Quartana se habet. **10.28** Haec moderanda, nec libera linquenda est, non raro enim cum vitae discrimine indomabilis accrescit. Anodyna, si unquam, certe heic indicantur. Initium illorum faciendum est, quamprimum anxietates & inquietudines nocturnae in conspectum prodeunt. **10.29** In infantibus SYDENHAMUS illis uti non ausus fuit; nos vero Syrupum e Meconio Londinensem in adultis, pariter ac infantibus, feliciter adhibuimus, praecipue si diarrhoeae obnoxii fuere aegri. Illi tamen, Elixir Paregoricum Londinense a gtt. 30. ad 50. adultis propinatum, palmam facile praeripere, quatenus praeter vim, qua gaudet, anodynam, pectori & diaphoresi simul consulit, haud diffiteri ausim. **10.30** Purgantium genuinum in hac febri debellanda usum, plurimis experimentis demonstravit J. FREIND per totam suam epistolam, de horum necessitate ad *Richard* MEAD missam.

10.31 Inflammatione itaque variolarum in benignam abeunte suppurationem, subito remitti debet febris, si morbus ordinem naturae suetum sequatur. Hoc vero constanter in benignis obtinet; at in confluentibus non semper ita agitur; casu posito posteriore, pro certo signo haberi potest, vel suppurationem non rite procedere, vel pus e pustulis debito modo non evacuari, verum in sanguinem resorberi, novumque adeo addi calcar febri currenti. **10.32** Haec puris e pustulis resorptio frequentissima est variolis Confluentibus. Quid enim in praxi frequentius, quam circa finem stadii tertii novas turbas ortas videri? Quanta saepius non excitatur febris! Quid putredinis! **10.33** Febris sane denuo mutata, & loco inflammatoriae, putridae scenam ludere visa; ea tamen ratione, ut exacerbationes febri secundariae adjudicatae minime sedentur, sed potius deliriis & aliis infaustis symptomatibus vitam miseri dejiciant. **10.34** Dicas mihi ad quam, positis his, sacram confugiendum anchoram, & magnus mihi eris Apollo! Venaesectionis interdum magna vis, quam tamen saepius vetant contraindicantia. Pulveres Nitrosi & camphorati, succi & syrupi acidi saepe efficaces se probant, saepe etiam nihil valent. **10.35** Nec semper sufficiunt Paregorica, quamvis quavis 7. hora hausta. In casu tam desperato ad Chinchinam, quasi ad magnum antiputredinosum confugimus, idque summo cum fructu.

10.24 But if the fever is too high, with hard, inflammatory pulse, there is no reason to consider giving China, as this increases the burning in the blood, and brings with it much evil. On the contrary, extensive bloodletting, clysters, nitrous preparations, and acid juleps should be adhibited. **10.25** But if the fever is moderate and nature has enough power to bring about an even suppuration, all medicine is superfluous, diluants and paregorics only, in the evening, will solve everything.

10.26 *Secondary fever* should now be discussed. It begins mostly on the sixth day in confluent pocks, but in benign pocks it is not observed before the eighth day. It resembles the amphemerous fever in a way, by its nightly aggravations, but distinguishes itself thus, that the nightly aggravations which appear on the critical days are far more vehement. **10.27** The critical days are 8, 11, 14, 17, 20, etc. On any night in one of these days, thus, the fever is more increased, and if I may put it that way, it behaves in the same way as a quotidian fever combined with a quartan fever. **10.28** This must be diminished, and not left free, as it does not seldom, with danger to life, grow untamable. Here, if ever, analgesics are certainly indicated. The initiation of these should be effected as soon as the fits of anguish and nightly unrest show up. **10.29** With children SYDENHAM did not dare to use these; but I have used *Syrupus e Meconio Londinensis* with success, with adults as well as with children, especially if the patients have been suffering from diarrhoea. I would not dare to deny, however, that *Elixir Paregoricum Londinense*, when given to adults in a dose of 30 to 50 drops easily beats that remedy, inasmuch as it above the analgetic power, which is has, at the same time helps the chest and the perspiration. **10.30** That purging remedies are truly useful in defeating this fever has J. FREIND showed, by several experiments, in a whole letter on the need for these remedies to *Richard* MEAD.

10.31 Thus, as the inflammation of smallpox passes on to a benign suppuration, the fever should at once decrease if the disease follows the normal, natural course. This is fully correct in benign smallpox, but in confluent it does not always happen; when the latter case is present, it could be regarded as a certain sign, either of the suppuration not duly proceeding, or of pus not being properly evacuated from the pustules, but being resorbed in the blood, a new incitement thus being provided for a fever already in full development. **10.32** This resorption of pus from the pustules is most common in confluent smallpox, for what is more commonly seen in practice than new disturbances towards the end of the third stage? What a high fever is not often brought about? What putrefaction! **10.33** The fever is truly altered anew, and seems to be acting as a festering fever instead of an inflammatory fever, in such a way, however, that the exacerbations ascribed to the secondary fever do not wear off, but rather, by deliriums and other ominous symptoms, precipitate the life of the wretched. **10.34** In this condition, tell me, to what safe haven one could escape, and you are truly the great Apollo! At times, bloodletting has great effect, but it is often contraindicated. *Pulveres Nitrosi et Camphorati*, sour juices and syrups often prove effective, but often are also without effect. **10.35** Neither are the paregorics always sufficient, even if taken every seventh hour. In such a desperate case, I take to *Chinchina* as the great remedy for festering, and with great success, too.

10.36 Binos tantum afferamus casus. Studiosus 10. ann. tenuis debilisque complexionis, dolore capitis, febri, ceterisque variolarum symptomatibus, *die 29 martii 1753 p.m.* aegrotare incipiebat. **10.37** *d. 30 M.* Emeticum, & sola diluentia propinavimus, cum febris non adeo fortis esset. *d. 31 M.* Febris magis aestuans pulverem Nitrosum & Julapium acidulum postulavit; & dolorem dorsi acutissimum fotu e Mentha crispa cum vino, mitigavimus. **10.38** *d. 1 A.* Fotus e speciebus emollientibus pedibus admovimus. Haemorrhagia narium satis larga hodie morbo se junxit. Inclinante die indicia variolarum erumpentium invenimus, quae per totam noctem subsequentem adeo multiplicata, ut variolae *d. 2 A.* agmine satis magno faciem & pedes occuparent. **10.39** Febris cum debilitate corporis manebat. Totam fere diem dormiendo consumebat aeger, quare de epispastico pedibus applicando cogitaverimus, quod itidem aegro praescripsimus, id tamen vitio curam gerentis supine omissum videbamus. **10.40** *d. 3 A.* Variolae majori numero eruptae conspiciebantur, forte e sero lactis vinoso cum floribus sulphuris usitato. *d. 4 A* Variolae in facie parvae & confluentes; genae roseae erant. **10.41** *d. 5 A.* Nocte praecedenti inquietudines ortas fuisse deprehendebamus. Facies tumere incipiebat. Variolae depressae sed paulo elatiores erant. Alvum nigris & pessime olentibus scybalis exoneravit. **10.42** *d. 6 A.* Saliva circa meridiem fluere incipiebat. Vesperi elixir Paregoricum Londinense gtt. XXX prima vice propinavimus. *d. 7 A.* Alvum iterum deposuit. **10.43** Pustulae genarum corium pergamentum contrahere incipiebant. Ptyalismus pleno fluebat rivulo, *dieque 8 A.* continuabat; *die* vero *9 A.* paulo erat diminutus. Tumor manus patebat. **10.44** *d. 10 A.* Salivationem penitus sedatam videbamus. Pustulis oleo amygdalae dulcis & decocto Avenae illivimus. Sed quam subita metamorphosis! Nescivimus sane qua de caussa hora 8. vespere aegrotum inveniebamus laborantem pulsu cito, ingenti siti, calore immodico &c. **10.45** Syrupum igitur e Meconio larga dosi propinavimus, quem post 7. horas repeti jussimus. *d. 11 A.* Febrem & cetera symptomata vehementiora, cum delirio vago, magna debilitate, odore summo putredinoso, conspeximus. **10.46** Clysma igitur, & Julapium refocillantem *Illustris* PRAESIDIS sine vino, subito praescripsimus. Clysma, sine effectu applicatum, iteravimus, effectu autem ut antea frustraneo. Tandem de Cortice Chinae propinando consilium cepimus, eumque ad scrupulum I quavis hora, exceptis nocturnis, quarum quavis syrupum e Meconio sorberet, ordinavimus. **10.47** *d. 12 A.* aegrotem 4 tantum Pulveres deglutiisse, ceteris intactiis audivimus. Pulsus durior, & putredo summa. Pulveres Robe Sambuci immixti, ut faciliores deglutiti forent. **10.48** Ante meridiem deliravit, unde tamen ab instituto nos deterreri non passi fuimus. Clysma iterabatur, adjecto copioso sale, unde plurima excreta biliosa excernebat. Versus vesperam pulsum molliorem, magisque plenum, nec adeo citum experiebamur. **10.49** *d. 13 A.* Urina priori die sumta sedimento albo dimidium fere vitrum implebat. Febris nulla. Putredo vix sensibilis. Pustulae flaccidae & rugosae erant pelliculae, liquore nullo aut pultaceo repletae. **10.50** *d. 14 A.* Urina pellucida absque sedimento. Chinchina postmodum indies repetita, quavis vero nocte. Paregorica, donec aegrum periculi expertem cognoverimus.

10.36 I will merely put forth two cases. A ten-year-old schoolboy, of slender and weak constitution, suffering from headache, fever and other symptoms of smallpox, began to feel ill in the afternoon of *March, 29th, 1753*. **10.37** On *March 30th*, I offered emetics and diluants only, as the fever was not yet high. On *March 31st*, it was more burning; and demanded *pulveres Nitrosi* and acid julep; the sharp pains in the back I mitigated by a foment of mint with wine. **10.38** On *April 1st*, I applied a fomentation of emollient spices to the feet. This day a rather profuse nose bleed joined the disease. Towards the end of the day, I discovered signs of erupting pocks, which during the whole night after were multiplied to such extent that, on *April 2nd*, quite a large number of them had occupied the face and feet. **10.39** The fever remained, with feebleness of the body. The patient spent almost the whole day sleeping, wherefore I considered applying an epispastic to the feet, which I also prescribed to the patient, but which I saw was carelessly neglected by fault of the nurse. **10.40** On *April 3rd* a larger number of erupted pocks was seen, perhaps from use of whey with wine and flowers of sulphur. On *April 4th* the pocks in the face were small and confluent; the cheeks were rose-red. **10.41** On *April 5th* I learned that there had been unrest during the night before. The face began to swell. The pocks were depressed, but slightly more raised. He emptied his bowels of black and evil-smelling faeces. **10.42** On *April 6th* the saliva started to run about mid-day. In the evening I offered *elixir paregoricum Londinense*, 30 drops, for the first time. On *April 7th* he evacuated his bowels again. **10.43** The pustules on the cheeks started to contract a parchment-like coating. The saliva flew in a profuse stream; on *April 8th* it continued, but on *April 9th* it was somewhat decreased. The swelling of the hands was manifest. **10.44** On *April 10th* I saw that salivation had stopped totally. I poured *oleum amygdalae dulcis* and a decoction of oat on the pustules. But what a sudden transformation! At eight o'clock in the evening I found the patient for unknown reasons labouring under a quick pulse, a vehement thirst, an immoderate heat, etc. **10.45** Consequently I offered a large dose of *syrupus e meconio*, which I ordered to be repeated after seven hours. On *April 11th* I observed that the fever and the other symptoms were more vehement, together with a general confusion, great feebleness and a very rotten odour. **10.46** Thus, I at once prescribed a clyster, and the refreshing julep of the *famous* PRAESES, without wine. The clyster, adhibited without effect, was repeated, but, as before, without any result. At last I decided to offer china bark, of which I prescribed one scruple every hour, except for the hours of night, when he should take *syrupus e meconio* every hour. **10.47** On *April 12th* I learned that the patient had only taken four powders while the rest were untouched. The pulse was harder, and the stench very strong. The powders were mixed with *rob sambuci* to be easier to swallow. **10.48** A. m. the patient was delirious, which I however did not allow to deter me from my intentions. The clyster was repeated, with a large quantity of salt added, whence it washed out much bilose excrement. Towards the evening the pulse felt softer, more full, and not as quick. **10.49** On *April 13th* the urine sampled the day before filled about half the glass with a white sediment. No fever. The stench hardly discernible. The pustules had flaccid and wrinkled membranes, filled with no liquid or pulp. **10.50** On April *14th* the urine was clear, without sediment. Chinchina was used again, only once a day, but in the evening. Paregorics, till I knew that the patient was beyond danger.

10.51 *Anno 1753 die 13 Augustii.* Puerum biennem die 11:mo morbi visitare incipiebamus. Variolae confluentes erant; tumor faciem & manus reliquerat; per totum morbi cursum diarrhoeam ad 3 evacuationes quotidie passus fuerat. **10.52** Aegrotum maxime debilem inveniebamus; diarrhoea adhuc continuans, scybala grisea evacuabat; respiratio laboriosa valde erat, anhelosa & cita; Febris vehemens; pustulae variolosae fere vacuae; urina sponte & aegro invito in lecto semper evacuabatur; putredo intolerabilis; stridor dentium fere continuus. **10.53** In casu adeo ancipiti, ne dicam desperato, ad Corticem Chinae propinandum, tandem nos accinximus, quamvis probe conscii, in casibus, ubi respirationi vis infertur, usum ejus a quibusdam Auctorum impugnari. vide HUXHAM *loco citato p 196.* Corticem ad scrupuli β quavis integra hora porreximus, ita ut Drachmas II hoc die consumeret parvulus. **10.54** *die 14 Augustii.* Pulsus moderatus erat, & aeger cibum appetebat. Hodie Corticis scrupulos IV deglutiebat. Excreta per alvum grisea erant & foetida. *die 15 Augustii.* Corticem repetebamus, cum per nycthemerum propinatus non fuerit. Pulsus paulo citatior, quam antea erat. Putredo adhuc fortis. Pustulae indurari videbantur & decidebant. **10.55** *die 16 Augustii.* Per totum diem pulveres assumere noluit aeger. Versus vesperam symptomata aucta deprehendebamus. Nocte sequenti pulveres cum saccharo commisti gustum aegri adeo elusere, ut illos deglutierit. **10.56** *die 17 Augustii.* Melius erat aegroto quam praecedenti die, & symptomata magna parte remissa. Jam facies a variolis fere liberata. Excreta per alvum brunneum exhibebant colorem, forte ex China tincta. Pulsus naturali similis. Putredo hodie nulla, adeo ut nec spiritus, neque excreta alvi ullum odorem putridum sparserint. Depositiones alvi non ita urgebant, ut antea. Respiratio in integrum restituta non fuit, longe tamen facilior quam ab initio, dum arcessiti adveniebamus. **10.57** *die 18 Augustii.* China neglecta fuit. Versus noctem syrupum meconii Londinensem sumebat, qui placidum conciliabat somnum. *die 19 Augustii.* Nescimus qua de caussa loco Corticis, nonnullos pulveres Nitrosos sumsisset. Tres habuit sedes mucosas. **10.58** Stragilectionem hodie exercuit. Versus vesperam magna ei supervenit debilitas, cum pulsu cito, sudore, inquietudine & jactationibus, maxima difficultate respirandi, agrypnia, quae per totam noctem durabant, quamvis paregorica non omissa fuerint. **10.59** *die 20 Augustii.* Symptomata, paulum tamen remissa, continuabant. Excreta per alvum flava, mucosa & repetita erant. Putredo rursus se manifestabat. Variolae e toto fere corpore deciderant. Ad Chinchinam iterum confugimus, ex qua symptomata sensim leviora apparuerunt. **10.60** Deinde Chinam quotidie, omnibus tamen vesperis Paregoricum, diebus autem criticis dosi duplo majori, illud propinavimus, usque dum de felici exitu morbi certissimi essemus. Sic tandem sanitati restitutus aeger, cum diarrhoea, aliisque infaustis symptomatibus, per totum morbi cursum conflictatus.

10.51 *1753, August 13th,* I started visiting a two year old boy on his eleventh day of sickness. The pocks were confluent; the swelling had left the face and hands; throughout the course of the disease he had suffered from diarrhoea with up to three evacuations a day. **10.52** I found the patient very weak; the diarrhoea was still continuous, and he evacuated grey excrement; the breathing was very laborious, panting, and quick; the fever was vehement; the pustules were almost empty; the urine passed spontaneously and without the patient's will, always in bed; the stench was unbearable; the grinding of the teeth almost continuous. **10.53** In such an uncertain, not to say desperate, case, I at last prepared myself to offer china bark, even though I am well aware of its use being criticized by some authors in cases where the respiration is attacked: see HUXHAM, *the work quoted, p.196.* I offered the bark, half a scruple each hour, so the little boy should take two drachms that day. **10.54** On *August 14th* the pulse was moderate, and the patient wanted to eat. This day he took four scruples of the bark. The excrement was grey and nasty-smelling. On *August 15th* I offered bark again, as it had not been given in 24 hours. The pulse was slightly quicker than before. The stench was still strong. The pustules seemed to harden and fell off. **10.55** On *August 16th* the patient did not want to take any powder during the whole day. Towards the evening I noticed that the symptoms had increased. The following night powders mixed with sugar fooled the patient's sense of taste so that he swallowed them. **10.56** On *August 17th* the state of the patient was better than on the day before, and the symptoms were to a large extent decreased. The face was by now almost free from pocks. The excretion of the bowels showed a brown colour, perhaps coloured by the china. The pulse like the normal one. No stench this day, inasmuch as neither breath nor excrement spread any foul odour. The evacuations of the bowels were not as urgent as before. The respiration was not completely restored, but much easier than in the beginning, when I was sent for and arrived. **10.57** On *August 18th* the china had been neglected. Towards the night, he took *syrupus meconii Londinensis,* which provided a quiet sleep. On *August 19th* he had taken several *pulveres Nitrosi* instead of the bark, for unknown reasons. Three mucous evacuations. **10.58** Today he was floccitating. Towards the evening a great feebleness overwhelmed him, with quick pulse, sweating, unrest and agitation, great difficulty to breathe, sleeplessness, which lasted the whole night, even as the paregorics had not been omitted. **10.59** On *August 20th* the symptoms, although somewhat decreased, continued. The evacuations were yellow, mucous and frequent. The stench was again manifest. The pocks fell off from almost the whole body. I took to china once more, whereby the symptoms little by little seemed more lenient. **10.60** Then I offered china daily, but every evening paregorics; on the critical days, however, in a more than doubled dose; I gave this until I was quite certain of a happy outcome of the disease. Thus, at last, was the patient, who had been tormented throughout the entire course of disease by diarrhoea and other ominous symptoms, brought back to health.

10.61 Hactenus de resorptione puris. In variolis cum Petechiis, cum pustulis aut punctis nigris, quae gangraenam adesse monstrant, usus forte Corticis, aeque ac in casibus modo recensitis, felix esse posset. De utilitate Chinchinae in Gangraena & Sphacelo plurimi testimonia dederunt. **10.62** RUSHWORTH illam in sphacelo ex caussa interna, & ubi febris intermittit, commendat. AMYAND in 7 aegrotis semper cum effectu illam se dedisse narrat, J. DOUGLAS in omni sphacelo usum ejus admittit, propinata Drachmae β quavis hora 4. SCHIPTON ad scrupulos ij sub ipsis insultibus febris illam praescribit. *vide Philosophical Transactions, N:o 426, § 5.* **10.63** J. HUXHAM *loco citato p. 89 seqq* curiosum affert casum cortice curatum *cf The Medical Essays volume 2 article 34; volume 3 observation 5 p 35 & article 6 p 43 volume 4 observation 10 p 47. Si,* itaque ut verbis utar HUXHAMI *de Morbis epidemicis vol 1 p 109, in singulari Gangraena valeat Quinquina, quidni in universa humorum corruptione?* **10.64** Periculum certe nos hisce in casibus non fecimus; celebribus tamen viris, qui propria edocti experientia Chinchinam & hic commendant, fidem habere non dubitamus. Sic HUXHAM *de Morbis epidemicis vol 2 p 122* illa cum acidis, e.g. ᴧ Vitrioli aut vinum rubrum Gallicum instar omnium in variolis *nigris* usus fuit. *Richard* MEAD *loco citato cap 3 p 37* spem dat optimi successus in variolis cum pustulis sangvineis, ex Cortice admixto Alumine. **10.65** J. WALL *Philosophical Transactions N:o 484 § 4* plurimis demonstrat experimentis Chinchinae usum in variolis, quibus Gangraena, Haemorrhagiae, Petechiae & Maculae pessimi generis semet adjunxerunt. Acidum semper adjecit plerumque alumen, ut magis stypticum inde emergeret medicamentum. In ipso stadio 1 corticem adhibuit, quoties aliquid ex enumeratis symptomatibus adfuit. **10.66** Sed quid rei tot fide dignis observationibus extra controversiam positae, diu immoremur? Antequam autem stadio huic finem faciamus, verbo tantum nominabimus, quod serio aegrotos adhortari debemus, ne oblivioni tradant genua saepius saepiusque flectere; vidimus enim casum, ubi, hoc neglecto, contractus fere evasit aeger, & non nisi summa cum cura, scilicet unguentis emollientibus externe genibus applicatis, & sensim aucta genuum motitatione, in sanitatem restitutus.

§**11.1** STADIUM IV. Stadium hoc ingrediuntur variolae, cum pustulae exsiccari incipiunt. Quae de febri secundaria, resorptione puris & ceteris symptomatibus supra diximus, ea omnia etiam de hoc stadio, quum paria in illud incidunt symptomata, dictum volumus. **11.2** Ut exsiccatio placidior procedat, praesertim in facie, oleosis, e.g. oleum amygdalae dulcis vel Liliorum alborum illiniri possunt pustulae, interposito decocto avenaceo. Laxantia e Mercurio dulci non negligenda sunt, praesertim in variolis confluentibus quibus ulcera sordida plurimaque mala praecaventur. **11.3** Debilitas periodica (§ 5 st. 4) propinato Cortice Chinae feliciter cedit. Sed manum de tabula.

10.61 Thus far on resorption of pus. In smallpox with petecchia, with black pustules or dots, which show that gangrene is about, the use of the bark perhaps could be as successful as in the cases just put forth. Several authors have given testimony of the usefulness of chinchina in gangrenes and necroses. **10.62** RUSHWORTH commends it in necroses from internal causes and with intermittent fever. AMYAND says that he has given it in seven cases, always with good results, J. DOUGLAS accepts the use of it in all necroses, given in a dose of half a drachm every fourth hour. SCHIPTON prescribes two scruples of it during the very attacks of fever, see *Philosophical Transactions Nr.426, §5.*; **10.63** J. HUXHAM, *the work quoted, p.89* and following, reports a scientifically interesting case, cured with cortex, *cf. The medical essays, vol. 2, art. 34; vol. 3, obs. 5, p. 35, and art. 6, p. 43; vol. 4, obs. 10, p. 47. If* – to use Huxham's words, then, from *De Morbis epidemicis, vol 1, p. 109* – *Quinquina has effect in a distinct gangrene, why should it not in a universal corruption of the fluids?* **10.64** I certainly have not brought about any danger in these cases; I have no doubts against trusting the famous men who from their own experience commend *Chinchina* here also. So did HUXHAM *De Morbis epidemicis vol 2 p 122* use it, with acids, e. g. *Spiritus Vitrioli* or French claret, rather than anything else, in *black* smallpox. *Richard* MEAD, *the work quoted, chapter 3, p.37*, gives hope for optimal success in smallpox with bloodfilled pustules, by bark added with alum. **10.65** J. WALL, *Philosophical Transactions nr.484, §* 4, shows, from several experiments, the usefulness of Chinchina in smallpox, where gangrenes, bleedings, petecchia and spots of the malignant kind have shown up. He always adds an acid, and mostly alum, so that the medicine thus will come out more adstringent. He made use of the bark in the first stage itself, every time any of the enumerated symptoms were present. **10.66** But why dwell any longer upon things which from such credible observations are indisputable? But before I put an end to this stage, I will shortly put forth that we should seriously exhort the patients not to forget to flex their knees again and again, as I have seen a case where, this being neglected, the patient became almost contractured, and could be brought back to health only with great effort, i. e. by application externally on the knees of an emollient salve and little by little increased movements of the knees.

§ **11.1** STAGE IV. The smallpox comes to this stage as the pustules start to dry up. All that, which has been said above about secondary fever, resorption of pus, and other symptoms, I maintain is also applicable to this stage, as the same symptoms come to show here. **11.2** To make the exsiccation easier, especially in the face, the pustules could be smeared with an ointment of one grain of *oleum amygdalae dulcis* or *oleum liliorum alborum*, alternatingly with a decoction of oat. Especially in confluent smallpox, laxatives from calomel, by which bad ulcers and much evil could be prevented, should not be neglected. **11.3** Periodical feebleness (§ 5, st 4) will recede if china bark is given. But enough!

Commentary, Bergius

1.1 *inflammatiunculis*] See *Inflammatio and inflammatiuncula*, Latin word list, p 42.

1.2 *Bubones*] Greek word list, p 32.

anthraces] Greek word list, p 31.

1.3 *Miliariae*] See *Miliaria*, Latin word list, p 43.

papulae] See *Papula*, Latin word list, p 44.

1.4 *Rubeolam*] See *Rubeola*, Latin word list, p 47.

1.5 *uredinem*] See *Uredo*, Latin word list, p 51.

1.6 *Petechias*] See *Petechiae*, Latin word list, p 45.

1.7 *Bullosam*] See *Bullosa*, Latin word list, p 40.

SAUVAGES] François Boissier de Sauvages (1706–67), professor of medicine at Montpellier, France, who in his *Nouvelles classes de maladies* (1731–34) had worked out a classification system for diseases, adopted by Linnaeus, among others. It became the basis for the Linnaean dissertation *Genera Morborum* from 1759 (resp. J. Schröder).

1.8 *Erysipelas*] Greek word list, p 34.

2.1 *Species*] The small catalogue of smallpox varieties found in this paragraph is a characteristic feature of this time, with its fancy for systematic categorisation in the Linnaean fashion; cf. **7.6**, *e regno animali* below; cf also **Martin 5.1–5.2**.

SYDENHAMUS] Thomas Sydenham (1624–89), British physician; the reference here is probably to his *Observationes medicae* (1676); cf. my commentary to **Martin 17.2**.

pagina mea] A common expression meaning 'page … in my copy'.

2.2 *MORTON Pyretologia de variolis*] The English physician Richard Morton (1637–98) published the first part of his *Pyretologia: seu exercitationes de morbis universalibus acutis* in 1693. The abbreviated title here would mean "*Pyretologia*, the chapter on smallpox", which is chapter 10 of part two: *exercitatio de febribus inflammatoriis universalibus*, 1694.

2.4 *Variolae … nigrae*] i.e. smallpox with blood-filled pustules.

2.5 *durae ovales*] According to Murray's *Historia insitionis variolarum in Suecia*, p 13, these are not genuine smallpox.

WERLHOF de Variolis & Anthracibus] The title is *Disquisitio medica et philosophica de variolis et anthracibus, ubi de utriusque affectus antiquitatibus, signis, differentiis, medelis disserit* (1735).

2.6 *J.G. HAHN de variolarum ratione*] Johann Gottfried von Hahn's *Variolarum ratio* *exposita*, published in 1751.

morbillis] See *Morbilli*, Latin word list, p 43.

G. HARRIS] This is in all probability Walter (Gualterius) H. Harris (1651–1725) whose *Observationes medicae* were published in 1726; that this Dr Harris was known to Rosén is evident from the catalogue of Rosén's library which was printed for an auction after his death, where, as No. 375 among the books in *octavo*, is recorded a 1736 edition of Walter Harris' *De morbis acutis infantum*, originally published in 1689.

Haemorrhagiis] See *Haemorrhagia*, Greek word list, p 35.

Haemoptoë] Greek word list, p 35.

2.7 *Crystallinae*] According to Dorland, this is not smallpox, but rather chicken pox.

SCHENCK] Probably Johannes Schenck von Grafenberg (1530–98), a German physician, who published Παρατηρήσεων *sive observationum medicarum rararum, novarum, admirabilium et monstrosarum volumen* (1584–97).

2.8 *pustulis*] See *Pustula*, Latin word list, p 46.

sanguine plenis] Cf. **2.4** above.

HILDANUS] Wilhelm Fabricius Hildanus (1560–1634), German surgeon and anatomist, inventor of several surgical instruments.

2.9 *J.H. SCHULZ*] Johann Heinrich Schulz (1687–1744), German physician.

2.10 *historiam dare*] *Historia* meaning 'description' or 'account' as used in ancient Latin, e.g. in Pliny's *Naturalis historia*. The word *historia* in this sense is very common in book titles from the Renaissance on; cf. e.g. Alessandro Benedetti's *Anatomice sive de Hystoria corporis humani libri V*, 1528; Jean Bauhin's *Historia Plantarum Universalis* (1650-1651); Valerius Cordus' *Historia plantarum* (1561–63).

3.2 *quot fere … Medici, tot … varietates sententiarum*] This is of course an adaption of Terence, *Phormio* 454, *Quot homines, tot sententiae*.

3.3 *LIDDELIUS*] Duncan Liddel (1561–1613), Scottish physician, professor of mathematics, astronomy and geography in Helmstädt.

WILLIS] Thomas Willis (1621–75); the work referred to is probably *Diatriba de febribus, seu de motu earumdem in sanguine animali* (1659).

FORESTUS] Probably Pieter van Foreest (1522–97), Dutch physician.

3.4 *GENTILIS de FULGINEO*] Gentile de Fuligno (?–1348), Italian physician, professor in Perugia.

MERCURIALIS] Geronimo Mercuriale (1530–1606) Italian, most known for his editions of ancient medical texts, e.g. Hippocrates and Galen.

3.5 *SYLVIUS*] Probably Franz de le Boë/Dubois/Sylvius (1614?–72)

ETMÜLLER] Michael Etmüller (1644–83), German profesor of botany and surgery.

biliosa] See *Biliosus*, Latin word list, p 40.

lympha] Greek word list, p 36.

WOODWARD] John Woodward (1665–1728), English geologist and physician. The work referred to might be *The state of physick and diseases, with an inquiry into the causes of the late increase of them, but more particularly of the small pox* ... (1718), which seems to be the only medical work of any importance published by Woodward.

3.6 *Salia ...fixa*] The plural *salia* (n) for the classical *sales* (m) is mentioned (and disapproved of) by Krebs-Schmalz II, p 480: *salia, wie man im* N.L. *die* Salze *zu benennen pflegt*.

Since the plural *sales* in ancient Latin never seems to indicate chemically different substances but, at the most, different varieties of common salt, as e.g. in Varro, *RR* 2.11.5: *Qui aspargi solent sales, melior fossilis quam marinus*, it seems probable that *salia* at some point has been introduced as a technical term by alchemists/chemists as a useful collective denomination; it is used e.g. by the German Petrus Kertzenmacher in *Alchimia. Wie man alle farben, wasser, olea, salia, unnd alumina ...machen soll* in 1546.

Furthermore, there are examples of a singular *salia* (f) declined according to the 1ˢᵗ declension, e.g. in Quiricus' *Lumen Apothecariorum* (1494), where, in the recipe for *Salia Muscata* on fol. XXr, it is stated that *salie omnes species sunt subtilissime terende*.

The term *sal fixum*, finally, is used about a salt, which *magna ignis vi non avolat*, according to Blancardus, s.v. *sal*.

SIDOBRIUS] Antoine Sidobre (?–?), who published a *Tractatus de variolis et morbillis* in 1699.

3.7 *M. LISTER*] Martin Lister (1638–1711), English scientist, otherwise best known as an entomologist.

3.8 *Sideribus aliquam inesse vim*] The idea that the positions of stars and, above all, planets, could bring forth diseases once was a generally accepted scientific truth; one might, however, consider Fracastoro's *De contagione* (1546), where it is stated that the connexion between celestial phaenomena and diseases must be an indirect one: *Sed certe (quando nihil a coelo huc demitti potest, quod proxime tangat, nisi spirituale aliquod, seu lumen, seu tale aliud) ... videmus a coelo nullas contagiones per se fieri posse, per accidens autem nihil prohibet quasdam ab ipso fieri* (1.12); what actually happens, according to Fracastoro, is that the heat of the celestial bodies – especially of planets in conjunction – makes vapours rise from earth. These vapours may then putrefy, thus producing various kinds of contagion.

arrisit] Cf. **10.12**

N. CHESNEAU] Nicolas Chesneau/Quercetanus (1601?–?), Frenchman, whose *Observationum libri quinque* …were published in 1672.

3.9 *renum succenturiatorum*] See *Renes succenturiati*, Latin word list, p 46.

Ph. VIOLANTE de variolis et morbillis] Philippo de Violante of Naples, according to the book in question, *De variolis et morbillis tractatus physico-mechanicus* (1750), PhD and MD, *archiater et consiliarius* to the king of Poland; the book is listed as number 143 of the titles in quarto of the auction catalogue mentioned in **2.6** above.

3.10 *vasa sangvinea*] See *Vasa*, Latin word list, p 51.

3.12 *scabiei*] See *Scabies*, Latin word list, p 47.

4.1 *invadere*] Regarding military metaphors, see p 79sqq.

BORELLI] Alfonso Borelli (1608–79), Italian physician and physiologist.

5.1 *Ultra limites …excurremus*] As Östlund points out (p 65), this kind of metaphor is quite common in dissertations; the writing of the dissertation – and probably even more the oral defence – is metaphorically regarded as a journey (probably not as much a walk in the park as rather a *Pilgrim's progress*), upon which the traveller in this case wants to keep a straight course. See also "Style: Metaphors", p 78.

5.2 *adoriuntur*] Another military metaphor, see p 79sq.

HUXHAM] John Huxham (1694–1768), English physician; his *Essay on fevers, with their various kinds, as depending on different constitutions of the blood, with dissertations on putrid, pestilential spotted fevers, on the small pox, and on peripneumonies* was published in 1739.

5.3 *CLEGHORN*] George C. Cleghorn (1716–89), Scottish military physician stationed mainly in Minorca. Published his *Observations on the epidemical diseases in Minorca from 1744 to 1749* in 1751.

5.4 *Stupor*] Latin word list, p 48.

Hydroas] See *Hydroa*, Greek word list, p 35.

5.5 *Insultus*] Latin word list, p 43.

epileptici] See *Epilepsia*, Greek word list, p 34.

eclampsia] Greek word list, p 34.

variolas in procinctu esse] A military metaphor, see p 79sq.

5.6 *inflammatoria*] See *Inflammatorius*, Latin word list, p 42.

5.7 *Delirium*] Latin word list, p 41.

5.8 *nisi febris status nimis depressus sit*] The principles for body temperature as a diagnostic means were not generally accepted until 1868, when Carl Wunderlich put forth his *Über das Verhalten der Eigenwärme in Krankheiten*, where he stated that "fever" is not a *disease* but a *symptom*, furthermore that a record of the body temperature would show different, characteristic fluctuations during different diseases.

In his book, Wunderlich credited Herman Boerhaave with having introduced the bedside use of the thermometer; Boerhaave did indeed include increased body temperature among the symptoms of fever, as put forth in *Aphorismi*, 563: *In omni Febre ... horripulatio, pulsus velox, calor vario febris tempore vario gradu, adsunt*, and made use of the thermometer (cf. Lindeboom, p 294ff; cf also van Swieten, *Commentaria in Hermanni Boerhave Aphorismos*, T 1, § 370, p 626: *In loco autem inflammato majorem ignis copiam adesse, docent thermometra*); on the other hand, heat was regarded just as *one* of the common symptoms of a fever, and, apparently, not always regarded as possible to measure exactly, cf. Schacht p 13: *Calor, cujus accuratus gradus neque sensu ... neque Thermoscopio determinari potest.*

The predecessor of the thermometer, the thermoscope (the difference between these is defined by Knowles Middleton (p 4) as a matter of the scale, which the thermometer has, but not the thermoscope), seems first to have been used for scientific purposes by the Italian Santorio, professor of medicine in Padua, at least from 1612 (*Commentaria in artem medicinalem Galeni*, 85.10). In 1632, the French physician Jean Rey writes (Knowles Middleton, p 27) that he sometimes makes use of a thermoscope of his own design on fever patients.

All early thermoscopes and thermometers, as they were of the open air type, reacted not only to temperature change, but also to atmospheric pressure, which made them less reliable, as stated by Pascal in 1648 (Knowles Middleton, p 28).

In 1654, however, the Grand Duke Ferdinand II of Tuscany sent out standardized, sealed wine spirit thermometers, probably invented by himself (Knowles Middleton, p 28sq), to several cities in order to make the keeping of a comparative air-temperature record possible, thus becoming a meteorological pioneer.

Still the only method for standardization of scales was the manufacture, by a skilled artisan, of several instruments at the same time, as nearly identical as possible with regards to dimension, which ought to have made any attempt at setting an international, or even national, standard fruitless. Nevertheless, the "Florentine thermometer" of the Grand Duke was spread across the continent.

In 1665, however, the famous English scientist Robert Hooke described his method of standardization, which consisted in placing all his thermometers in water, just about to freeze, thereby getting a common starting point for the scales, regardless of the size or shape of the specific instrument, whereupon he heated the water, at intervals making a mark on each thermometer. His method seems, however, to have been virtually unknown outside of his own laboratory.

In 1672, professor Sebastiano Bartolo in Naples suggested that the freezing point and the boiling point of water be used for the endpoints of the scale; the space between these points was then to be divided in eighteen equal parts, with special marks for "normal air temperature" and body temperature. Evidently, scales divided in 100 degrees had been thought of by, among others, Réaumur, but never actually used, until Celsius, in 1742, put forth his proposition of a scale ranging from 100° at the freezing point of water to 0° at its boiling point. In 1750, the scale of Celsius was replaced by an inverted scale. The actual idea of this inversion can probably, according to Knowles Middleton, be attributed to Linnaeus, and not later than 1745.

Cf. W. E. Knowles Middleton, *A History of the Thermometer ...*, 1966.

5.9 *critica*] See *Crisis*, Greek word list, p 33.

5.11 *miasma*] Greek word list, p 36.

orificium ventriculi] Latin word list, p 44.

Cardiam] See *Cardia*, Greek word list, p 32.

Illud … aggrediuntur] Yet another military metaphor, see p 79sq.

5.12 *plexus nervosi*] Latin word list, p 45.

a pari Nervorum octavo] At this time, ten pairs of cranial nerves had been described; the terminology differs somewhat between different authors – cf. e.g. Zedler, s.v. *Nerve*, and Blancardus – but the 8ᵗʰ pair is always that, which we today call the 10ᵗʰ pair, i.e. the *nervus vagus*.

5.13 *intra horarum paucas*] The partitive genitive with infinite numerals is mentioned in Sz § 52.a.β and K-St § 84.2.d; cf. also § 84.3.b, *anmerkung* 7.

5.14 *DIEMERBROEKI*] Ysbrand van Diemerbroeck (1609–74), Dutch physician, professor of anatomy and medicine in Utrecht. His *Opera omnia* were published in 1685.

5.19 *in binis reliquis*] *Bini* for *duo* occurs in ancient Latin (cf. Sz § 113.b with further references; K-St § 121.5), and is a common feature in Neo-Latin, cf. Östlund, p 50. One might also note that Petri Gothus, even as he indicates *Bini* as *Adjectivum numerale distributivum*, gives the Swedish translation *Twå* (two), while the German translation is *Je zween* (two each).

Variolaeque … verrucosae … evadant] for *evadere* in this sense, cf. my commentary to **Martin 4.9**.

5.20 *diarrhoea*] Greek word list, p 34.

spasmodica] See *Spasmodicus*, Greek word list, p 38.

5.21 *scrobiculi cordis*] See *Scrobiculum cordis*, Latin word list, p 47.

5.23 *carotides … & temporales … pulsent*] The *aa carotides externae* and *aa temporales superficiales*, respectively.

peripneumonia] Greek word list, p 37.

5.24 *potulenta*] This noun (npl, from adj. *potulentus*), meaning 'drink' as a collective, is found in Cicero *Nat. deor.* 2.141: *gustatus … habitat in ea parte oris qua esculentis et potulentis iter natura patefecit* (some edd. have *posculentis*), and in Apuleius *de Platone* 1.15: *ne esculenta et potulenta sese penetrarent*.

Since both these authors use the phrase *esculenta et potulenta*, one might suspect that the word in ancient Latin has been used only in this combination, as a set phrase; it might further be noted that the same phrase is also found in Medieval Latin, e.g. in Philippus de Leydis *Tractatus de cura rei publicae* ..., 65.12 (c. 1355): *qui recipere possunt esculentum et poculentum* (cf. *Lexicon latinitatis Nederlandicae medii aevi*, s.v. *potulentum*). As regards Neo-Latin, the sg *potulentum* is found in Petri Gothus, translated to Sw. *Allahanda dryck som drickas kan* (Eng. "every kind of drink that can be drunk") Cf. also **Schröder 11**.

oesophagum] See *Oesophagus*, Greek word list, p 37.

certocertius] This phrase, here written as one word, is known from Plautus' *Capt.* 644: *Quin nihil, inquam, invenies magis hoc certo certius*, further from Apuleius, e.g. *Met.* 2.7: *felix et certo certius beatus*.

5.25 *raro periculum effugiunt aegroti*] Cf. Cicero *Phil.* 12.30: *tanta pericula si effugero*; Caesar *BG* 4.35: *celeritate periculum effugerunt*; cf. also OLD s.v. *effugio* 2 b.

5.26 *suppurantibus*] See *Suppuratio*, Latin word list, p 49.

5.27 *pleuritis*] Greek word list, p 38.

5.28 *sanies salsum praebeat saporem*] One might note that this method of examining the pustules is merely mentioned by the way, thus likely not to be very unusual. Cf. also **10.20** below, s.v. *linctu*.

5.29 *sputa*] See *Sputum*, Latin word list, p 48.

tumorem] See *Tumor*, Latin word list, p 50.

ptyalismus] Greek word list, p 38.

5.30 *abscessus*] Latin word list, p 40.

Abscessus ... si maturantibus ad suppurationem redacti ... fuerint] This kind of construction, where an absolute ablative pertaining to the subject of the clause against the general rule takes the place of a *participium coniunctum* is known from Classical Latin, e.g. Cicero *Phil* 3.36: *nobis vigilantibus ... erimus ... liberi*; cf K-St § 140.9, SZ § 85.a.β.

6.1 *En itaque curam ... paucis tradendam momentis.*] See "Style: Exclamations", p 83sq.

6.2 *amuleto*] A word of unknown etymology, *Amuletum* is known from Pliny *NH*, e.g. 37.118: *totus...oriens pro amuleto gestare eas* [*iaspidas*] *traditur*.

moscho] See *Moschus*, Pharmacological word list, p 68.

7.2 *regimen frigidiusculum*] The adj. *frigidiusculus* is in ancient Latin found only in Gellius 3.10.16: *sed alia quoque ibidem congerit frigidiuscula*, where the sense seems to be 'unimportant', 'irrelevant', etc; for the Neo-Latin period, Hoven lists altogether some forty diminutives of this type; among these is the adv. *frigidiuscule*, explained as *d'une manière assez froide*, thus in a figurative sense; here, however, the meaning is with all probability that the patient and his room are to be kept rather cool in the literal sense.

a primo invasionis momento] Also a military metaphor, see p 79sq.

7.6 *diaeta*] Greek word list, p 33.

e regno animali] The division of *Naturalia* into three kingdoms, as seen e.g. in the Linnaean dissertation *De curiositate naturali* (1748, resp. O. Söderberg): *Naturalia … in tria divisa sunt Naturae regna, in Regnum nimirum Lapideum … in Regnum Vegetabile … Et in Regnum Animale* (In *Amoenitates academicae*, I, p 431) fits in well with the general tendency to categorisation at this time, even if it is based upon an overarching division of the Universe into *Astra, Elementa* and *Naturalia*, which to great extent is derived from ancient sources, most notably Seneca's *Naturales quaestiones*, book 2. Cf. also **2.1** above.

facile alcalescunt] *Alcalesco*, 'to become alkaline', is an important conception in the iatrochemical theories, which basically consist in the idea that "fermentation" is the fundamental principle of life; one further feature of this system is the thought that sickness is generally caused by an improper balance between acidous and alkaline fluids.

The inchoative verb *alcalesco* is not found in ancient Latin, but Hoven lists forty-six verbs of the type.

7.7 *infusum Theae, decoctum Coffeae*] The use only of the words *thea* and *coffea*, respectively, would, especially in this context, indicate the actual plant drugs; in a medical prescription, the method of preparation would also have to be indicated, as it is here. It might also be noted that 18th century Swedes apparently still understood that coffee actually should be *boiled* to be really salutary.

7.8 *Liquores spirituosi*] The following approval of a more moderate use of alcohol seems to indicate that this is not to be translated as 'alcoholic beverages' in general; I have taken the message to be that strong liquor is to be avoided, while a limited amount of e.g. wine might be consumed; hence the suggested translation.

autoptae] Plural of Gr. αὐτόπτης, 'eye witness'; not found in ancient or mediaeval Latin.

8.1 *filum tractationis*] For this kind of metaphor, see p 81.

8.2 *evacuantibus, an corrigentibus*] See "Drug categories", s. v. *Evacuantia* and *Corrigentia*, respectively.

morbo occurrendum] Another case of military metaphor, see p 79sq.

8.3 *cephalalgiam*] See *Cephalalgia*, Greek word list, p 32.

vena … amplo vulnere secanda est] Bloodletting had been considered one of the most beneficial medical treatments since antiquity; Celsus remarks (2.10) that the method is used in almost all diseases.

Throughout the Middle Ages bloodletting came to be regarded as almost the quintessence of medical or surgical treatment; cf. also **PHLEBOTOMIA**, Greek word list, p 37, and **VENAESECTIO**, Latin word list, p 52.

8.4 *Andreas HOFFART*] Andreas Hoffart, doctor of medicine and of *artes liberales*, published *Consideratio physico-medica variolarum Vratislaviae anno mdccxl epidemice grassantium* in 1742 (*Vratislavia* is of course Breslau, and not the Bratislava of today, which still was known only as Preßburg or, in Latin, *Presburgum, Posonium, Bosana* etc.).

Lucas TOZZI] Luca Tozzi (1638–1717), Italian physician, the successor to Malpighi as physician-in-ordinary to the Pope in 1695; his commentaries, *In Hippocratis aphorismos commentaria, ubi universae medicinae, cum theoreticae tum practicae celebriores quaestiones perpenduntur ...*, were published in 1693.

J.G. a BERGER] Johann Gottfried von Berger (1659–1756), German, published *Dissertatio de usu venaesectionis & clysterum in curatione variolarum* in 1711.

8.5 *Phlebotomia*] Greek word list, p 37.

globuli sanguinis rubri] Cf. **Martin 7.2**.

8.6 *scopo*] In Classical Latin rare, in Neo-Latin however a common word for 'aim', both of marksmanship etc., and, as in this case, in the sense of 'purpose', cf. e.g. Pufendorf, *De rebus a Carolo Gustavo ... gestis*, p 384: *Ad quem scopum obtinendum ipsos nunquam omittere omnia machinari in nostrum exitium*, and Svedberg, *Lefwernes beskrifning* (ed. Wetterberg), p 276: *ut ita scopum, ad quam tam rite, tam legitime vocati et missi sunt, felices adsequantur.*

Pulveres e Nitro purissimo crystallino] See *Pulvis e nitro purificato crystallino*, Pharmacological word list, p 69.

sale Ammoniaco] See *Sal ammoniacum*, Pharmacological word list, p 71.

Morsuli Citri] Pharmacological word list, p 68.

syrupi Acidi] See *Syrupus acidi*, Pharmacological word list, p 73.

Cerasorum Nigrorum] See *Cerasus niger*, Pharmacological word list, p 62.

Acetositatis citri] See *Acetositas citri*, Pharmacological word list, p 59.

Ruborum Idaeorum] See *Rubus idaeus*, Pharmacological word list, p 71.

clysma] See "Drug categories", p 57.

8.7 *cum grano salis*] cf. Pliny *NH* 23.149.

urina cruda] here 'not processed by digestion', see TLL s.v. *crudus* 1235,32 ff; cf. Celsus 2.7 *Urina tenuis et cruda.*

ichore] See *ichor*, Greek word list, p 35.

8.8 *refrigerantia*] See "Drug categories", p 58.

excitantia] See "Drug categories", p 57.

vesicatoria] See "Drug categories", p 59.

aquam Alexiteriam spirituosam Londinensem] See *Aqua alexiteria spirituosa Londinensis*, Pharmacological word list, p 60.

Contrayervam] See *Contrayerba*, Pharmacological word list, p 63.

Serpentariam Virginianam] See *Serpentaria virginiana*, Pharmacological word list, p 72.

floris Sambuci] See *Flos sambuci*, Pharmacological word list, p 66.

propinandas] *Propino* in the medical technical sense of 'offer to drink as a remedy'; cf. **Martin 15.2**.

Chinchinam] See *Cortex chinae*, Pharmacological word list, p 63.

MONRO] Alexander Monro (1697–1767), Scottish physician, published from 1732 *Medical essays and observations by a Society at Edinburgh*.

8.9 *Emetica*] See "Drug categories", p 57.

8.10 *nausea*] Greek word list, p 37.

8.12 *tubercula*] See *Tuberculum*, Latin word list, p 50.

denso agmine] A military metaphor, see p 79sq.

8.13 *tubercula disparuerint*] *Dispareo* for 'disappear' is not uncommon in Neo-Latin, which, as Hans Helander points out in *Swedish Neo-Latin literature 1650–1720* (in *Mare Balticum – Mare Nostrum*, pp 38–52), is due to its (dubious) occurrence in Lactantius and hence in contemporary dictionaries (p 49, note 18). In Krebs-Schmalz the word is said to be *nicht nachzuahmen für* evanesco *u. ä.* (I, p 415).

8.14 *plethoricis*] See *Plethoricus*, Greek word list, p 38.

sonticas ob caussas] *sonticus* (normally *sonticus morbus* or *sontica causa*) seems to be an originally legal term, indicating lawful excuse because of disease or from some other reason. The earliest occurrence is in Cato the elder: … *caussam sonticam* (*Orat. frag.* 58, ed. Jordan); the term is otherwise rather frequent in Julianus' *Digesta*. One might also note that Petri Gothus misinterprets the word, giving the Swedish translation *Skadelig*, German *Schadhaft* (Eng. 'harmful' – a disease would indeed have to be harmful to be *sonticus*!). In Bergius' text, however, the sense is clearly closer to that of the ancient usage, albeit modified to simply mean 'valid' in a general sense.

8.15 *radix Ipecacuanhae*] Pharmacological word list, p 71.

drachmae ß] 'Half a drachm'; the symbol is, in spite of its appearance in the original print, probably rather intended as an 'ss'-ligature than as a Greek β (which in Grun's

Schlüssel, p 102, actually is indicated as meaning *semis*, as is 'Ss' on p 105); it is also found in *Oraculum*, p 28; for *drachma*, see p 55.

Vinum Ipecacuanhae Londinense] Pharmacological word list, p 75.

8.16 *catharsi*] See *Catharsis*, Greek word list, p 32.

8.17 *Laxantia*] See "Drug categories", p 58.

obstipatio] Latin word list, p 44.

scybala] Greek word list, p 38.

8.18 *Cathartica*] See "Drug categories", p 56.

Decoctum Tamarindi cum senna] Pharmacological word list, p 65.

Cassia] Pharmacological word list, p 62.

Salibus catharticis] See *Sal catharticum*, Pharmacological word list, p 72.

Senna] See *Decoctum tamarindi cum senna*, Pharmacological word list, p 65.

Mercurio dulce] See *Mercurius dulcis*, Pharmacological word list, p 67.

8.19 *Diluentia*] See "Drug categories", p 57.

8.20 *corio …inflammatorio*] See *Corium*, Greek word list, p 33.

salivationi] See *Salivatio*, Latin word list, p 47.

pus] Latin word list, p 45.

8.21 *phrenesis*] Greek word list, p 37.

8.22 *saponaceis*] See *Saponacea*, "Drug categories", p 58.

Oxymel …Mororum &c.] The general meaning of *oxymel* is that of honey mixed with vinegar only. The genitive forms of various acidous berries etc. indicate several varieties of the preparation.

oxymel] Pharmacological word list, p 69.

Acetosae] See *Acetosa*, Pharmacological word list, p 59.

Berberis] Pharmacological word list, p 62.

Ribium] See *Ribes*, Pharmacological word list, p 71.

Mororum] See *Mora*, Pharmacological word list, p 68.

8.23 *quoad ejus fieri potest*] This expression, roughly 'as far as [anything of] it can be done', occurs in Petri Gothus, where examples of the construction of *quoad* with the partitive genitive *eius* are given e.g. from Cicero, *Ep ad fam*, 3.2.2: *Si eam (quoad eius facere potueris) quam expeditissimam mihi tradideris*, which of course renders the construction perfectly unassailable at this time.

In 1879, however, Jordan, in his *Kritische Beiträge zur Geschichte der lateinischen Sprache*, p 336sqq, declared the reading *quod eius* to be the correct one in every occurrence, which is assented to by Krebs-Schmalz (II, p 422) and indicated as the predominant opinion by K-St, § 84.3.c.β.

symptomatibus maturo occurrere auxilio] Also a military metaphor, see p 79sq.

Camphora] Pharmacological word list, p 62.

Laryngi] See *Larynx*, Greek word list, p 35.

Theriacam Andromachi] See *Theriaca Andromachi*, Pharmacological word list, p 74.

8.25 *Topica*] See "Drug categories", p 58.

Balsamum Embryonale] Pharmacological word list, p 62.

lacte cum Croco] See *Crocus*, Pharmacological word list, p 64.

aqua Cinnamomi] Pharmacological word list, p 61.

8.26 *ausimus*] Cf. **10.29**

epispasticis] See *Epispastica*, "Drug categories", p 57.

8.27 *ADOLPHI*] Christian Michael Adolphi (1676–1753), German physician.

mala …succedanea] *Succedaneus* or *succidaneus*, which is originally a sacrificial term meaning 'killed as a substitute or an addition', e.g. in Cn. Gellius (late 2nd century B.C.) *Historiae*, 4.6.5: *succidaneae … hostiae … appellatae, quoniam, si primis hostiis litatum non erat, aliae post easdem ductae hostae caedebantur*, is later to be found also in the sense 'exposed to a danger etc. in another's place', e.g. in Fronto (c.100–166) *ad Aurelium* 1 p 86: *succidaneum se pro vestris periculis subdidit*.

In Neo-Latin the sense has been modified to simply mean 'replacing' in general, cf. Petri Gothus, s.v. *succedaneus*, where the word is translated as *Then som sätties i ens annars stadh eller ställe* (Eng. 'He who is put in another's place or position').

The construction here, with the dative, is not known from ancient Latin, where the genitive seems to have been the norm, to judge from the very few extant occurrences, e.g. Ulpinianus *Digesta*, 26.7.3.8: *nec patiuntur succidanei esse alieni alieni periculi*.

FISCHER] Daniel Fischer (1695-1745), Hungarian physician; the title of his book would in English be "Report on the smallpox, which in 1740, -41, and -42 were raging in Hungary, during a rampant outbreak of genuine plague"

8.28 *speciebus emollientibus*] See *Species emollientes*, Pharmacological word list, p 72.

e facie revellendam] *Revello* in the more technical sense of 'pull up' etc, used in ancient Latin about skinning, e.g. in Ovid, *Met.* 9.168: [*cutis*] *haeret membris frustra temptata revelli*, and Columella 2.3.1: *pellem revellat nec patiatur corpori adhaerere*, but also in a medical context by Celsus: *resina subinde tempora revellere et imposito sinapi exulcerare ea quae male habent* (4.2)

sinapismis] See *Sinapismus*, Pharmacological word list, p 72.

8.30 *J. HAARTMAN*] Johan Johansson Haartman (1725–87), from Finland, studied at Uppsala University from 1748 to 1754. In 1753 he published *Indelning i Ört-Riket*, a Swedish translation of Linnaeus' *Systema Naturae* (2nd enlarged ed. 1777).
Haartman was to become professor of medicine at Åbo University in 1764, and is considered the pioneer of smallpox inoculation in Finland.

vesiculas] See *Vesica, vesicula*, Latin word list, p 53.

ingentem … copiam pedes occupasse] Military metaphor, see p 79sq.

8.31 *Difficultatem deglutiendi … profligavimus*] Military metaphor, see p 79sq.

Gargarismate] See *Gargarisma*, "Drug categories", p 58.

Herba] See *Herba rutae*, Pharmacological word list, p 66.

Menthae crispae] See *Mentha crispa*, Pharmacological word list, p 67.

Salviae] See *Salvia*, Pharmacological word list, p 72.

8.32 *aqua Vitrioli caerulea Londinensi*] See *Aqua vitriolica caerulea*, Pharmacological word list, p 62.

Alumine crystallino] See *Alumen crystallinum*, Pharmacological word list, p 60.

Vitriolo Martis] See *Vitriolum martis*, Pharmacological word list, p 75.

8.33 *cataplasmate*] See *Cataplasma*, "Drug categories", p 56.

Recipe …misceatur] As is seen from the *invocatio* (the imperative *recipe*, sometimes written as a ℞, which, acc. to Bendz, *Latin för medicinare*, 1950, p 339, originally was the ♃-sign, indicating the invocation of Jupiter, later of God), from the *praescriptio*, with the amounts of each substance involved being indicated, and from the *subscriptio* (the hortative subjunctive *misceatur*) regarding method of preparation, this is a genuine prescription.

Salis Absinthii vere alcalinis] See *Sal absinthii vere alcaline*, Pharmacological word list, p 71.

Aquae stillatitiae menthae crispae] See *Aqua stillatitia*, Pharmacological word list, p 61.

8.34 *expellentibus*] See *Expellentia*, "Drug categories", p 58.

9.1 *ambitum petiit miasma*] For *ambitus* in the sense of 'periphery' or 'surface', cf. TLL 1860.4, where it is indicated that Caelius Aurelianus uses *ambitus* in a medical context, e.g. in *Chron.* 2.6.91 [*convenit*] *spongiarum … admotio gutturi per ambitum faucium, quem anthereona vocant*, and 5.4.65: *quoniam non solo ex ambitu vesicae fluor iste fiet, sed etiam ex collo.*

9.2 *Febrem semper normae & regulae instar sequamur*] This might indicate that the fluctuations of the body temperature were actually recorded, however not necessarily compared to any standard value; cf. also **5.8**, above.

flores Sulphuris] See *Flos sulphuris*, Pharmacological word list, p 66.

Ulmaria] Pharmacological word list, p 75.

9.3 *Decocta alba Londinensia Rhabarbarina*] See *Decoctum album Londinense Rhabarbarinum*, Pharmacological word list, p 64.

Diascordium Fracastorii] Pharmacological word list, p 65.

9.4 *nuchae*] See *Nucha*, Latin word list, p 44.

9.5 *screatu*] *Screatus* seems to be known only from Terence, *Heautontimorumenos*, 373: *gemitus, screatus, tussis, risus abstine*; it occurs in Petri Gothus.

9.6 *frigus cane angueque pejus vitetur*] From Horace *Ep.* 1.17.30f: *alter Mileti textam cane peius et angui vitabit chlamydem, morietur frigore …* Cf. A. Otto, *Die Sprichwörter und sprichwörtlichen Redensarten der Römer*, s.v. *canis*, p 69f.
     One detail of no particular relevance for this context, by the way, is that in both Horace and Bergius, *frigus* is mentioned in the context.

siphone injiciantur] The *siphon* is by Zedler, V, col 561, s.v. *canola*, said to be a tube used by early Christians for the distribution of wine in the Holy Communion; thus probably much the same as the normal sense of Eng. 'siphon' today; probably this is also the sense in this text, particularly since the other alternative, the "soda" siphon bottle – which indeed would serve the purpose well – seems not to have been invented until the 1830:es.

spiritu salis] See *Spiritus salis*, Pharmacological word list, p 73.

9.7 *ptyalismum fluxisse vidit* FISCHERUS] A case of abstractum pro concreto; cf. **10.43** below.

10.1 *van* SVIETEN] Gerard van Swieten (1700–72), Dutch physician who studied and graduated (1725) under Boerhaave. His *Commentaria in H. Boerhaavii aphorismos de cognoscendis et curandis morbis* were published in 1742.

10.2 *Resolutio*] In this case probably used as a technical term, meaning the resorption of inflammatory matter without any suppuration.

gangraena] Greek word list, p 35.

10.3 The reasoning of this paragraph might serve as an illustration to the iatromechanical way of thinking; the suppuration is thus thought to be brought about by the purely mechanical pressure exerted by the bodily fluids.

10.4 *Myrrha*] Pharmacological word list, p 68.

10.5 *variolae erumpebant die 2 ab invasione*] Another military metaphor, see p 79sq.

10.6–10.8 Judging from its overall structure, this part of the text seems to be a translation of an authentic case sheet.

From contemporary case records by, or under the supervision of, Nils Rosén, kept in Uppsala University Library (ms. D 708b) it is evident that such records, quite naturally, generally consisted of the kind of notes present here – as a rule written in Swedish, though – recording specific observations and prescriptions day by day in short clauses, a structure which probably would not be kept in the Latin if a case were related in any other way than by exact translation (cf. **10.9–10.10**, which is also a case description, however probably not an authentic case record).

10.6 *per tres sedes*] Even as this exact phrase is not to be found in ancient Latin, nor, as it seems, in medieval Latin, one could note that Marcellus empiricus in *De medicamentis liber* makes use of the verb *sedeo* in a similar sense: (28.58) *Laborantibus tenesmo, id est qui de perfrictione adsidue sedere cupiunt* and that he uses the synonymous *sella* e. g. (30.17) [*veratri sucus albi*] *detrahit pituitam et per vomitum et per sellas.* Cf. also **10.57**.

Pulveres nitrosos] See *Pulvis nitrosus & camphoratus*, Pharmacological word list, p 70.

10.7 *Corticem Chinae*] See *Cortex chinae*, Pharmacological word list, p 63.

punctum maturationis] cf. **5.26**.

10.8 *Anodyna*] See "Drug categories", p 55.

quavis vespera] There are eight instances of this common Neo-Latin feature in this text, all pertaining to temporal intervals, e.g. *Quavis …nocte* (**10.27**) and *quavis 7. hora* (**10.35**), cf. also **Martin 15.2**.

10.9 *deliquiis*] *Deliquium animi* is in Krebs-Schmalz I, p 374, said to be a Neo-Latin synonym for *defectio animi/animae*, which is also stated by Petri Gothus, who furthermore adds that *Medici Syncopen vocant.* The only sense of the word known from ancient usage, however, is that of an eclipse of a celestial body, e.g. in Pliny, *NH* 2.54, while one instance in Plautus' *Captivi*, taken to mean 'loss', nowadays generally seems to be read as *deliquio*.

10.10 *cortice profligabatur*] Regarding this military metaphor, see p 79sq.

10.11 συνεχέως] 'continuously', from συνεχής, continuous (to συνέχω, hold together).

10.12 *si haec minus arrideret*] Cf. **3.8**

10.14 *Illustris Dominus* PRAESES] Cf. **Martin 16.1**.

10.15 *Si pustulae retrocedant*] A military metaphor, see p 79sq.

res... altioris est indaginis] The use of *indago* for *indagatio*, originally a term from hunting, meaning the act of 'tracking down', 'encircling', etc, is not classical, but is found in Gellius' (c. 123–165) *Noctes Atticae* VI.16.6: *Hanc … peragrantis gulae … industriam atque has undiqueuorsum indagines cuppediarum maiore detestatione dignas censebimus.*

The transferred sense of 'investigation' or 'scrutiny', as here, occurs in Late Latin, e.g. in Ammianus Marcellinus 15.5.30: *consilium occulta scrutabamus indagine* and in Ambrosius *De Abraham* 1.6.47: *descende indaginis studio, ne quid sit quod fallat* ....

The exact expression used by Bergius is also found in a letter from the famous Swiss mathematician Jean Bernouilli in 1733: *Vix est ut credam Problema … solutum fuisse eo etiam casu, de quo dixi, videri rem esse altioris indaginis.*

Krebs-Schmalz I, p 659, mentions the phrase as a Neo-Latin construction, upon which the judgement is, that *diese Künstelei ist unnötig.*

10.18 *lethargus*] Greek word list, p 36.

cardiacis] See *Cardiaca*, "Drug categories", p 56.

pro re nata] 'In accordance with the circumstances', etc; this phrase is found in at least three instances in Cicero's letters to Atticus, viz. in 7.8.2: *animadverteram posse pro re nata te non incommode ad me in Albanum venire*; in 7.14.3: *cum ea praedia … habeamus cui ego praesum ut in iis pro re nata non incommode possint esse*, and in 14.6.1: *Antoni colloquium cum heroibus nostris pro re nata non incommodum.* Cf also **Schröder 14**.

10.20 *si oculos servare volupe fuerit apertos*] Cf. **Martin 18.2**.

linctu] *Linctus* as a medical term would normally mean an electuary, i.e. a preparation of a pulverized drug with syrup or honey, made viscous as to enable its effect to last longer by means of a slower passage through the mouth and throat. As the word is used here, it might have a widened denotation of a viscous preparation in general, not necessarily intended to be taken orally, but rather applied to e.g. the eyelids.

One possibility would of course also be, that what is meant here is the actual act of licking the eyelids, a thought which perhaps wouldn't be quite as nauseating in the 18th century as it would be today; cf. e.g. **5.28**.

10.21 *J.Z.* PLATNERUS] Johann Zacharias Platner (1694–1747), German; the *Institutiones Chirurgiae rationalis tum medicae, tum manualis in usum discentium* were published in 1745.

10.23 *Parentes … religioni duxerunt palpebras dimovere*] *Religio* in the sense of 'misgivings' or 'scruples' is known e.g. from Cicero *Off.* 2.51: *nec tamen … est habendum religioni nocentem aliquando … defendere*; cf. also K-St § 77.4.b.

10.24 *phlogosin*] See *Phlogosis*, Greek word list, p 37.

Nitrosa] Probably, *nitrosa* means preparations made with, or with qualities like, saltpetre. Cf. *Pulvis nitrosus & camphoratus*, Pharmacological word list, p 70.

Julapia acidula] See *Julapium acidulum*, Pharmacological word list, p 66.

10.25 *paregorica*] See "Drug categories", p 58.

10.28 *indomabilis*] An unusual word, known from Plautus *Casina*, 811: *si equos esses, esses indomabilis*; to be found in Petri Gothus, however not explicitly in this transferred sense.

10.29 *Syrupum e Meconio Londinensem*] See *Syrupus e Meconio Londinensis*, Pharmacological word list, p 73.

Elixir Paregoricum Londinense] Pharmacological word list, p 65.

qua gaudet] *Gaudere* in the mere sense of 'have' is quite common in Neo-Latin; cf Krebs-Schmalz I, p 564.

diaphoresi] See *Diaphoresis*, Greek word list, p 34.

haud diffiteri ausim] *Ausim* in the sense of 'go so far as', etc, is known from e.g. Plautus *Aul* 474: *hunc non ausim praeterire*; Lucretius 2.178: *hoc … ausim confirmare*; Tacitus *Dial* 8.1: *ausim contendere*. Cf. also **8.26**.

10.30 *in hac febri debellanda*] Another military metaphor, see p 79sq.

J.FREIND] John Freind (1675–1728), English physician, philologist and politician, who among other things published editions of Greek speeches and of Ovid; the letter to Mead mentioned in the text, *De purgantibus in secunda variolarum confluentium febri adhibendis epistola*, was written in 1719; in 1722 Freind was elected an MP, only to be imprisoned in the Tower in 1723 for political reasons. During his imprisonment, Freind wrote another letter to Mead, *De quibusdam variolarum generibus*, and also started working on *The history of physic from the time of Galen to the beginning of the 16. century*, which was published 1725–26.

10.31 *novumque … addi calcar febri curranti*] Expressions denoting 'the exciting of sb/sth already in action' are found in ancient Latin, e.g. in Cicero, *Phil.* 3.8.19: *Quamquam ille non eguit consilio cuiusquam, sed tamen currentem, ut dicitur, incitavi*, where it obviously is regarded as a proverbial expression; Otto, s.v. *currere*, p 102sq, lists several varieties, such as *ut currentem … instigem* (Pliny *Ep.* 3.7.15); *quo currentem impellam* (Jerome *Ep.* 66.13), etc; similar expressions have also been used e.g. by Homer: τί με σπεύδοντα καὶ αὐτὸν|οτρύνεις (*Il.* 8.293sq).

Otto further notes that the expression often is amplified by including the horse-and-rider metaphor, as in this case; of this type, there are occurrences e.g. in Ovid. *Rem. am*, 788: *Non opus est celeri subdere calcar equo*, and in Pliny *Ep.* 1.8.1: *addidisti ergo calcaria sponte currenti*, which might be Bergius' immediate pattern.

10.32 *Quid … videri?*] Cf. "Style: Rhetorical questions", p 84.

Quanta … febris! Quid putredinis!] Cf "Style: Exclamations", p 83sq.

198

10.33 *scenam ludere*] For this metaphor, see p 81.

10.34 *Dicas ... et magnus mihi eris Apollo!*] cf. Virgil *Ecl.* 3.104sq: *Dic quibus in terris – et eris mihi magnus Apollo – tris pateat caeli spatium non amplius ulnas*

10.36–10.60 Two more case studies, cf. **10.6–10.8**.

10.38 *variolae ...agmine ...magno faciem & pedes occuparent.*] You've guessed it! A military metaphor, see p 79sq.

10.39 *supine*] This adverb is in ancient Latin known only(?) from Seneca, *de beneficiis*, 2.24: *alius [accipit] supine, ut dubium praestanti relinquat, an senserit*. It is found in Petri Gothus, where it is translated as Sw. *Laatligha*, Germ. *Liederlich/hinlässiglich* with a reference to Seneca.

10.43 *Ptyalismus pleno fluebat rivulo*] Cf. **9.7** above.

10.44 *oleo amygdalae dulcis*] See *Oleum amygdalinum*, Pharmacological word list, p 68.

Sed quam subita metamorphosis!] Cf. "Style: Exclamations", p 83sq.

10.46 *refocillantem*] *Refocillo* is a Late Latin word, known from Jerome and the Vulgate; according to e.g. Petri Gothus and Forcellini it occurs in Seneca, *de beneficiis*, 3.9, which is no longer believed to be the case.

frustraneo] *Frustraneus* is quite a common Neo-Latin word for *inutilis, irritus*, etc. cf. Krebs-Schmalz I, p 558.

10.47 *Robe Sambuci*] Se *Rob sambuci*, Pharmacological word list, p 71.

10.53 *ad ... propinandum ... nos accinximus*] A military metaphor, see p 79sq.

10.54 *nycthemerum*] From Gr. νύξ, 'night' + ἡμέρα, 'day', i.e. 'the space of twenty-four hours'; the compound is in Greek usually spelled νυχθήμερον and occurs e.g. in *2 Ep. Cor.* 11.25 and in Galen 7.508.

10.55 *pulveres cum saccharo commisti*] The pf. ptc. *commistus* for *commixtus* is by Petri Gothus given as the only form, while, s.vv. *mistura* and *mistus*, the forms *mixtura* and *mixtus*, respectively, are also provided.

10.56 *brunneum*] *Bruneum* or *brunneum* for 'brown' is mediaeval Latin, known e.g. from Johannes Busch (1399–1479), *Liber de reformationibus monasteriorum diversorum I*, 27 p 476: *birretum bruneum capiti suo imposuit*, acc. to *Lexicon latinitatis Nederlandicae medii aevi*.

10.57 *tres habuit sedes mucosas*] Cf. **10.6** above.

10.58 *Stragilectionem...exercuit*] From *stragulum* + *lectio*, 'collecting' or 'picking'; probably the same as 'floccilation' or 'floccilegium', i.e. 'The picking at the bedclothes by a delirious patient' (Dorland); cf. also Zedler, s.v. *Flocken sammlen oder lesen*, where it is said, that *dieser Zufall ist gemeiniglich ein gar schlimmes Zeichen*.

agrypnia] Greek word list, p 31.

10.60 *conflictatus*] This is also a military metaphor, see p 79sq.

10.61 *sphacelo*] See *Sphacelus*, Greek word list, p 39.

10.62 This passage is based upon *Philosophical Transactions*, 426, §§4–5, where §4 is an abstract of John Douglas' (see below) book *A short Account of MORTIFICATIONS, and of the Surprising Effect of the BARK, in putting a Stop to their Progress* ... and §5 is an account of the experience of *cortex peruvianus* in gangrene treatment, written by John Shipton.

RUSHWORTH] John Rushworth (1669–1736); this man is mentioned by Douglas as *Mr. Rushworth, a Surgeon in Northampton*, who is said to have discovered the effect of *Cortex Peruvianus* on gangrene.

AMYAND] Claudius Amyand (?–1745), Englishman, *sergeant-surgeon* to the king of England; also mentioned as having tried the *cortex* therapy.

J. DOUGLAS] John Douglas(?–1743), surgeon in London; his brother James Douglas (1665–1742), physician, published the abstract in *Philosophical Transactions*.

SCHIPTON] John Shipton (1680–1748), surgeon in London.

⌣] This sign stands for *spiritus* acc. to *Oraculum*, p 29.

10.65 *J. WALL*] John Wall (1708–76), a physician in Worcester, England; this contribution to the *Philosophical transactions* was written in 1746–7.

10.66 *Sed quid rei ...diu immoremur?*] see "Style: Modifying expressions", p 87.

ne oblivioni tradant genua saepius saepiusque flectere] Even if 'physiotherapy' as a concept is a relatively recent phaenomenon, the idea of motion and massage as a part of medical treatment can be traced as far back as to Hippocrates.

Of more immediate interest for the period dealt with here is, possibly, that Thomas Sydenham (see **2.1** above) reintroduced motion as a treatment by recommending riding for patients suffering from consumption, thus inspiring a colleague, Francis Fuller, to publish *Medicina Gymnastica* (1705).

One should, on the other hand, note that genuflection might well have been prescribed in considerably earlier ages, then, however, probably more as a means to promote spiritual than physical health.

11.2 *oleum ...Liliorum alborum*] See *Oleum liliorum alborum*, Pharmacological word list, p 69.

11.3 *manum de tabula*] This expression is used by Cicero, in *Ad fam.* 7.25: *heus tu, manum de tabula! Magister adest citius quam putaramus;* further by Pliny in *NH* 35.80: *[Apelles] dixit ... uno se praestare, quod manum de tabula sciret tollere.*

200

De epilepsia infantili, resp. Petrus Sundius,
text and translation

DISSERTATIO MEDICA
DE

EPILEPSIA INFANTILI

QUAM
CONSENSU EXPERIENTISSIMAE FACULTATIS MEDICINAE
IN REGIA ACADEMIA UPSALIENSI

PRAESIDE

VIRO NOBILISSIMO atque EXPERIENTISSIMO

DOMINO DOCTORE NICOLAO

ROSÉN

SACRAE REGIAE MAJESTATIS **ARCHIATRO**
MEDICINAE AC ANATOMIAE **PROFESSORE** REGIO ET ORDINARIO
ACADEMIAE REGIAE SCIENTIARUM ET SOCIETATIS REGIAE SCIENTIARUM
UPSALIENSIS **MEMBRO**
DIE XXVIII SEPTEMBRIS ANNI MDCCLIV
HORIS ANTE ET POST MERIDIEM SOLITIS
IN AUDITORIO CAROLINO MAJORI
PRO
OBTINENDIS DOCTORIS MEDICI HONORIBUS
PUBLICE DEFENDET

PETRUS SUNDIUS NICOLAI FILIUS

STOCKHOLMIENSIS
STIPENDIARIUS WREDIANUS ac REGIAE ACADEMIAE ADSCRIPTUS

—

UPSALIAE
Excudit LAURENTIUS MAGNUS HÖJER Regiae Academiae Typographus

A MEDICAL DISSERTATION
ON
CHILDREN'S
EPILEPSY
WHICH
WITH THE APPROVAL OF THE MOST EXPERIENCED MEDICAL FACULTY
IN THE ROYAL UNIVERSITY OF UPPSALA
UNDER THE PRESIDENCY OF
THE MOST NOBLE and EXPERIENCED
DOCTOR NILS
ROSÉN,
ARCHIATER TO THEIR SACRED ROYAL MAJESTIES
PROFESSOR REGIUS ET ORDINARIUS OF MEDICINE AND ANATOMY
MEMBER OF THE ROYAL ACADEMY OF SCIENCES AND THE ROYAL SOCIETY OF
SCIENCES IN UPPSALA
ON SEPTEMBER, THE 28TH, 1754
AT THE USUAL HOURS AM AND PM
IN THE MAJOR CAROLINE AUDITORIUM,
FOR
OBTAINING THE DEGREE OF MD
WILL BE DEFENDED IN PUBLIC BY
PETRUS SUNDIUS, SON OF NILS
FROM STOCKHOLM
HOLDER OF THE WREDE SCHOLARSHIP AND ASSOCIATE OF THE ROYAL ACADEMY

———

UPPSALA
Printed by LAURENTIUS MAGNUS HÖJER Typographer to the Royal University

Upon Him, that not only Royal favour, but also the extent of knowledge acquired at home and abroad, as well as the preservation of the health of so many human beings, has placed among our country's foremost practicioners of the Machaonic art; upon *You, most Noble Man,* we bestow well-deserved reverence and veneration, from a far distance we observe *Your* example, we depend upon *Your* advice, finally, we contend to prove our diligence and obedience to *You,* all of us who direct our energies towards the science of health. Among us I, overwhelmed by tokens of your benevolent affection, in return for *Your* merits dare to offer you this, albeit insignificant, pledge from an affectionate mind, and I will consider myself happy, if I in the future will benefit, as hitherto, from your protection. May You live, *Illustrious man,* may You live for King, citizens and science! May You live long and happily!

YOUR Most Noble NAME'S

most humble ward
PETRUS SUNDIUS

Regii Collegii Medici
ADSESSORI,
Urbis Metropolitanae
PHYSICO,
ut &
Regiae Academiae Scientiarum
MEMBRO,
Amplissimo atque Experientissimo DOMINO,
DOMINO DOCTORI ZACHARIAE
STRANDBERG,
PATRONO OPTIMO

Diu est, *Vir Amplissime,* ex quo in aere *Tuo* coepi esse. Inde enim ab ipsis meorum studiorum primordiis eo me apud *Te* loco esse voluisti, quo solent ii, quibus optime cupis. Digna tanto favore quum rependere non valeam, accipe tamen eodem, quo ipsum me semper beasti, vultu affectuque, hoc aeternae in *Te* pietatis meae quantumvis exile monumentum, meque *Tibi,* ut coepisti, commendatum habe. Praeclarissima in artem nostram & hominum salutem merita *Tua,* non hac voce dicenda, sciens praetereo, utpote quae jam diu immortali cum laude *Tua* in ore famae & prudentum conscientia versantur. Cum publicis vero mea privatim vota conjungo, ut qui tot mortalium vitam diris fatis eripuisti, felicissima vita diu adhuc fruaris, illustre sic eximiae artis *Tuae* experimentum ipse futurus.

Amplissimi NOMINIS TUI

cultor humillimus
PETRUS SUNDIUS

To the ASSESSOR
of the Royal Medical Board,
The City PHYSICIAN
of the Capital
as well as
MEMBER
of the Royal Academy of Sciences,
The Most Prominent and Experienced GENTLEMAN,
DOCTOR ZACHARIAS
STRANDBERG
THE BEST OF BENEFACTORS

It has been a long time, *Most Prominent Man,* since I began to belong to *Your* friends. For from the very beginning of my studies, *You* wanted me to have the position, which is due to those *You* love. Since I cannot justly return such great a favour: accept, with the same countenance and affection as that, by which *You* have always made me happy, this, albeit slight, token of my eternal respect to *You,* and appreciate me as *You* have done before. *Your* splendid merits regarding our art and the public welfare, impossible to display in these words, I will deliberately pass over; they are long since, as is *Your* fame, spread by rumour and known to wise men. But I will add to the public prayers my personal wish, that *You,* who have saved so many human lives from a sad fate, will enjoy a happy life for many years yet, and thus yourself become a splendid proof of *Your* excellent art.

YOUR Most Prominent NAME'S

most humble admirer
PETRUS SUNDIUS

Ecclesiae Almungensis
PASTORI,
Vicinique Contractus
PRAEPOSITO,
VIRO Admodum Reverendo atque Praeclarissimo,
DOMINO JOHANNI SUNDIO:

Officinarum Ferrearum
INSPECTORI,
VIRO Spectatissimo Prudentissimoque,
DOMINO

CHRISTIANO SUNDIO:

PATRUIS omni pietatis genere suspiciendis

Dum *Nominibus Vestris, Patrui Optimi,* multis de caussis praecipue mihi colendis, hanc Dissertationem inscribo, non tam consuetudini obsequor, quam pietati meae, & officio fungor, quod & sanguinis jura & plurimorum in me beneficiorum *Vestrorum* animo penitus infixa memoria exigit. Nolite vero, *Patrui Carissimi,* ex hujus munusculi tenuitate meum erga *Vos* adfectum metiri. Multo potiora & vellem & deberem. Sed felicium dona *Vos* dare sueti a me non expectatis: venerabundum animum, quo solo gratus esse possum, meritissimo jure a me postulatis. Hunc nullo unquam tempore apud me desiderabitis, in pia vota effusum, dignetur rerum vitaeque nostrae Arbiter Summus ingravescenti aetati vestrae divino robore adesse, ut de sacro grege, de bonis omnibus, deque nobis, felici necessitudine *Vobis* junctis, quemadmodum soletis, diutissime adhuc bene mereri possitis

Carissimorum NOMINUM VESTRORUM

cultor observantissimus
PETRUS SUNDIUS

To the
VICAR
at the church in Almunge,
and DEAN
of the surrounding Deanery,
The Most Venerable and Illustrious
Mr JOHANNES SUNDIUS:

To the
INSPECTOR
of the Iron Works,
The Distinguished and Wise
MR

CHRISTIAN SUNDIUS:

My UNCLES, worthy of all kinds of respect.

As I write *Your Names,* for so many reasons worthy of my admiration, my *Good Uncles,* in this dissertation, I do not so much follow tradition as I obey my own affection and fulfil the obligation, which both ties of blood and *Your* many good deeds towards me have planted in my memory. Do not, however, *My dear uncles,* judge my affection for *You* by the insignificance of this small gift. I would, and should, have given much more. But you do not expect from me gifts of the happy which you are used to give to others: *You* could justly demand of me a grateful mind, by which alone I can show my gratitude. *You* will always find in me this mind, exhibited in pious prayers, that the Supreme Judge over our lives and conditions may deign to be present in *Your* increasing age with his divine power, so that *You* for a long time yet may deserve well of the congregation, of the public welfare, and of all of us who are tied to *You* by a fortunate relationship

YOUR *Beloved NAMES'*

most respectful admirer
PETRUS SUNDIUS

Ecclesiarum, quae Deo in Nora, Skog & Biertråd
Angermanniae colliguntur,
PASTORI,
Admodum Reverendo atque Praeclarissimo DOMINO
NICOLAO SUNDIO,
PARENTI INDULGENTISSIMO.

Pia mente saepissime recordor, *Tibi, mi Pater,* non illud modo, quod in humanis maximum est, vivendi beneficium debere me, sed & innumera tenerrimi amoris benignissimaeque de salute mea curae documenta, quibus propemodum alterius vitae auctor mihi exstitisti, accepta referre. Quae cogitatio sicut obaeratum animum intimo officii sensu afficit, ita sollicitum pariter reddit, quo modo digna quaedam pietatis in *Te* meae indicia exhibere *Tibi* queam. Video enim ipsa meritorum de me *Tuorum* magnitudine ac numero omnem in me, non referendae modo gratiae, sed vocis etiam calamique in iis praedicandis, conatum vinci et superari. *Tu* vero, *mi Pater,* gratuiti amoris non aliam a me mercedem requiris, quam venerabundam gratissimamque beneficiorum *Tuorum* memoriam, non nisi cum spiritu ipso a me dimittendam: cujus ut monumentum aliquod publice exstaret, hosce studiorum meorum fructus *Tibi* sacros esse volui. Servet *Te* Aeternum Numen Ecclesiae usibus, cujus in ardua cura vitam viresque consumis, servet nobis, quorum *Tuae* innexa salus est; *Tuam*que senectam omni felicitatis genere florentissimam reddat.

PARENTIS INDULGENTISSIMI

Filius Obsequentissimus
PETRUS SUNDIUS.

To THE VICAR
of the churches, which are gathered for God's sake, in Nora, Skog and Biertrå,
in the province of Ångermanland,
The Most Venerable and Illustrious

NILS SUNDIUS,

MY MOST BENEVOLENT FATHER.

With pious mind I often remember that I am obliged to repay to *You, my Father,* not only for that, which is the foremost to human beings, the blessing of being alive, but also for the innumberable proof of tender affection and benevolent care for my preservation, by which *You* to me almost appear as the founder of a second life. This thought, just as it has provided my indebted mind with a profound sense of duty, has also left this mind anxious, as to in which way I might be able to give *You* a worthy token of my affection to *You,* for I realise that every attempt, spoken or written, not only to thank *You,* but also to announce them, will be surpassed by *Your* great and numerous merits. But *You, my Father,* do not ask for any other reward for *Your* altruistic love, than the respectful and grateful memory of *Your* charitable deeds, which I will not leave unless together with my very life: in order that there will be at least some monument of it, I wanted this fruit of my labour to be dedicated to *You.* May the Eternal Deity keep *You* to serve the Church, in the ardent care of which you spend *Your* life and energy, may He preserve us, whose welfare is connected to *Yours,* may He make *Your* old age bloom with all happiness.

MY MOST BENEVOLENT FATHER'S

Most Obedient Son
PETRUS SUNDIUS.

Singulari, quo res humanae reguntur, fatorum ordine ac consilio evenit, ut quos eadem terra, idem parens progenuit, longissimis haud raro locorum intervallis disjungantur. Id cum & nobis acciderit, ego, ut sangvine, sic animo, *Tecum, mi Frater,* omni tempore conjunctissimus, *Tui* desiderium gravissime ferrem, nisi & Magni REGIS gratia in eo *Te* honoris ac fortunae gradu collocasset, ad quem ingenio & industria viam *Tibi* raro exemplo paravisti: & *Tu Ipse,* quamvis procul patrio lare remotus, non mutati tamen fraterni adfectus meique memoris animi luculentissima documenta mihi exhibuisses. Accipe jam exiguum hoc, quod *Tibi* offero, mei vicissim in *Te* amoris & observantiae pignus, *Tibi*que persuade, neminem praesente rerum *Tuarum* florentissimo statu me vel suavius adfici posse, vel diuturnitatem ejus ardentioribus votis exoptare.

Exoptatissimo NOMINI TUO

addictissimus
PETRUS SUNDIUS

By the extraordinary ways of the fate, by which the conditions of human life are governed, it quite often happens, that those, which the same earth, the same parents, have procreated, are separated by a long distance. Since this has also happened to us, I, always closely tied to *You, my Brother*, by blood as well as by spirit, would hardly sustain *Your* absence, were it not that the grace of a Great KING had placed *You* in the position of honour and fortune, to which talent and diligence in a unique manner have paved *Your* way: and were it not that *You Yourself* had, albeit far away from your native country, given great testimony of your perpetual brotherly affection, and of your rememberance of me. Now, accept this small token, that I offer *You*, of my love and reverence for *You*, and be assured, that noone could be more happy for *Your* present flourishing position than I, neither wish for it to last in more ardent prayers.

YOUR Beloved NAME's

most affectionate
PETRUS SUNDIUS

0.1 Infantibus sensibiles admodum seu facile mobiles nervos esse experientia edocet. Horum magnitudo, ad exile corpus comparata, proportione multum excedit eam, quae in adultis reperitur. Cumque humoribus abundent infantes, major in eis nervorum mollities est, qui cum & tenuissimis membranis tegantur, subtiliorem inde tenerioremque sensum habent. Hinc fit, ut infantes facile adeo spasmis obnoxii sint. Qui si in uno alterove membro accidant, *Convulsiones* dicuntur: sin autem in corpore toto, cum faciei livore, existant, a recentioribus Medicis *Epilepsia infantilis*, ab Hippocrate *Eclampsia* appellantur. At morbum hunc Epilepsias genuinam esse speciem cuivis de hujus indole edocto facile patet.

0.2 Gravis profecto & difficilis est morbi facies, quem aditu prohibueris facilius, quam admissum expuleris. Plurimum igitur interest, praevidere posse, ubi metuendus sit. Huic timori locus est, si sub somno saepius riserit infans, si subitum & vehementem clamorem ediderit, si sopitus subinde expavescat: inprimis si eadem haec vigilanti acciderint. Haec tamen signa sola non sufficiunt. **0.3** Si vero infans simul adstrictiore alvo, aut febri, aut torminibus, aut mingendi difficultate, aut nascentium dolore dentium, aut vermibus laboraverit, vel nutricem vehementius animo commotam, aut externa scabiei remedia infanti adhibita fuisse, constet; jam non dubia imminentis Epilepsias indicia adsunt.

0.4 Si deinde ludentes errantesque oculos versus nasum aut frontem torquere coeperit infans, & in facie livor notetur, morbus jam incipit. Spasmus vel totum simul corpus adficit, vel per singula membra succedit: comprimuntur maxillae: os muco oppletur. Sequitur post breviorem longioremve moram quies & altus deinde sopor, ex quo expergefactus infans bene quodammodo valere videtur. Sed nisi caussa morbi interea tollatur, sequentis diei eodem tempore, & tertio pariter die, similis paroxysmus plerumque redire solet. Dein per aliquod tempus ut plurimum cessat morbus, sed rediturus quamprimum caussa eadem aut similis nervos stimulare coeperit.

0.5 Epilepsias infantilis plures sunt caussae, adeoque & species. Ei igitur ut felix medicina adhibeatur, in quolibet casu singillatim cognoscenda est caussa, ex qua tum oriatur. Neque enim Epilepsia universim, sed in certo quodam infante, ex determinata caussa proficiscens, curanda est. Enumeratis igitur diversis morbi hujus caussis vel speciebus, quo modo explorandae, & singulae earum quibus remediis tollendae sint, breviter exponam.

0.1 Experience teaches that children have more sensitive, or more easily ecxitable, nerves. The size of these, with respect to the small body, to large extent exceeds, proportionally, that which is found in adults. And as children abound in fluids, the weakness of the nerves is greater among these. As these nerves are also covered by thinner membranes, they have for that reason more accurate and delicate senses. Hence, the result is that children are more exposed to spasms, which, when they appear in one or another of the specific members, are called *convulsions*: if they appear in the whole body, accompanied by a bluish colour of the face, however, they are, by modern physicians, called *Epilepsia infantilis*, by Hippocrates they were called *Eclampsia*. But to anyone who has knowledge of the nature of this it is quite clear that this disease is a genuine kind of epilepsy.

0.2 The characteristic appearance of the disease, which you will more easily prevent from appearing, than expel when it has appeared, is truly grave and severe. It is of great importance, thus, to be able to see beforehand, in which instances there is reason for fear. Reason for this fear is present, if the child often smiles in his sleep; if he gives a sudden and vehement cry; if he is now and then scared while asleep, and especially if these same things happen to him while awake. These signs alone are not sufficient, though. **0.3** But if the child at the same time is suffering from constipated bowels, or fever, or colic, or difficulty in urinating, or pains from teething, or intestinal worms, or if it is manifest that the wet nurse is vehemently upset, or some external remedy for scabies has been used on the child, then it is obvious: there are unmistakeable signs of imminent epilepsy present.

0.4 If the child then begins to direct his wandering eyes towards his nose or forehead, and a bluish colour of the face is noticed, the disease is already beginning. The spasm either afflicts the whole body at the same time, or passes through one member at a time; the jaws are pressed together; the mouth is filled with mucus. After a shorter or longer interval, there follows quietude, and then heavy sleep, and as the child is awaked from this, he seems to feel quite well. But if the cause of disease is not meanwhile removed, a similar paroxysm usually appears at the same time on the following day, and likewise on the third. Then the disease most often will recede for some time, but will return as soon as the same, or a similar cause begins to stimulate the nerves.

0.5 There are several causes of children's epilepsy, and, above that, there are several kinds of it. Thus, for a successful cure to be adhibited, the cause for each specific case must be found out. And it is not epilepsy in general that is to be cured, but epilepsy in one certain child, and originating from a decided cause. After enumerating the various causes for, or kinds of, this disease, I will briefly put forth how they are to be examined, and by which remedies the specific kinds of it are to be expelled.

1.1 EPILEPSIA INFANTILIS *a Meconio retento vel alvo adstricta.* Si recens nati infantis alvus primis diebus ter aut quater quotidie soluta non fuerit, meconio sic plene non egesto, in corpore id retinetur, acre fit & intestinis stimulos, Epilepsiam efficientes, admovet. Ex iis quae dicta sunt, haud difficulter constat, ubi locum haec caussa inveniat, quae facile etiam tollitur clysmate ex lactis tepidi cochlearibus sex, olei olivarum quattuor, & sacchari pauxillo parato; & cui melius adhuc occurras Electuario e Manna, juxta quae in Calendario Stockholmensi Anni 1753 a Nobilissimo Domine Praeside allata sunt.

1.2 Accidit etiam, ut provectiorum infantum adstringatur alvus, dum excrementa partim indurescunt, partim acredinem concipiunt, & in utroque casu pressione sua ac stimulo Epilepsiam excitant. Quod dum fit, ex iis, quibus cura infantis commissa, cognoscendum est, an uno vel pluribus diebus occlusa alvus fuerit, simulque manu exploranda abdominis conditio, quod si intumuisse deprehendatur, aut in eo durities quaedam hinc inde sentiatur, clysma ad modum supra praescripti confectum confestim adplicetur, quo facto Electurii de Manna, aut tertia quavis hora syrupi cichorei cum rheo aequali parte olei amygdalarum dulcium recentis & frigide expressi vel olei olivarum & pauxillo saccharo, mixti, cochlearia pro theae sorptione usitata unum duove, exhibeantur, donec ventris borborygmi solvendae alvi indicium praebuerint. Rhabarbarum intestina corroborare novimus & efficere, ut facultate polleant excrementa, saccharo quod in syrupo est, emollita, exprimendi, quibus per intestina, olei beneficio laevigata, facilior via patet. Unde infantibus laxandae durioris alvi utilissimum adminiculum, nonnihil electi olei, per aliquod tempus quolibet mane dari suevit.

2.1 EPILEPSIA INFANTILIS *a Torminibus.* Et haec quidem Epilepsias infantilis frequentissimam caussam praebent. Ea vero apud infantes vel ex lactis, quo utuntur, vitio, vel nimia ejus accepti copia, vel ventriculi & intestinorum imbecillitate oriuntur. Quod infirmus infans sine culpa nutricis, torminibus laborare possit, evidenti experimento Nobilissimi Domini Praesidis constitit, cum bini infantes eadem nutrice uterentur. **2.2** Neuter plus lactis, quam opus erat, acceperat, & firmior unus bona valetudine utebatur, dum alter imbecillior perpetuis torminibus adfligebatur & viridis coloris excrementa dejiceret, acceptaque dein etiam propria nutrice plerumque tamen aegrotaret. Quare & nutrici ipsi & infanti huic adhibenda saepe medicamenta fuere, quorum ope servata ipsi vita, nec tamen valetudo prius, quam aucto paulatim corporis robore, confirmata fuit.

2.3 Torminum apud infantes signa in Calendario supra memorato exponuntur. Dum ex hac caussa oritur Epilepsia, sub ipso paroxysmo clysmate alvum sollicitare oportet, & si fieri possit, infanti cochlearia nonnulla minora olei amygdalarum dulcium recentis & frigide expressi infundere. Postquam autem praeteriit paroxysmus, diebus subsequentibus aliquot nutrix quater vel quinquies quotidie drachmam dimidiam sumat *Pulveris pro nutrice* Nobilissimi Domini Praesidis in Calendario nuper allato praescripti. Infanti vero in infuso theae cum lacte mixto vel aqua foeniculi pauxillum porrigatur sequentis *Pulveris infantum:*

216

1.1 EPILEPSIA INFANTILIS *from retention of meconium or from constipated bowels.* If the bowels of the newborn child have not been evacuated three or four times a day during the first days, and the meconium thus is not wholly discharged, it is kept in the body; it gets sharp, and applies to the intestines stimuli which bring about epilepsy. From what has been said, it will easily be quite clear, whereto this cause should be referred, which is also easily removed by a clyster, prepared from six spoons of luke-warm milk, four spoons of olive oil, and a pinch of sugar, and which you will counteract even better with an electuary of manna, in accordance with that which is put forth, in the Stockholm calendar for the year 1753, by the Honourable Praeses.

    1.2 It also happens, that the bowels of older children are to costive, while the excrements partly harden, partly assume a sharpness, and in both cases incite epilepsy by their pressure and stimulation. When this happens, it should be investigated, by inquiring of those, in whose care the child has been committed, whether the bowels have been closed for one, or several days. At the same time, the state of the abdomen is to be examined by hand, and if it is found to be swollen, or if some induration is felt in one part or another, a clyster, made in accordance with the one prescribed above, should be applied as soon as possible. As this has been done, electuary of manna, or, every third hour, a teaspoon or two of *syrupus cichorei cum rheo*, mixed in equal parts with fresh and cold-pressed *oleum amygdalae dulcis*, or with olive oil and a little sugar, should be given, until rumbles of the stomach indicate that the bowels are loosening. We know that rhubarb strengthens the intestines, and makes them more powerful in discharging the excrement, which has been softened by the sugar of the syrup, and for which the passage through the bowels, which have been smoothened by the beneficial oil, has been facilitated. Hence very useful help to loosen constipated bowels, namely, a certain amount of choice oil, has been given to children every morning for some time.

2.1 EPILEPSIA INFANTILIS *from colic.* This also brings about a very common cause of children's epilepsy. It originates in children, either from some flaw of the milk from which they benefit, or from too large a quantity of it being swallowed, or from a weakness of the stomach and intestines. That a weak child might suffer from colic without any fault of the wet nurse is clear, from the reliable experience of the Honourable Praeses, as two children had the same wet nurse. **2.2** Neither of them got more milk than necessary, and one was stronger and enjoyed good health, while the other, weaker one was beset with continuous colic, and excreted green-coloured excrement. Even after he then had got his own wet nurse, he was often sick. Therefore, both the wet nurse herself and the child often had to take medicine, by which his life was saved, while his health was not stabilized until the strength of his body had gradually been increased.

    2.3 The signs of colic among children are put forth in the above-mentioned calendar.

When epilepsy arises from this cause, the bowels should be stimulated by a clyster during the very paroxysm, and if it is possible, the child should receive several small spoons of fresh and cold-pressed *oleum amygdalae dulcis*. When the paroxysm has passed away, however, the wet nurse should, during a couple of the following days, four or five times a day take half a drachm of the *pulvis pro nutrice* which is prescribed by the Honourable Praeses in the just mentioned calendar. To the child should be given, in tea mixed with milk, or in *aqua foeniculi*, a little of the following *pulvis infantum*:

2.4 Recipe Magnesiae albae drachmam, seminum anisi scrupulos duos, Croci scrupulum dimidium, sacchari albi drachmas binas; Probe trita & mixta dentur & serventur usui. Horum remediorum usum continuare & nutrix ipsa & infans debent, donec excrementis debitus color redierit. Interea, ne in eundem morbum recidat infans, diaeta, in Calendario Stockholmense hujus anni nutrici praescripta, accurate observanda est.

3.1 EPILEPSIA INFANTILIS *ab affectibus animi nutricis.* Si nutrix vehementius animo commota infanti mox ubera praebuerit, plerumque Epilepsia inde oritur. Nec ullus sane animi motus ira nutricis gravior infanti accidit tristioresque in eo effectus producit. Hunc affectum ipsa quoque melius fere, quam ceteros, occultare novit. Ejus vero gravem suspicionem praebet inusitatus in ea oculorum splendor, alternus faciei rubor & pallor, vox cita & perturbata; inprimis si sani paulo ante infantis facies repente flavescat, aut is, lacte accepto, ad vomitum subito sollicitetur, mox dolere incipiat, & quiete intermissa, subinde expavescat, qui motus in Epilepsiam denique erumpunt. Alioquin enim oneratus nimia lactis copia ventriculus vomitu levatur.

3.2 Optime autem & certissime facti veritas ex ceteris, qui in domo sunt, intelligitur. Plurimis vero infantibus vitam adimeret irritatarum nutricum animi perturbatio, nisi huic fere medela mox succederet ex contrario affectu, metu nempe, ne detecta culpa domo expellantur. Ejus enim timoris beneficio magna ex parte conquiescunt a priori affectu oriundi motus.

3.3 In Calendario Stockholmense hujus anni indicatur, quomodo irritatae, aut perterritae, nutrici subveniendum sit, ne infantis inde salus periclitetur. Si vero ex hac origine jam Epilepsia exstitit, mox clysmate injecto, cochlearia quaedam olei amygdalarum dulcium dentur. Paroxysmo exantlato alvi facilitas promovenda, id quod eo, quo saepius ante diximus, modo fieri potest. Nutrix vero illis uti debet remediis, quae huic casui apta commendantur in Calendario, cujus mentionem nuper fecimus. Si nihilominus insequente nocte inquietus infans subinde expavescat, detur ei nonnihil syrupi de Meconio Londinense cautione qua dictum fuit in Calendario Gothoburgensi Anni 1753 & sequenti die adplicetur clysma tribus ante illud tempus horis, quo priori die invaserat Epilepsia.

4. EPILEPSIA INFANTILIS *a Dentitione.* Ex nascentium dolore dentium, cum alvi duritie conjuncto, pariter Epilepsia affici solent, quamvis hoc in casu intra faciem plerumque spasmi subsistant. Haec species quo modo dignosci possit, in Calendario Gothoburgensi Anni 1753 docetur. Ubi modus simul ostenditur, quo & occurrere huic malo, & eidem mederi queamus. Sub ipso enim paroxysmo non alii locus est remedio, quam clysmati, & intus exiguae portioni olei amygdalini.

2.4 Take one drachm of *Magnesia alba*, two scruples of aniseed, half a scruple of saffron, and two drachms of white sugar: it should be given well pestled and mixed, and be kept for further use. Both the wet nurse and the child should continue the use of this remedy until the due colour returns to the excrement. Meanwhile, the diet prescribed for the wet nurse in the Stockholm calendar for this year is to be kept rigorously, so that the child will not relapse into the same disease.

3.1 EPILEPSIA INFANTILIS *from disturbances of the wet nurse's mind.* If the wet nurse becomes vehemently disturbed in her mind, and then immediately afterwards gives the child her breast, epilepsy is often brought about. No mental excitement more unpleasant than the anger of the wet nurse can overcome the child, and none brings about more sad consequences. She also, mostly, knows better how to conceal this emotion than any other. However, an unusual gloss of her eyes, alternating redness and pallor of her face, fast and agitated speech, give grave reason for suspicion, especially if the face of a child, until then healthy, suddenly turns yellow, or if he, by receiving his milk, at once is incited to vomit, subsequently starts to be in pain, and, his quiet being interrupted, suddenly is startled, which disturbance then breaks out into epilepsy. For in other cases, the stomach, burdened with too much milk, is relieved by the vomiting. **3.2** The true facts are, however, best and most reliably learned from the others who live in the house. But the mental disturbance of irritated wet nurses would deprive more children of their lives were it not that something like a remedy at once comes about from the opposite emotion; namely, from the fear that she would be expelled from the house, if her guilt were detected. From the beneficient effects of this fear, the disturbances arising from the former emotion to great extent settle.

3.3 In the Stockholm calendar for this year is pointed out, how irate or terrified wet nurses should be helped, so that the well-being of the child is not endangered. But if epilepsy has already been brought about from such causes, a clyster should immediately be given, and subsequently a few table spoons of *oleum amygdalae dulcis*. When the paroxysm has been endured the readiness of the bowels should be improved, which could be done in the way that frequently has been indicated above. The wet nurse should however use the remedies which are commended as being the appropriate ones in this case in the just-mentioned calendar. If the child nevertheless becomes restless and is suddenly startled during the following night, some *syrupus de meconio Londinensi* should be given, with regard to what was said in the Gothenburg calendar for the year 1753. The following day, clysters should be given three hours before the time of day when the epilepsy attacked on the day before.

4. EPILEPSIA INFANTILIS *from teething.* From the pains of teeth forthspringing, in combination with constipation, children are often afflicted by epilepsy, even if the spasms in this case mostly restrict themselves to the face. By which method this kind could be distinguished is told in the Gothenburg calendar for 1753, where also is shown the means, by which we can both work against this disease, and cure it. But during the very paroxysm no other remedy is needed than the clyster, and internally, a small amount of *oleum amygdalinum*.

5.1 EPILEPSIA INFANTILIS *a Scabie retropulsa.* Epilepsias infantilis ex hac caussa origo facile intelligi potest. Si enim affectum scabie infantem frigori expositum, aut ungventa illita, eoque modo scabiem magis minusve pulsam fuisse, constet, vix dubitari potest, quin hac ex caussa natus sit morbus. Sub ipso paroxysmo ea unice, quae in alia qualibet specie epilepsias, adhiberi possunt: eo autem praetereunte, necesse omnino est, ut nutrici quotidie detur Floris sulphuris drachma dimidia in lacte calido, mane & vesperi, &, si fieri possit, infanti semel vel bis de die Moschi grana bina cum sacchari albi granis decem optime trita. Si scabies dein prodierit, illa vice periculo functus est infans. **5.2** Nec incommode capiti, si achoribus intempestive inde fugatis originem morbus debeat, capillis prius caesis, imponitur emplastrum quoddam emolliens pauxillo emplastri vesicatorii admisto, aut simile attrahens: quo facto, intra exiguum temporis spatium rubescente cute, humores acres denuo prodibant, haud sine aegri solatio. Quo autem pacto curari porro scabies debeat, in Calendario Gothoburgensi hujus anni descriptum reperias, simulque indicatum, quo modo caveri queat.

6.1 EPILEPSIA INFANTILIS *a Febribus exanthematicis.* Accidit nonnumquam, ut Variolis, Morbillis, Febre scarlatina affectos infantes paulo ante, quam erumpant pustulae, invadat Epilepsia. Quae tamen hoc in casu periculo fere caret & indicio est mitiorem morbum futurum. Ei igitur non alia opponuntur remedia, quam quae morbo primario apta sunt. **6.2** Ad hanc vero epilepsias caussam intelligendam sufficit nosse, infantem antea variolis &c. non laborasse, iisque hoc loco & tempore jam frequentibus, contagione quadam in domum illam aditum fieri potuisse, infantem praeterea per triduum febri adfectum fuisse, adjunctis aliis indiciis, quae aliquam febrium illarum exanthematicarum significare solent. Aequo autem & tranquillo animo ferenda est haec epilepsia, lenioris morbi praenuncia.

7.1 EPILEPSIA INFANTILIS *a Vermibus.* Quae hisce originem debet Epilepsia infantilis, admodum vehemens solet esse, & repetitis accessibus saevire. Salutaris autem humano generi naturae benignitas in eo conspicitur, quod teneri infantes, solo adhuc nutricis lacte viventes, ab hoc malo immunes sint. Vermium quippe in eis vestigia, priusquam esculentis simul uti coeperint, nulla unquam observavimus. Haec epilepsias species omnium difficillime dignoscitur. Saepe enim infantes, forma & viribus florentes, emisisse vermes vidimus, ita ut ex facie hac in re tutum ferri judicium non possit.

5.1 EPILEPSIA INFANTILIS *from scabies being driven back.* The origin of childrens epilepsy from this cause can easily be understood. If it is evident that the child who is affected by scabies has been exposed to cold, or that a salve has been applied, and that the scabies in this way has been more or less expelled, it could hardly be doubted, that the disease originates from this cause. During the paroxysm itself, only that which is used in any other kind of epilepsy can be used: as this passes, however, it is absolutely necessary, that the wet nurse be given, every day, half a drachm of flower of sulphur in hot milk, every morning and evening, and that the child, if possible, be given two grains of musk once or twice a day, carefully pestled together with ten grains of white sugar. If the scabies then reappears, the child is, for this once, out of danger. **5.2** If the origin of the disease is to be referred to the scabies unseasonably having been driven away from the head, it would not be out of the way to apply, after cutting the hair, some kind of mollifying plaster mixed with a little of vesicatory plaster, or with something equally drawing. As this has been done, after a short while, the sharp fluids, while the skin is reddening, will again advance to the area, not without relief for the patient. How the scabies then should be cured, you might find described in the Gothenburg calendar for this year, and at the same time it is pointed out how it could be avoided.

6.1 EPILEPSIA INFANTILIS *from exanthematic fevers.* At times it happens that epilepsy attacks children who are infected with smallpox, measles, or scarlet fever, just before the pustules erupt. In such a case, however, it is usually harmless, and indicates that the disease will be more mild. No other remedies should thus be used against it than those appropriate for the primary disease. **6.2** To recognize this cause for a case of epilepsy, it is sufficient to know, that the child has not before been suffering from smallpox, etc.; that those already are prevailing on the place at this time, and that they possibly could have been given access to the house through some kind of contagion; that the child, above this, has been afflicted by fever for three days, together with other signs that usually indicate one of these exanthematic fevers. This epilepsy, portending a more mild disease, should thus be endured with equanimity and calmness.

7.1 EPILEPSIA INFANTILIS *from worms.* The kind of children's epilepsy that is referred to this cause usually is rather vehement, and rages in recurrent fits. The curative goodness of nature towards mankind is seen thereby, though, that small children still living on the milk of the wet nurse only are immune to this disease. I have never seen any traces of worms in them until they just have begun to make use of ordinary food. This kind of epilepsy is the most difficult of all to distinguish. I have often noticed that children who are prosperous with respect to looks and strength emit worms, wherefore a certain judgement in this matter could not be brought about just by this external evidence.

7.2 Si vero infantem observaveris prurientes nares saepius scalpere, dormientem pavoribus infestari, in somno glutire volentis speciem referre, foetidum & acrem halitum emitere; si mane expergefacti os humore abundet, si colorem saepius mutet facies, si nunc fastidium, nunc appetitum cibi adeo vehementem ostendat, ut eo non statim accepto, proximus deliquio videatur; si appropinquante solito cibi capiendi tempore indurescat regio ventriculi & quasi tumeat; si sacchari aliorumve dulcium usus tormina illi adferat; si ex statu sano ad morbidum subito transeat; si de ventris doloribus, aut torminibus circa umbilicum queratur; si febris repente accedat aut vomitus, brevis utplurimum morae, sed alia vice, sine notabili caussa, aeque inopinato rediens: veri admodum simile est, vermibus eum laborare. Quos si antea eum dejecisse apparuerit, res dubio caret. Multis vero experimentis & propria oculorum fide constat nobis, quamplurimos infantes ex hac caussa in epilepsiam incidisse, quorum sub paroxysmo prominuisse umbilicum semper observavimus.

7.3 Quam vehemens haec epilepsia deprehenditur, tam facile paroxysmus ipse tollitur, si infantibus tantum adplicetur clysma ex lacte tepido, cui addendum nonnihil salis, si adstricta alvus fuerit: alioqui sal omnino omittendum. Neque vero olei quidquam, aut mellis, aut sacchari admiscendum: fugientes enim ingrata sibi haec remedia vermes altius per intestina adscendunt. Ceterum eo, quo diximus, modo praesens quidem paroxysmus vincitur, non tamen sine reditus periculo, donec plane extincti aut expulsi vermes fuerint. Quamprimum enim intestina perreptare dein & mordere, aut fugere coeperint, hoc stimulo novum excitant paroxysmum. **7.4** Nec praeterea sine noxa differtur idonea necandis ejiciendisque intestinis hisce hospitibus meddela; mora enim magisque numerus eorum & magnitudo crescit. Prolixiorem curandi hujus morbi descriptionem a Nobilissimo Domino Praeside expectamus; id unum monuisse jam contenti, teneris infantibus utilissimum esse edendi quotidie mellis & recentium radicum Dauci ubi reperiri possunt usum: provectioribus vero commendandam aquam mineralem, inprimis vero Seidlizensem, palato quidem valde ingratam, ad quam tamen bibendam invitari possunt injectis aquae in eodem vitro sapidis ejusmodi, quibus maxime delectantur, utpote confectio seminum Anisi &c, quae fundum petit, addita conditione, ut epota aqua, ubi fundum attigerint, his demum fruantur. **7.5** Ab ascaridibus, exiguis illis albisque vermibus, qui in parte intestinorum infima versantur, facillime infantes liberantur adhibito clysmate ex aqua minerali tepida, cui, si alvum solvere sola non valuerit, non nihil salis adjiciendum. Saepius autem repeti haec remedia debent: nam semel tantum usurpata pellendis omnino vermibus haud sufficiunt.

7.2 But if you have noticed that the child often scratches his itching nostrils, that he is startled in his sleep, that, while sleeping, he looks as if he were trying to swallow, or that he emits a foul and sharp breath; if his mouth is full of saliva when he is woken up in the morning, if the colour of his face often shifts, if he now shows disgust, now appetite for food so vehement, that he seems on the verge of fainting if he does not get it at once, if the stomach region gets hard and almost swollen towards the usual time for food, if the use of sugar or other sweet things brings about colic, if he suddenly, after being in a state of good health, turns sick, if he complains about pains in the stomach, or colic around the navel, if fever suddenly appears, or vomiting, mostly of short duration, but returning equally surprisingly on another occasion without known cause; then it is likely, that he is suffering from worms. If it appears that he has emitted such before, there is no doubt. From much experience, and by the reliable testimony of my own eyes, it is clear to me, that very many children have contracted epilepsy from this cause. I have noticed that their navels have always protruded during the paroxysms.

7.3 As vehement as this epilepsy is observed to be, the paroxysm is just as easily cured, if only the children are given a clyster of luke-warm milk, to which at times salt should be added, if the bowels have been constipated: otherwise salt should be omitted altogether. Neither should any oil, or honey, or sugar be added: for the worms, keeping away from these remedies that are disagreeable to them, will ascend higher up in the intestines. Furthermore, by the described method the acute paroxysm certainly is cured, but not without risk for relapse, until the worms are totally extinct or expelled. For as soon as they then begin to crawl through, and bite the intestines, or try to escape, by this irritation they provoke another paroxysm. **7.4** Furthermore, it is harmful to delay the use of appropriate remedies for the killing, and expelling of these hostile guests: by any delay both their number and their size will increase. I expect a more elaborate prescription for the cure of this disease from the Honourable Praeses: for the time being, it may be enough only to point out that, to small children, the habit of eating, everyday, honey and fresh carrots, when those can be found, is most useful: to older children, however, mineral water should be commended, and especially Seidlitzer, certainly most disagreable to the palate, but to the drinking of which the children could be attracted by adding, in the same glass, something tasty, of which they are particularly fond, namely sugar-coated aniseeds, etc, which sink to the bottom, with the condition, that these might be enjoyed only when the children after drinking the water reach the bottom. **7.5** From ascarids, those small white worms which live in the lowest part of the intestines, the children are most easily relieved by using a clyster of luke-warm mineral water, to which, if it has not on its own the power to loosen the bowels, some salt might be added. These remedies should, however, be reiterated: used only once, they are hardly enough to wholly expel the worms.

8. EPILEPSIA INFANTILIS *a Febre intermittente.* Exempla quoque infantum observavimus, quos sub paroxysmo febris intermittentis epilepsia adflixit. Quae cum toties redierit, quoties febris ipsa, hac vero curata, mox cessaverit; hujus epilepsias originem a Febre intermittente haud immerito repetimus. Adhibitum clysma insultum mox levavit, post paroxysmum vero febrilem redintegratis nonnihil infantis viribus, in hujusmodi casibus feliciter successit datum mox, justa cum cautione, lene emeticum, eo paratum modo, quo docetur circa finem Calendarii Londinensis hujus anni. Finitum vomitum secutus est celebris Peruviani corticis usus.

9.1 EPILEPSIA INFANTILIS *a Calculo.* Nec desunt omnino exempla infantum, hoc malo laborantium, quorum doloribus epilepsia conjuncta fuit. Ea est patriae nostrae felicitas, ut raro heic apud infantes calculus reperiatur, quod dum accidit, exploratu admodum difficilis est, quum ipsi doloris sui indolem & caussam describere nondum possint. Morbi hujus suspicionem praebet querulus clamor infantis urinam missuri, & hujus, sub continua doloris significatione, guttatim fluentis, aut subito impeditae prorsus cessantisque mora. Crescit conjecturae fides, si articulari morbo, podagra aut calculo, laborare parentes constet: magis vero adhuc, si digito in intestinum rectum immisso & ad vesicam usque producto, objici durum quid & simul mobile senseris. Certissime autem idonei instrumenti (Catheteris) indicio calculus cognoscitur.
9.2 Sub paroxysmo vena incidi debet & clysmata injici, quae prima vice ex cochlearibus aliquot tepidi lactis, tantundem olei & exigua sacchari portione, deinde ex oleo solo parantur. Duas pariter vesicas contusis lini seminibus, cum lacte & croci portione simul coctis ad dimidium usque impletas, unam superius, alteram inferius, adflictae parti adhiberi oportet, & ut renovetur calor, quamprimum refrigescere coeperit, mutare. Nec fructu suo tepida carent balnea. Interne commendatur lenientis emulsionis usus, quae paratur ex infuso florum Malvae, oleo amygdalino, ovi vitello & pauxillo syrupi e Meconio Londinensis ea scilicet lege, ut hujus infusi librae dimidiae admisceantur olei amygdalini frigide expressi uncia, vitelli ovi dimidium, & syrupi nominati drachmae binae. Ex hisce in vitro conquassatis facta emulsio infanti paulatim bibenda traditur, donec morbi dolores demum conquieverint.
9.3 Eam epilepsias infantilis speciem, quae ex venerea acrimonia oritur, scientes praetermisimus. Prolixiorem quippe curationem postulat, quamque describere loci angustia non permittit. Eam pariter silentio praeteriimus, quae ex alimenti defectu, ubi lactis inopiam celat nutrix, proficisci solet, detegenda facile, & novae nutricis copiosiore lacte brevi tollenda. Aliam adhuc morbi hujus speciem Medici commemorant, deglutito sanguini, qui ex praeciso lingvae vinculo, frenulo dicto, profluat, tribuendam. Haec remedio, vomitum leniter ciente, aut syrupo Rhei & clysmate, superatur.

8. EPILEPSIA INFANTILIS *from intermittent fever.* I have also seen instances of children, whom the epilepsy has afflicted at the beginning of a fit of intermittent fever. Since the epilepsy has returned, as often as the fever itself, the epilepsy will also disappear when the fever has been cured: it is not without reason that I derive the origin of this epilepsy from the intermittent fever. An applied clyster has immediately cured the fit, and after the fit of fever, when the child's powers have often been restored, a mild emetic, prepared in accordance with what is said towards the end of the Lund calendar for this year, given immediately, with due caution, has been successful in such cases. As the vomiting has ceased, the use of the famous *cortex Peruvianus* has followed.

9.1 EPILEPSIA INFANTILIS *from stone.* Nor do we completely lack examples of children suffering from this evil whose pains are accompanied by epilepsy. It is a benefit to our country that bladder stones are seldom found among children here, which ilness, when it occurs, is quite difficult to ascertain, as the children cannot yet themselves describe the nature and cause of their pains. Plaintive crying of the child when about to pass water, or the urine flowing drop by drop, accompanied by continuous signs of pain, or its suddenly being hindered and totally stopping, arouse suspicion about this disease. The credibility of this conjecture increases, if the parents are known to suffer from any articular disorder, from gout, or from bladder stone, but even more, if you have noticed that something hard and at the same time movable meets the finger, when introduced into the rectum and all the way to the bladder. A stone is, however, most reliably discovered by investigation through a suitable instrument (the catheter).
9.2 During the paroxysm, a vein should be opened, and clysters should be given: the first time prepared from a couple of spoons of luke-warm milk, with the same amount of oil and a little sugar added; thereafter, they should consist of oil only. At the same time, two bladders, half filled with crushed linseed, boiled with equal parts of milk and saffron should be applied to the afflicted region, one above and one below, and to keep the warmth, they should be changed as soon as they begin to get cool. Neither do warm baths lack their advantages. Internally, the use of a mild emulsion, which is prepared from an infusion of mallow flowers, *oleum amygdalinum*, yolk, and a little *syrupus e meconio Londinensis*, in such a way, that is, that with half a pound of this infusion is mixed one ounce of cold-pressed *oleum amygdalinum*, half a yolk, and of the syrup mentioned two drachms. Of the emulsion, made by shaking these in a glass, a little at a time is offered to the child to drink, until the pains of the disease have been subdued.
9.3 The kind of children's epilepsy that has its origin in veneric acridity I will deliberately pass over, as it demands a more thorough treatment, the description of which this limited space does not permit. I will likewise pass over in silence the kind that is brought about by lack of nourishment, when the wet nurse is concealing shortage of milk, but which is easy to disclose, and quickly cured, by the more abundant milk of another wet nurse. Physicians talk about yet another kind of this disease, which is due to swallowing of the blood, which runs from cutting the ligament of the tongue, the so-called frenulum. This kind is defeated by a remedy that gently provokes vomiting, or by *syrupus Rhei* and clysters.

9.4 In genere notamus

1:o. Secundam, tertiam, quartam & septimam epilepsias infantilis species frequentissime occurrere.

2:o. Venaesectionem fieri debere, si infans corpore sit bene nutrito, & ultra annum vixerit, nec alio morbo antea debilitatus fuerit.

3:o. Ori aperto inserendum aliquid, ne ex compressis dentibus vitium lingva patiatur.

4:o. Clysmata, ut felicissimum remedium, sub paroxysmo optime adhiberi. Cetera enim quae dantur, plerumque per os statim effluunt. Sub maxima paroxysmi vehementia officium gula detrectat.

5:o. Calefactum linteum, vino Rhenano calido madidum, infantibus sub paroxysmo circumdatum, mirifica virtute saepe pollere visum.

6:o. Excludendae epilepsiae gestandam ab infantibus amuleti loco *Verbenae radicem* frustra commendari. Plurimos enim infantes eam gerentes, epilepsia tamen saepius adflictos ipsi vidimus.

9.5 In solatium vero parentum illorum, qui de liberorum suorum salute anxii metuunt, ne repetitis ictibus infesta ipsis Epilepsia in habitum denique transeat, nec dissimulandum est crescente aetate ac viribus hunc morbum plerumque cessare, diminuta in fortioribus nervis irritabilitate illa, quae, ut praediximus, teneriores adhuc infantes eidem facile adeo obnoxios reddit. Parentes interim ad officia sua pertinere judicent diligenter notare quaecunque infanti vel ante paroxysmum, vel sub eodem, vel postea denique accidant: in vomitumne, an laxam alvum desinat: an in victu, cibo, potu, vel cura infantis &c. observetur quidquam, quod graviores aut leniores paroxysmos vel majorem minoremve eorum frequentiam moramque efficiat. Haec enim aliaque hujusmodi vocato Medico indicata plurimum ei lucis & adjumenti ad vincendum facilius morbum adferunt. **9.6** Si vero Medici copia non detur, ex his tamen observationibus parentes ipsi facile colligere possunt, quibus a rebus infanti cavendum sit, & quid praeterea facto sit opus. Sic, e.g., si decimo quarto quolibet die redeuntem paroxysmum vomitu aut laxata alvo finiri animadvertant, facili negotio intelligitur decimo aut undecimo post ultimum paroxysmum die, remedium, in priori casu leniter laxans, per duos aut tres dies continuandum, in posteriori, vomitorium pari modo infanti exhiberi debere. Pariter si docuerint observationes, quarta qualibet hebdomade epilepsia affici infantem, caussa inde nascitur explorandi, an illis temporibus nutrici mensium fluxus redierit, quo casu haec statim mutanda est, utpote quae vitio non voluntario, levissima saepe ex re animo commota & irritata, gravem infanti noxam adfert. Observatus item uno alterove ante quemlibet paroxysmum die foetidus infantis halitus, vermium praebet indicium, aut ventriculi vitium arguit, cui proinde accommodari tum cura morbi & vivendi ratio debet.

Solo Deo gloria

9.4 Generally, we could note,

1st: that the second, third, fourth, and seventh kinds of childrens epilepsy are the most commonly appearing.

2nd: that bloodletting should be done, if the child is well nourished, above one year of age, and has not before been weakened by any other disease.

3rd: that something should be put into the open mouth, so that no injury to the tongue is suffered from pressing the jaws together.

4th: that clysters, being the foremost remedy, are what is preferrably given during the paroxysm, as other substances which are given most often immediately flow out through the mouth. During the most violent paroxysms, the gullet refuses to perform its duty.

5th: that a warm linen towel, moistened with heated Rhine wine, and wrapped around children during the paroxysm, has often been noticed to have a wondrous effect.

6th: that the recommendation, that *Verbenae radix* be worn by children, as an amulet to avoid epilepsy, is in vain. I have myself seen many children, wearing this, who have nevertheless often been afflicted by epilepsy.

9.5 As a consolation for those parents, who, anxious about the well-being of their children, fear that the menacing epilepsy, by its repeated attacks, will eventually become habitual, it should not be concealed that this disease, as age and powers increase, most often disappears, as the irritability is diminished, which, as is said above, while the children are still small, quite easily makes them disposed to this. In the mean time, parents should regard it as one of their duties to note carefully everything that happens to the child, before the paroxysm, or during the same, or even after: whether it ends with vomiting or with loosening of the bowels, or whether something regarding the life-style, food, drink, or care, etc. of the child is observed which makes the paroxysms more grave or more mild, or makes their frequence, or their duration, greater or smaller. By telling this, and similar things, to the physician sent for, they bring him much enlightenment and help, in order to defeat the disease more easily. **9.6** But if there is no physician at hand, at least the parents could themselves easily conclude from these observations, from what the child should abstain, and what has to be done in addition. Thus, if they notice, for example, that the paroxysms reappear every fourteenth day, and end with vomiting or with loosening of the bowels, it will easily be understood, that a remedy should be given to the child on the tenth or eleventh day after the last day of the paroxysm: in the former case, a mild laxative, which should be continued for two or three days, in the latter, an emetic, given in the same way. Likewise, if the observations have told that the child is afflicted by epilepsy every fourth week, there is reason to investigate whether the wet nurse has been menstruating during these periods, in which case she must at once be replaced, as she, by a non-intentional fault, often disturbed and annoyed by the slightest things, inflicts serious injury on the child. Furthermore, if foul breath has been observed one or two days before a paroxysm, this indicates worms, or shows a stomach disorder, in accordance with which the cure for the disease and the way of living should then be altered.

GLORY TO GOD ALONE

Commentary, Sundius

This dissertation contains basically the same information, and is organized in the same way, as Rosén's *Underrättelser*, ch. 10.

STIPENDIARIUS WREDIANUS] Holder of the Wrede scholarship, one of the largest of several "magnate scholarships" (as opposed to the Royal scholarships).

ABRAHAMO BAECK] The famous Abraham Bäck (1713–95) had taken his MD degree in Uppsala in 1740; he was a member of the *Collegium medicum*, professor of anatomy in Stockholm from 1749, and the first physician of the Serafimer hospital from 1752. Bäck's main medical interests were the promotion of rural health care and medical education. See Lindroth, p 442sqq, with further references.

Machaoniae artis … principes] *Ars machaonia* for 'medicine' of course refers to Machaon, Gr. Μαχάων, the son of Asklepios, who appears in Homer *Il.* e.g. 2.731sq and 4.193sq; cf. also Ovid *Ex ponto* 1.3.5sq: *utque Machaoniis Poeantius artibus heros lenito medicam vulnere sensit opem*; since *Poeantius* – i.e. Philoctetes, who is mentioned in *Il.* 2.718 and holds the title role of Sophocles' play *Philoctetes* – was not actually cured by Machaon, the adj. *machaonius* apparently meant 'medical' in general as early as Ovid's time.

ex magno intervallo] The phrase is known from ancient Latin, e.g. Livy 6.1.2: *res … obscuras velut quae magno ex intervallo loci vix cernuntur*. Cf. also Virgil *Aen.* 5.320.
   The purpose here might be the underlining, either of the distance between Sundius' and Bäck's positions, or of the qualities and reputation of Bäck's being such that they are observable even from a distance.

ZACHARIAE STRANDBERG] Zacharias Strandberg (1712–92), Swedish physician, who had studied in Uppsala, where he achieved the degree of MD in 1741, whereupon he was recommended by Nils Rosén to the position as *adjunctus*, but declined to become Admiralty physician with the Swedish galley fleet. In 1745, Strandberg was elected a member of the Royal Academy of Sciences, and in 1748 also of *Collegium medicum*.
   In 1748, he also declined an offer to become Royal physician-in-ordinary; instead, he held the position of City physician in Stockholm until 1776, when he retired, only to devote his remaining lifetime to studies in, and the development of, agriculture and gardening.

in aere Tuo … esse] An expression used e.g. by Cicero in *Fam.* 15.14: *multi enim anni sunt cum ille in aere meo est*, to indicate a close relationship or obligation, at least in Neo-Latin usage also with a nuance of close friendship, as indicated by Petri Gothus, who, s.v. *Aes* (11), writes: *In aere meo est, id est, meus est. Seu: inter amicos meos est.*

JOHANNI SUNDIO] Johannes Sundius (1694–1781), clergyman, vicar in Almunge (the province of Uppland).

CHRISTIANO SUNDIO] Regarding this man there does not seem to be much information available beyond that which is provided in Sundius' dissertation.

NICOLAO SUNDIO] Nils Sundius (1687–1761), vicar in Nora (the province of Ångermanland) from 1746/7, dean from 1754.

ABRAHAMO SUNDIO BURENSUND] Petrus Sundius' brother Abraham Sundius Burensund (1715–?), who combined the family names of his mother Catharina Burman and his father Nils Sundius to form his own; Burensund became a civil servant in Norway, where he later was joined by his brother.

0.1 *Cumque humoribus abundent infantes*] The distribution of human beings into different categories with respect to qualities such as lean/fat, hot/cold, or humid/dry is found e.g. in Celsus 1.3, and is based upon the so-called *humoralism*, or *humoral pathology*, which generally is regarded as having been introduced by Hippocrates (c. 450–370 BC), even if the Hippocratic Corpus does not provide an entirely univocal humoralistic theory; one of the main features, the definition of four bodily fluids, viz. blood, phlegm, black bile, and yellow bile, is thus found in περὶ φύσιος ἀνθρώπου, 4, while other texts, as e.g. περὶ πάθων, deal mainly with two fluids, bile and phlegm, as is pointed out by Vivian Nutton in *Humoralism*, p 285.

The theories from περὶ φύσιος ἀνθρώπου were adopted most notably by Galen (129–c. 200), who enlarged the system as to comprise nine natural temperaments; he further regarded the actual four fluids as being physically invisible; human blood, e.g, is not equal to the elementary blood, but rather consists of all four humours in combination, albeit a combination where the elementary blood constitutes the largest part.

In its Galenic shape, humoralism was spread throughout the Islamic world and Europe; the idea of the *res non naturales* (cf. my commentary to **Martin 19.1**) also contributed to the success of Galen's theories, since it facilitated a certain degree of "self-treatment" (*Humoralism*, p 289).

spasmis] See *Spasmus*, Greek word list, p 38.

0.3 *scabiei*] See *Scabies and Scabiosus*, Latin word list, p 47.

0.4 *paroxysmus*] Greek word list, p 37.

1.1 *alvo adstricta*] *Asstringo* or *Adstringo* in the sense of 'make costive' is found e.g. in Celsus 1 *pr.* 68: *quae ventrem aut asstringunt aut resolvunt*, and in Pliny *NH* 20.75: *stomachum dissolutum asstringit cocta* ...; cf. "Language: Variation", p 21.

Electuario e Manna] See *Electuarium diascordium*, Pharmacological word list, p 65, and *Manna*, Pharmacological word list, p 67.

in Calendario Stockholmensi] The privilege of publishing almanacs in Sweden from 1747 rested with the Academy of Sciences, which published four different editions each year, representing the horizons of Stockholm, Gothenburg, Lund, and Åbo, respectively.

Since the print at this time seems to have been ca. 180,000 copies a year altogether (Vahlquist, p 53, referring to Sten Lindroth), and since the price originally was only 9 *öre kopparmynt* (ca. $^1/_{10}$ of a *daler silvermynt*, see my commentary to **Martin**, *Stipendiarius Stieglerianus*), the almanacs were regarded as a suitable means for spreading information – Nils Rosén had indeed made use already of the Uppsala almanacs for

1737–39 to communicate information on some houshold remedies – and in 1752, the Academy of Sciences decided to publish Rosén's observations on children's diseases in the almanacs of 1753; the Stockholm almanac referred to in the dissertation thus contained remedies for several diseases of sucklings, while the Gothenburg edition dealt with teething, and the Lund edition treated thrush and cough.

The publishing of Nils Rosén's articles on children's diseases in the almanacs continued up to 1771, when altogether fifty treatises had been printed in this way (Vahlquist, p 54). Since the almanac articles had been well received (not only in Sweden: Vahlquist (ibid) quotes a passage from the *Göttingische Anzeigen*, 1757, where a separate German translation is proposed), the Academy of Sciences had, in 1763, decided to sponsor the printing of a monograph edition, consisting of 1000 copies; in 1771 a second, considerably enlarged edition appeared.

1.2 *syrupi cichorei cum rheo*] See *Syrupus cichorei cum rheo*, Pharmacological word list, p 73.

cochlearia pro theae sorptione usitata] Apparently, there was no Latin word for 'teaspoon' available at the time.

borborygmi] See *Borborygmos*, Greek word list, p 32.

durioris alvi] In ancient Latin, *durus* is used to describe excrement e.g. in Celsus 2.7.5: *venter nihil reddit nisi et aegre et durum*; in the sense as used here, of the bowels themselves rather than of their content, the word is known from Pliny *NH* 28.129: [*lac*] *asininum* [*infunditur*] … *durae alvo in febre*. Cf. Horace *S.* 2.4.27: *si dura morabitur alvus*; Martial 13.29.2: *sume: solent duri solvere ventris onus*; cf. further TLL, 2305, s.v. *durus*, I A 3. Cf. also "Language: Variation", p 21.

2.2 *nec … valetudo … prius, quam aucto … robore, confirmata fuit*] This kind of participle construction coupled with a temporal adverbial can be found in ancient Latin, e.g. in Cicero *Cat.* 1.10: *vixdum etiam coetu vestro dimisso*; Livy 8.14.6: *nec prius quam aere persoluto*; cf. K-St, § 140, *Anm.* 4; Sz, § 206, β.

2.3 *Pulveris pro nutrice*] See *Pulvis pro nutrice*, pharmacological word list, p 70.

3.3 *exantlato*] *Exanclo/exantlo* (Gr. ἐξαντλέω, 'draw out' or 'drain', figuratively 'endure') is found in ancient Latin, e.g. (in the literal sense) in Plautus' *Stichus* 273: *vinum poculo … exanclavit*, and (figuratively) in Cicero *Div.* 2.64: *tot nos ad Troiam belli exanclabimus annos* (in Cicero's own translation of a Greek poetical work), and *Tusc.* 1.118: *cum exanclavisset omnes labores*.

About a hundred years later, Quintilian (1.6.40) regarded *exanclato* as an obsolete word, but in Neo-Latin it is quite frequent; Petri Gothus has *exantlo* in both senses indicated above, and the word is frequently found in the texts, e.g. in Johannes Loccenius, 1637: *Tot vigiles curas non exantlare valeret* and Emanuel Swedenborg, 1745: *ut exantlati operis praemium reportarent, urgebat*. (unpublished material by Hans Helander, 03). (In Souter, by the way, *exanclo* is said to be a medical term, meaning 'to drain of blood', which is entirely irrelevant here, of course.)

ante illud tempus, quo … invaserat Epilepsia] Another military metaphor, see p 79sq.

4 *modus … quo … occurrere huic malo*] This is also a military metaphor, see p 79sq.

5.1 *Epilepsias ... ex hac caussa origo facile intelligi potest*] It is not self-evident for a modern reader, but the general idea seems to be – even if **Bergius 3.12** refers to a probable external cause – that the *scabies* is thought to emanate from a process within the body, and thus could not be "pushed back" without other symptoms, in this case the epileptic fits, appearing; cf. also what is said about the necessity of the smallpox pustules e.g. in **Martin 8.2**. Cf. also Linnaeus, *Diaeta naturalis*, p 46: *Smolandi epileptici a repulsione scabiei capitis frigida* [*aqua*].

The widespread use at this time of vesicatories etc, is of course footed on very much the same idea, as is indicated in **5.2**.

5.2 *achoribus intempestive inde fugatis*] For the military metaphor, see p 79sq; for *achor*, see the Greek word list, p 31.

6.1 *Febre scarlatina*] See *Scarlatina*, Latin word list, p 47.

7.2 This entire paragraph was later to appear, in an almost literal Swedish translation, in Rosén's *Hus- och Rese-Apoteque*, 1765, p 83.

7.4 *Prolixiorem ... descriptionem ... expectamus*] Maybe a kind of advertisement for some forthcoming article by the *Nobilissimus Praeses*?

aquam mineralem ... Seidlizensem] See *Aqua mineralis Seidlizensis*, Pharmacological word list, p 61.

confectio seminum Anisi] Pharmacological word list, p 63.

7.5 *ascaridibus*] From the description of the worms in question, this is in all probability not what is understood by "ascarid" today, but rather the *Oxyuris vermicularis*.

9.1 *Calculo*] See *Calculus*, Latin word list, p 40.

mora] It is uncertain, whether *mora* here has its usual meaning of 'delay' etc, or if it should be interpreted as a more physical obstacle, which might be indicated by *subito impeditae ... cessantisque* in the context; *mora* in this sense is known e.g. from Caesar *Civ.* 1.64.7: *magna ... fluminis mora interposita* and from Pliny *NH* 10.84: *parva aliqua opposita mora*; however, no indications of *mora* seem to exist in any specifically medical sense.

Catheteris] See *Catheter*, Greek word list, p 32.

9.2 *emulsionis*] *Emulsio*, from *emulgeo*, 'milk out', denotes a milk-like substance, consisting of minute particles of the *emulgendum*, some insoluble substance, which by means of the *emulgens*, a soluble substance which gives the emulsion its somewhat viscous consistency, e.g. yolk or gum arabic, is suspended in the *menstruum*, typically distilled water. The term *menstruum* is, acc. to G&L I p 76, an old term from alchemy, indicating that certain substances by alchemists were believed to take one full month to dissolve completely. *Emulsio* is not found in any Classical or Mediaeval Latin dictionaries, neither in Petri Gothus; in English, the first occurrence, then spelled "emulction", is from 1612, cf. OED, s.v. *emulsion*.

librae] see "Weight units", p 55.

9.3 *ex venerea acrimonia*] This might be either an example of iatrochemical usage of language, in which case *venerea acrimonia* would mean "acridity [of the bodily fluids] due to venereal infection", or a case of *acrimonia* meaning 'excitement', which might have developed from the sense of 'vigour' etc, found e.g. in Cicero *Inv.* 2.143; Petri Gothus has *acrimonia* as synonymous to *vehementia*, which perhaps could support the latter interpretation; the sense indicated in Zedler, I, col 378, s.v. *Acrimonia*, is also mainly *Schärfe des Geblüts*.

On the other hand, "acrimony" in English can denote a particular quality of the blood, e.g. in Francis Fuller's *Medicina Gymnastica* (1711): "When the Blood of a Poor Consumptive Wretch is … loaded with Acrimony" (OED); since the text furthermore is dealing with epilepsy in small children, and since hereditary syphilis was not an unknown phaenomenon, I consider the most likely sense to be the iatrochemical 'acridity'.

Prolixiorem quippe curationem postulat, quamque describere loci angustia non permittit] See "Style: Modesty of the author", p 88.

Eam … silentio praeteriimus] See "Style: Metaphors of travel and movement", p 78.

frenulo] See *Frenulum*, Latin word list, p 41.

9.4 *virtute*] Cf. **Martin 13.3**

Excludendae epilepsiae … gestandam … commendari] *Excludendae epilepsiae* could, theoretically speaking, be a *genitivus finalis* in accordance with K-St I, § 132, *Anm.* 3, a, but is probably a *dativus finalis*, since the genitive form throughout this text is *epilepsias*.

As is pointed out e.g. by Alf Önnerfors (*Pliniana*, p 70sq), the usage of this dative was largely extended in Post-classical Latin; even if *commendo* is not explicitly indicated in this respect, it certainly would be a construction close at hand.

Verbenae radicem] See *Radix verbenae*, pharmacological word list, p 71.

9.5 *In solatium … parentum … nec dissimulandum est, crescente aetate … hunc morbum plerumque cessare … Parentes … ad officia sua pertinere judicent … notare quaecunque infanti vel ante paroxysmum, vel sub eodem, vel postea denique accident … Haec … Medico indicata plurimum … ad vincendum facilius morbum adferunt.*] The consideration for the parents, as well as the involvement of them in the therapy, is most certainly an important part of the qualities which rendered Rosén his good reputation as a physician; it is also quite in line with his ambitions regarding popular education.

De morbis infantum, resp. Johannes Schröder,
text and translation

[*A. S. M.*]

DISSERTATIONIS MEDICAE

DE

MORBIS

INFANTUM

PARS PRIMA

QUAM

INDULTU NOBILISSIMO NEC NON EXPERIENTISSIMO ORDINE MEDICO

IN SUPREMO AD SALAM LYCAEO

PRAESIDE

viro experientissimo

DOMINO DOCTORE NICOLAO

ROSÉN,

SACRAE REGIAE MAJESTATIS **ARCHIATRO**

MEDICINAE ET ANATOMIAE **PROFESSORE** REGIO ET ORDINARIO

REGIARUM ACADEMIARUM SCIENTIARUM STOCKHOLMENSIS ET UPSALIENSIS

MEMBRO

IN AUDITORIO CAROLINO MAJORE AD DIEM XXIII DECEMBRIS MDCCLII

HORA ANTE MERIDIEM SOLITA

MEDICINAE STUDIOSIS EXAMINANDAM OFFERT

JOHANNES SCHRÖDER

GOTHOBURGENSIS

———

UPSALIAE

[*A.S.M.*]
OF A MEDICAL DISSERTATION
ON

CHILDREN'S
DISEASES,

THE FIRST PART,
WHICH,
BY COURTESY OF THE MOST NOBLE AND EXPERIENCED MEDICAL ORDER
IN THE SUPREME *LYCAEUM* AT SALA,
UNDER THE **PRESIDENCY** OF
the most experienced
DOCTOR NILS
ROSÉN,
ARCHIATER TO THEIR SACRED ROYAL MAJESTIES,
PROFESSOR REGIUS ET ORDINARIUS OF MEDICINE AND ANATOMY
MEMBER OF THE ROYAL ACADEMIES OF SCIENCES OF STOCKHOLM AND UPPSALA,
JOHANNES SCHRÖDER
FROM GOTHENBURG
PUTS FORTH FOR EXAMINATION BY MEDICAL STUDENTS
IN THE MAJOR CAROLINE AUDITORIUM ON DECEMBER 23RD 1752
AT THE USUAL HOUR, AM

———

UPPSALA

TO

The most Honourable

SIR

DOCTOR NICOLAS

ROSÉN

ARCHIATER to His Majesty
the King of Sweden
PROFESSOR in Medicine and Anatomy
at the University of Upsale
MEMBER of the Royal Society
in Stockholm and Upsale

SIR

Great Experience together with kindness of mind are the true qualities, that render the renown of a Physician as immortal, as his Person universally belov'd and respected. If the Ancients have transmitted to us the Name of HIPPOCRATES, in spite of the Injurys of time, through a Course of so great a while ago; Our last Posteriority will not fail to pay YOUR Merits an equal Honour for being a SECOND RESTORER of that very Science amongst us. 'Tis therefore no Wonder if a great Number students of Medicine do seek for this renown'd Academy in Hope to reap a rich Harvest of their labours from the Skill of so excellent a Guide, as YOU are. For as the sick may recover his Health from YOUR Hands, so your Disciples wait for their Improvement from YOUR brighting Light. May it please YOU, SIR, to suffer these Lines, so to be inlighten'd by YOUR noble Name, as YOUR Worth and Favours have kindled my Devotion and burning Zeal, with which putting up to Almighty GOD dayly Prayers for YOUR uninterrupted Prosperity in many Years and that of YOUR dear and ever honoured FAMILY, i remain with a very profound respect

SIR

Your most humble
and obedient servant
John Schröder

TO

The most Honourable

SIR

DOCTOR NICOLAS

ROSÉN

ARCHIATER to His Majesty
the King of Sweden
PROFESSOR in Medicine and Anatomy
at the University of Upsale
MEMBER of the Royal Society
in Stockholm and Upsale

SIR

Great Experience together with kindness of mind are the true qualities, that render the renown of a Physician as immortal, as his Person universally belov'd and respected. If the Ancients have transmitted to us the Name of HIPPOCRATES, in spite of the Injurys of time, through a Course of so great a while ago; Our last Posteriority will not fail to pay YOUR Merits an equal Honour for being a SECOND RESTORER of that very Science amongst us. 'Tis therefore no Wonder if a great Number students of Medicine do seek for this renown'd Academy in Hope to reap a rich Harvest of their labours from the Skill of so excellent a Guide, as YOU are. For as the sick may recover his Health from YOUR Hands, so your Disciples wait for their Improvement from YOUR brighting Light. May it please YOU, SIR, to suffer these Lines, so to be inlighten'd by YOUR noble Name, as YOUR Worth and Favours have kindled my Devotion and burning Zeal, with which putting up to Almighty GOD dayly Prayers for YOUR uninterrupted Prosperity in many Years and that of YOUR dear and ever honoured FAMILY, i remain with a very profound respect

SIR

Your most humble
and obedient servant
John Schröder

à

monsieur

CHARLES

LINNAEUS

PREMIER MEDECIN du Roi de Suede
PROFESSEUR en Medecine & de la Bo-
tanique à l'Université d'Upsal
MEMBRE des Academies des Sciences de
Montpellier, de Berlin, de Toulouse, de Stock-
holm, de la Societé Literaire d'Upsal &
de celle de Nurnberg.

MONSIEUR

Les Eloges, que VOUS *donne tout le Monde savant, & les avantages, que nôtre Patrie a tiré de* VOS *Lumieres & de* VOS *travaux, fournisent de matiere trop ample aux plus eloquens, pourque j'ose y toucher par des foibles louanges; Car ayant ouvert à nos yeux le sein de la Nature,* VÔTRE *merite ne sauroit être assez étalé, que par ceux, qui en connoissent tout le prix, ou par un genie aussi vaste, que le* VÔTRE. *Puisqu' il n' y a presque rien au monde de si petit, ou de si peu d'usage en apparence, dont* VOUS *ne comprenez l'utilité;* VOUS *ne sauriez gueres apperçevoir quelque chose digne de* VOUS *dans ces sortes de Declarations de respêt. Voila pourquoi j' attend plus de* VÔTRE *Discretion, que de mes talens à* VOUS *plaire, ou à* VOUS *faire des homages dignes de* VÔTRE *illustre Nom. Il ne me reste donc, que d'avoir recours aux prieres, que j'adresse à Dieu, souhaitant qu'il lui plaise de* VOUS *conserver pendant longues années en toute sorte de Prosperité pour la gloire de* DIEU, *pour l'avantage du public, pour l'honneur des Lettres & pour l'appui de* VÔTRE *Famille. Je suis avec une profonde veneration*

MONSIEUR

Vôtre trés humble & trés
obeissant serviteur
JEAN SCHRÖDER

239

VIRO *Nobilissimo*
DOMINO ERICO
SCHRÖDER,
CAPITANEO Legionis Pedestris
Strenuissimo,
PATRUO summa animi pietate
colendo

VIRO *Admodum Reverendo atque*
Praeclarissimo
DOMINO MAGISTRI MARTINO
KIERULFF,
Ecclesiarum Tranemoënsium
PASTORI
Fidelissimo,
AVUNCULO aeternum colendo

VIRO *Consultissimo,*
DOMINO ARWIDO
KIERULFF,
Summi Dicasterii COMMISSARIO &
SENATORI apud Gevalienses
Aequissimo,
AVUNCULO summa pietate colendo

VIRO *Solertissimo*
DOMINO FREDERICO
KIERULFF,
MERCATORI in civitate Sanct Ybes
Prudentissimo,
AVUNCULO maxime honorando

Dissertationem hanc, ob maxima in se collata beneficia, cum omnigenae felicitatis voto, TIBI, Patrue
Carissime, *nec non* VOBIS, Avunculi Amantissimi *consecratam, voluit, debuit*
Nobilissimorum Admodum Reverendorum Consultissimorum nec non
Prudentissimorum
NOMINUM VESTRORUM

Cultor humillimus
JOHANNES SCHRÖDER

To the most Honourable,
Mr ERIC
SCHRÖDER,
A Brave Infantry CAPTAIN,
A paternal UNCLE worthy to be
piously honoured.

To the Most Venerable and Illustrious
MAGISTER MARTIN
KIERULFF,
Most pious VICAR in the Church in
Tranemo,
A maternal UNCLE worthy of eternal
honour.

To the Juridically Skilled
MR ARWID
KIERULFF,
COMMISSARY to the *Supreme Court*
and Most Impartial
COUNCILLOR in Gävle,
A maternal UNCLE worthy to be
piously honoured

To the Skilled
MR FREDRIK
KIERULFF,
A Most Clever MERCHANT in Sankt
Ibb
A maternal UNCLE to be most
honoured.

For the sake of the many kind deeds bestowed upon him, the most humble Worshipper
of YOUR *Noble, Most Venerable, Skilled and Clever NAMES,*
JOHANNES SCHRÖDER
together with all kinds of good wishes wanted to dedicate, and was obliged to dedicate, this dissertation
to YOU, my Dear Uncles.

HERREN

HANDELSMANNEN uti Götheborg,

Herr LARS

SCHRÖDER

Min Huldaste FADER

At de Barn äro lycklige, som födas af friska Föräldrar, samt, då de ännu uti lindan äro inweklade, upammas af sina egna Mödrar, och icke utam trånnsmål öfwerlemnas åt Ammor, hwilka, såsom legde, merendels den anförtrodda skatten miswårda, tilstå almänt wåra tiders störste *Läkare;* ty de få då det, som af en blid Natur är dem tildelt til at bortföra de orenligheter, de i Moderlifwet samlat, hwilka, om de qwarhållas, tilskynda dem en sjuklig lefnad och ofta en hastig död. De späda telningar undgå ock då tillika den faran, at, medelst en odygdig Ammas mjölk, insupa uti sin menlöshet sin egen olycka. Denna saken är af stor wigt, och har så wäl af förnuftet som dagliga förfarenheten sin styrka. *Huldaste* FÖRÄLDRAR! när jag eftersinnar, huru stor EDAR omwårdnad warit för mig äfwen i detta målet; finner jag min skuld wara stor. Men EDAR godhet har ej med lindan lemnat mig, utan sedermera, til min upfostran och tilwäxt uti nyttiga Wettenskaper, haft all kostnad och möda ospard. Huru kan jag wäl emot så många wälgärningar wisa mig rätt tacksam? Såsom et ringa wedermäle af wördsam erkänsla frambär jag nu förstlingen af mitt Academiska arbete, hwarutinnan jag bjudit til at beskrifwa de *Sjukdomar, som owålige Mödrar sin lifsfrugt påföra.* Uptag, *Huldaste* FADER, densamma med wanlig ynnest, och tro för öfrigit, at, fast jag icke en gång med orden förmår afskildra EDAR huldhet och min Sonliga wördnad, skall jag dock icke förr uphöra at prisa EDAR ömhet, och anropa ALMAGTEN om EDAR och min kära MODERS beständiga wälgång, än blodet medelst sitt omlop i min kropp afstannar. Jag lefwer med wördnad

Min Huldaste FADERS

Lydige Son
JAN SCHRÖDER.

HERREN,
HANDELSMANNEN uti Götheborg,
Herr LARS
SCHRÖDER

Min Huldaste FADER

At de Barn äro lycklige, som födas af friska Föräldrar, samt, då de ännu uti lindan äro inweklade, upammas af sina egna Mödrar, och icke utam trånnsmål öfwerlemnas åt Ammor, hwilka, såsom legde, merendels den anförtrodda skatten miswårda, tilstå almänt wåra tiders störste *Läkare;* ty de få då det, som af en blid Natur är dem tildelt til at bortföra de orenligheter, de i Moderlifwet samlat, hwilka, om de qwarhållas, tilskynda dem en sjuklig lefnad och ofta en hastig död. De späda telningar undgå ock då tillika den faran, at, medelst en odygdig Ammas mjölk, insupa uti sin menlöshet sin egen olycka. Denna saken är af stor wigt, och har så wäl af förnuftet som dagliga förfarenheten sin styrka. *Huldaste* FÖRÄLDRAR! när jag eftersinnar, huru stor EDAR omwårdnad warit för mig äfwen i detta målet; finner jag min skuld wara stor. Men EDAR godhet har ej med lindan lemnat mig, utan sedermera, til min upfostran och tilwäxt uti nyttiga Wettenskaper, haft all kostnad och möda ospard. Huru kan jag wäl emot så många wälgärningar wisa mig rätt tacksam? Såsom et ringa wedermäle af wördsam erkänsla frambär jag nu förstlingen af mitt Academiska arbete, hwarutinnan jag bjudit til at beskrifwa de *Sjukdomar, som owålige Mödrar sin lifsfrugt påföra.* Uptag, *Huldaste* FADER, densamma med wanlig ynnest, och tro för öfrigit, at, fast jag icke en gång med orden förmår afskildra EDAR huldhet och min Sonliga wördnad, skall jag dock icke förr uphöra at prisa EDAR ömhet, och anropa ALMAGTEN om EDAR och min kära MODERS beständiga wälgång, än blodet medelst sitt omlop i min kropp afstannar. Jag lefwer med wördnad

Min Huldaste FADERS

Lydige Son
JAN SCHRÖDER.

Min HERRE.

De snillen kunna med skäl kallas lyckeliga, som jemte hastigt begrep, hafwa fådt mogen eftertanka til följeslagare, hwilken både öfwerwägar de förut fattade ting, som äfwen förer hwarje til sit rätta ändamål. Blir Guds ära och Samhällets wälstånd ögnamärket; hwad sällare än det rike, hwilket af många sådane lemmar öfwerflödar. Det ämne, I Min Herre, til lärospån utwalt, witnar ojäfaktigt både om Edert sinne och snille. Wår Ungdom wisnar ofta bort, innan den begynt wisa sin blomma, til så stor sorg för anhörige, som saknad för fäderneslandet. De mäste dö bort i yngre åren mera af okunnoghet än nödwändighet. Huru wäl gör då icke den, som uptäcker de mördare, som så många späda barns lif dräpa, och framwisar de läkwböten, genom hwilka en tidig död förekommes, och inbyggarnes tilwäxt befrämjas. At berömma Edra egenskaper och id Min Herre, kunde jag hafwa så mycket större skäl som jag warit dertil för någon tid et åsyna witne; men Eder dygd synes förbjuda mig instämma til et wälförtjänt lof. Himmelens Herre, hwars fruktan har städse warit grunden uti Edra wisdoms framsteg, ware än widare Eder anförare: säkert lära de återstående lärdoms delar snart winnas, och belöningen utaf Anföraren utdelas!

Stockholm den 26 November
    1752

JONAS AHLELÖF.
Apol. Scholae Cathedralis Gothoburgensis

Min HERRE.

De snillen kunna med skäl kallas lyckeliga, som jemte hastigt begrep, hafwa fådt mogen eftertanka til följeslagare, hwilken både öfwerwägar de förut fattade ting, som äfwen förer hwarje til sit rätta ändamål. Blir Guds ära och Samhällets wälstånd ögnamärket; hwad sällare än det rike, hwilket af många sådane lemmar öfwerflödar. Det ämne, I Min Herre, til lärospån utwalt, witnar ojäfaktigt både om Edert sinne och snille. Wår Ungdom wisnar ofta bort, innan den begynt wisa sin blomma, til så stor sorg för anhörige, som saknad för fäderneslandet. De mäste dö bort i yngre åren mera af okunnoghet än nödwändighet. Huru wäl gör då icke den, som uptäcker de mördare, som så många späda barns lif dräpa, och framwisar de läkwböten, genom hwilka en tidig död förekommes, och inbyggarnes tilwäxt befrämjas. At berömma Edra egenskaper och id Min Herre, kunde jag hafwa så mycket större skäl som jag warit dertil för någon tid et åsyna witne; men Eder dygd synes förbjuda mig instämma til et wälförtjänt lof. Himmelens Herre, hwars fruktan har städse warit grunden uti Edra wisdoms framsteg, ware än widare Eder anförare: säkert lära de återstående lärdoms delar snart winnas, och belöningen utaf Anföraren utdelas!

Stockholm den 26 November
    1752

            JONAS AHLELÖF.
                Apol. Scholae Cathedralis Gothoburgensis

§1. Ex Anatomia & Physiologia constat
a) Infantum quam adultorum plures esse glandulas & majores, pluraque vasa.
b) Haec vero magis pervia esse & flexilia.
c) Immo, viscera eorum facilius liquores injiciendos admittere.
d) Eorum etiam sanguinem magis esse tenuem, floridum, solubilem & nutritium.
e) Quodque circulatio fluidorum in his sit magis citata, citatior coctio & secretio, copiosiusque corporis incrementum.

§2. Mirum igitur mihi semper visum est, qui fiat, ut densiora sint, quam adultorum, infantum funera. Horum quidem magis sensiles sunt nervi, sed nec adeo hi exponuntur caussis externis ac adulti.

Matrum, nutricum, ministrorum maximam esse culpam verisimile est, praesertim quum aegrotorum Infantum curatio obstetricibus feminis plerumque committatur, quas illorum Medicos facit opinio vulgi; sed huic quaestioni immorari non licet, id enim Volente Deo agam, ut paucis exponam, qua ratione Infantum Morbi vel caveri, vel ingruentes superari possint.

§3. Utero exclusus INFANS, & ab obstetrice rite curatus, in ulnas deponitur feminae lactantis, ut ab hac, post justum jejunium, alimentum accipiat, sibi a provida natura destinatum.

§4. Quae lac praebet, est vel ipsa MATER, vel alia femina, quae ejus suscipit officia & partes, ac NUTRIX dicitur. Ut prius fieret, optimum & summopere optandum foret. Cum vero interdum Mater ubera praebere non possit, quod tamen paucis accidit, interdum non debeat, quod de paulo pluribus valet, plerumque vero non velit, quod plerisque nostris feminis vitio verti potest, apud bruta vero animantia non observatur; Cum, inquam, haec ita sint, tolerari potest adoptitia, quae tenello alimentum porrigat, & ejus gerat curam, ea tamen cum conditione, ut illis gaudeat facultatibus, & illa sancte teneat praecepta, quae sequentes proponunt canones, qui etiam MATRI, si ipsa huic officio vacat, hodegi ad modum esse possunt.

§5. Nutrix igitur mentis esto integrae, moribus morata, animi constantis, & turbatos hujus motus cohibere sciat, nec nimium sui juris sit sententiaeque.

§6. Corpore utatur sano, a morbis libero, qui in infantem traduci possint, tum optimis repleto humoribus, & bene constituto, non fragili, cui odiosa est quaevis offensio. Aetas illi sit florida, & laudabilis sit digestio, ut bene nutriatur & bene nutrire valeat. Succulenta magis quam sicca, non gracilis nimis, nec corpore natura solido & in multos labores durato, haec enim infanti tenerioris constitutionis minus accomodata est. Nec apta est Magnatum & bene habentium proli nutriendae plebeja, parvis olim aridisque alimoniis adsueta. Si vero alia haberi non potest, mutandum quidem est ejus vitae genus, sed ut sensim id fiat, necessum est. In genere Optima illa censetur, cujus temperies ad Matris quam proxime accedit.

§1. From anatomy and physiology it is clear

a) that children have more and larger glands than adults, and more blood vessels,

b) that these are more pervious and flexible,

c) that their intestines indeed more easily receive infused liquid,

d) that their blood is also thinner, more bright, more soluble, and more nutritious, and

e) that the circulation of fluids is quicker in them, that the digestion and excretion are quicker, and that the growth of the body is greater.

§2. Thus, it has always been astonishing to me why deaths of children are more frequent than those of adults; their nerves are certainly more sensitive, but they are not exposed to external causes as much as adults.

It is probable that the mothers, the nurses and the servants are those mostly to blame, especially as the care of sick children often is left to midwives, whom general opinion makes their physicians; but I must not dwell upon this question; for I am, God willing, about to explain, shortly, by which method the child's diseases can either be avoided, or, if they attack, be defeated.

§3. The CHILD, having come out from the uterus and having been duly taken care of by the midwife, is placed in the arms of the lactating woman, so that it after due fasting can obtain from her the nourishment which is intended for it by provident nature.

§4 She, who gives the milk, is either the MOTHER herself or another woman who undertakes the mother's duties and role, and who is called a WET NURSE. Best, and most largely desirable, would be that it were the former. But as the mother at times cannot give the breast, which however happens to few, and at times should not, which is applicable to a somewhat larger number, but mostly does not want to, which could be pleaded against most of our women as a fault, a behaviour which is not observed among the wild animals; this being the case, as I was just saying, an adoptive mother could be tolerated, who provides the little child with nourishment, and takes care of it, provided that she possesses the qualities, and strictly follows the prescriptions which the following guidelines stipulate, which could also serve as a kind of guide to the MOTHER, if she herself discharges this duty.

§5. Thus, may the wet nurse be clean-minded, well-mannered, with a firm mind, and may she know how to control its excitements, and may she not be too self-willed.

§6. She should have a healthy body, free from illnesses which could be transferred to the child, filled with the best fluids, of good constitution, not a frail one, that shuns every adversity. She should be in the prime of life, and her digestion should be good, so that she is well-nourished herself, and able to nourish well. Succulent rather than dry, neither too slender, nor with a body, robust by nature, and hardened by many labours, as this is less well adopted to the child as being of a more tender constitution. Neither is a plebeian woman, previously used to meagre and frugal nourishment, fit for nourishing the children of the upper class and well-to-do. But if no one else can be obtained, her lifestyle has to be changed, which however needs has to be done little by little. Generally, as the best should be regarded one, whose disposition most closely resembles that of the mother.

§7. MAMMAE sint ambae lactationi aptae, non pensiles vel flaccidae, nec nimis exiles. Papillae exstantes, & ejus magnitudinis, ut ab ore pusilli comprehendi commode & retineri possint. Erigi vero hae debent ex quavis titillatione, lac ceteroquin non daturae.

§8. LAC sufficienti copia semper adsit, dum mammae praeberi debent, optimi etiam habeat notas. Differt quidem pro eo ac differt feminae temperamentum, victus ratio & vitae genus. In genere vero bonum censetur id, quod subcaeruleum est, blandum, dulce & satis tenue, nec pingue nimis, nec salsum, vixque odorum. Tepidum igitur, oculo instillatum, nullum omnino excitare debet doloris sensum. Saporis dulcedo facile sentiatur oportet, nec ullo modo convenire debet cum sapore colostri vaccini, dum illud in verum lac mutatur. Decidens sphaerulam defluentem referat similitudine, tum enim justa ejus est spissitudo cum ungui instillatum nec statim defluit, nec reclinato illi immotum adhaeret. Coagulo addito quantum caseosae partis contineat innotescit. Quiete in vitro in quantitatem supernatantis cremoris inquiritur, quae etiam, pondus ipsius lactis explorando, aliquo modo deprehenditur, quo enim cremore magis abundat, eo etiam levius est.

§9. Ut vitae regimen nutrici praescribi possit, per sex res non naturales dictas eundo, quid in his illi utile, quid noxium videbimus.

§10. AËREM ut hauriat sanum, conclave inhabitet non angustum & sordidum, sed amplius & bene habitum, ubi multum & purum aërem trahere possit. Calor sit moderatus, non aestuans, frigus vero omni cura arceatur. Praecipue vero Mammas ab illo defendat, & dum camera egreditur hae tegantur, sique frigori forte patuerint, non nisi tepefactae iterum infanti praebeantur, ceteroquin Catarrho, Coryza, Tussi, malis a frigore oriundis, corripietur tener. De pedibus idem tenendum, ne illis nudis ambulet, aut quocunque eos modo frigori exponat.

§11. CIBUS & POTUS justo tempore nutrici porrigantur, nec unquam fame vel siti vexetur. Potulenta vero, majori quam ante lactationem consueta fuit copia assumat. Cibum probe dentibus terendo subigat. In ciborum speciebus, ubi & illa & infans bene valent, non minute nimis & anxie agendum, probe modo curetur, ut concoctio sit bona, & quae commeduntur laudabile praebeant nutrimentum. Consueta & grata facilius tolerantur etsi deteriora, quam insueta & ingrata. Si quae inprimis fugienda, erunt ea acida, quae lac acore possunt inquinare. Cibi etiam sale adspersi parcius sumantur, quibus lac salsedine imbui potest. Ita etiam ceparum & alliorum odor saporque in lacte recenti agnoscitur. Ex assumtis a nutrice cibis flatulentis minus belle habuisse infantes saepius vidimus, illosque in Diarrhoeas incidisse, epota a nutrice cerevisia, syrupo sacchari mixta, non insolens est.

§12. POTUS sit cerevisia bona, non tenuis nec meracisssima, minime quae inebriat, bene cocta, non recens nec nimis vetusta, non acore impraegnata, nec illa quae in dolio ultimo restitat, nec quae supra noctem cantharo fuit infusa. Si vini cyathus aliquando concedendus, sit illud ex meracioribus, & parca dosi sumatur, inebriari enim visus est infans, postquam lac ex Mamma nutricis suxisset, quae paulo ante vinum largius potaverat. THEÆ infusum rarius concedatur, COFFEÆ vero Decoctum nunquam. Spiritus autem vini etiam graviori constituta poena prohibeatur.

§7. Both BREASTS should be suited for lactation, not pendent and drooping, nor too small. The nipples should be protruding, and of such size, that they conveniently can be grasped by the child's mouth and held fast. They should be erected from any tickling, as they otherwise will not give any milk.

§8. There should always be a sufficient amount of MILK, when the breast is offered, and it should also present the signs of good quality. This varies, as the woman's temper, eating habits, and life style vary. Generally, however, that milk is regarded as good which is bluish, mild, sweet and rather thin, not too fat, nor salty, and almost scentless. Luke-warm, it should not, when dripped in the eye, bring about any sense of pain. The sweetness of the taste should easily be felt, and it should not in any sense resemble the taste of the cow's beestings, as this changes into real milk. Dripping, it should resemble a downwards flowing little sphere, as its due thickness is when it, dripped on a finger nail, neither flows down immediately, nor remains immobile when the nail is slanted. When rennet is added it shows how much of cheese-matter it contains. By leaving it in a test tube the quantity of floating cream is investigated. This quantity is also established by another method, by examining the weight of the milk itself; for the more it abounds of cream, the lighter it is.

§9. To be able to prescribe the guidance of the wet nurse's life-style, we shall see, by going through the six so called non-natural things, what is useful about them, and what is harmful.

§10. She should breathe fresh AIR, live in a chamber which is not small and dirty, but large and well-kept, where she could breathe much, and clean, air. The temperature should be moderate, not very hot, even if the cold is to be kept out by all means. She should especially protect the breasts against it, and as she leaves her chamber, they should be covered, and if she should happen to expose them to the cold, they should not be offered to the child until they are warm again, as the little one otherwise will contract catarrh, cold, and cough, evils which derive from the cold. As for the feet, it should likewise be observed, not to walk about barefoot, or to expose them to the cold in any way.

§11. FOOD and DRINK should be provided for the wet nurse on due time, and she should never be tormented by hunger or thirst. She should have larger quantities to drink than what has been usual before lactating. She should process the food duly by chewing. As for kinds of food, one should not, as long as she and the child are well, be too strict, as long as it is properly seen to, that the cooking is good, and that the food eaten provides good nourishment. The ordinary and liked is more readily accepted, even if of inferior quality, than the unusual and disliked. If anything should especially be avoided, that would be those sour things which could taint the milk with sour taste. Salted food, by which the milk could receive a saltiness, should also be consumed with caution. Likewise the smell and taste of onions and garlic can be sensed in recent milk. That children have felt less well from flatulent food, eaten by the wet nurse, we have often seen, and it is not unusual that they contract diarrhoea when the wet nurse has drunk beer mixed with syrup of sugar.

§12. The DRINK should be good beer, neither weak nor absolutely unmixed, not at all inebriant; well-brewed; neither recent nor too old; not with a sour taste; neither that, which is left in the bottom of the keg, nor that, which has been left in the tankard over-night. If, once in a while, we are to grant a drink of wine, it should be of the purest kind, and be taken in a small amount, as the child seems to be intoxicated after sucking milk from the breast of a wet nurse who has just drunk a larger quantity of wine. Infusion of TEA should seldom be allowed, decoction of COFFEE never. Strong liquor should however be prohibited under an even more severe penalty.

§13. EXCRETIO quae per ALVUM fit proxime consideranda. Ea non nimis laxa fluat, & si Diarrhoea infestetur, mox illud indicabit, ut sumto Rhabarbaro & postea Diascordii Electuario, compesci queat. Nec contracta sit & dura, tum enim admoto e melle & sale parato suppositorio offici statim memor reddi debet. Purgantia fortiora semper vitentur, horum enim vis facile in lactentem traducitur. Tristem historiam narrant Acta Naturae Curiosorum de nutrice, quæ, ut Melancholiæ medicinam adferret, usa est parva copia succi radicis hellebori nigri. Post quartam horæ partem infanti exhibet mammas, unde is ad mortem usque purgabatur, nullo pharmaci effectu in ipsa nutrice edito. Si flatibus gravatur nutrix, iis mederi licet carminativis e. gr. Semine Anisi, Carvi &c, habito tamen caussarum respectu.

MENSES raro lactantibus fluunt, nec fluere debent. Sin accidat autem, debet id nutrix indicare, ut illis præsentibus lac ejus non sugat infans.

TRANSPIRATIO, quae ut integra sit tanti ad sanitatem interest, promovetur bono victu, & modica corporis exercitatione, quo & mundities cum corporis, tum vestimentorum, linteorum in primis, non minimum facit.

Veneris usus nutrici omnino interdicendus, adeoque si nupta sit, ab omni cum marito consuetudine, quae illius rei occasionem praebere queat, excludatur. Si vero stupere cernatur anxia, in unam rem defixa, vel in laetas cogitationes mens, sui impotens evagetur, nunc morosa, nunc hilaris, sed intempestive; tum scire licet illam perdite amare. Quumque tot inter jactationes integra servari illi sanitas non possit, ab infante lactando arceatur. Quod si concepisse se ipsa animadvertit, nequaquam id reticeat, noxium enim esse infanti lac gravidae non semel observavimus.

§14. EXERCITATIONES corporis, cujus tanta est vis ad bonam constitutionem comparandam, immo ad universi corporis valetudinem tuendam, non omnino nulla in nutrice habenda est ratio. Aliis hac in re multo feliciores sunt ruricolarum pusiones, lac enim in corpore exercitato elaboratum sugunt, & dubium non est, quin princeps haec sit caussa, cur plebeculae infantes bono corporis habitu & recta valetudine optimatum tenellis antecellant. Exerceat igitur corpus moderate nutrix, pro re nata, ambulando in aëre puro, sereno, qualis esse solet in umbrosis, per loca acclivia ascendendo & descendendo, & dum occasio fert leviora munera, quae in domo gerantur, obeundo, aliove modo, ne otio hebescat corpus & laudabili progignendo succo nutritio, in acidum non nimis prono, fiat ineptum. Instituatur vero omnis corporis motio vel ante vel longius post sumtum cibum, ne chylus crudus lacti commisceatur.

§15. SOMNUS sit moderatus & quietus, justumque illi impendatur tempus. Si vero insomnes noctes in tenello curando agere necessum habeat nutrix, convenit valetudini ejus, ut horas aliquot diurnas damno reparando conficiat.

§13. Next, the EXCRETION of the BOWELS is to be dealt with. It should not be too loose, and if she is infested by diarrhoea, she shall tell this immediately, so it can be cured by taking rhubarb, and then *diascordii electuarium*. Nor should it be reduced in size and hard; in such case the bowels should at once be reminded of their duties by giving a suppository, made from honey and salt. Stronger purgents should always be avoided, as their effect is easily transferred to the suckling. *Acta Naturae Curiosorum* tells a sad story of a wet nurse who, to cure melancholy, took a little juice of the root of *Helleborus niger*. After a quarter of an hour she gave the breast to a child, whence he was purged to death, while no effect of the remedy was brought about in the wet nurse herself. If the wet nurse is troubled by flatulence, this can be cured by a carminative, for example aniseeds, seeds of caraway, etc., with regard, though, to the causes.

MENSTRUATION is rarely found in lactating women, and should not be. If this happens, the wet nurse should tell, so the child does not suck her milk during this period.

Good TRANSPIRATION, which means so much to health, is promoted by good nourishment and moderate exercise; to this also cleanliness, both of the body and of the clothes, especially of the underwear, largely contributes.

Sexual intercourse should be absolutely forbidden to the wet nurse, to such extent, that if she is married, she should be prohibited from every contact with her husband, which could give an opportunity to this. But if she is observed being stunned by uneasiness, stuck in one thing only, or if her mind wanders in happy thoughts, unable to control itself, now wayward, now merry, but out of season; then one may conclude that she is hopelessly in love. As her sanity cannot be kept intact in such agitations, she has to be kept from breast-feeding the child. But if she notices that she is herself pregnant, she must absolutely not keep this a secret, as we have observed more than once that the milk of a pregnant woman is harmful to the child.

§14. There is no reason why physical EXERCISE, having such power to bring about a good constitution and, indeed, to protect the health of the whole body, should not be practised by the wet nurse. In this respect, the children of the rural population are much more fortunate than others, as they suck milk which has been processed in an exercised body, and there is no doubt that this is the foremost reason why the children of the common people surpass the delicate offspring of the upper classes in physical appearance and good health. The wet nurse should thus moderately exercise her body according to the circumstances, by walking in pure and clear air, which is usually found in shadowy places; by walking up and down broken ground, and when opportunity arises, by undertaking lighter household work, or by other means, so that the body will not be weakened by inactivity and become incapable of producing praiseworthy, nutrient sap, which will not so easily become sour. All physical exercise should however be undertaken either before eating, or a long time after, so that raw chyle does not mix with the milk.

§15. SLEEP should be moderate and calm, and appropriate time should be set aside for it. But if the wet nurse is forced to spend sleepless nights taking care of the child, it will be profitable to her health if she spends some hours in day-time making up for the loss.

§16. Perturbationes tandem, tot mutationum cum animi tum corporis auctores, probe observentur & quoad ejus fieri potest fugiantur.

Iracundiæ igitur, a nullo illorum, qui nutricis fruuntur consuetudine, justa subministretur caussa. Si vero aliquando ira fuerit percita, exhibendus est ex aqua pulvis nitrosus, lac vero ex mammis exprimi non debet, ut moris est, sed ab alio exsugi, prius quam infans uberibus admoveatur, & ne tum quidem, nisi certo constet mente decessisse iram. Nutricem irae non fuisse potentem detexit interdum subsequutus in infante vel icterus, vel motus convulsivus.

Quae Terrere possunt sedulo vitentur. In terrorem vero conjecta nutrix sumat liquorem Cornus Cervi succinatum vel mixturam simplicem Syrupo floris Papaveris Rhoeadis mixtam, de cetero mammae ut modo dictum exsugantur.

Mœroris removeantur caussae vel occasiones, nec pertinax nimis sit mater in corrigendis moribus nutricis, haec enim alienos ad suos referre mores non statim discere potest.

Re Familiari si gaudet nutrix, ab illius cura sit immunis, nec permittatur, ut ad aures ejus perveniat, si quid in re domestica actum sit, quod animum ejus possit turbare.

§17. Hisce rite observatis spes est fore, ut integra maneat valetudo nutricis. Si vero, vel his neglectis, vel alia caussa in morbum implicatur, tum alii feminae lactanti permitti debet infans, haec vero recentius lac habeat priore, non tamen infra sex hebdomadas a partu assumatur, ceteroquin lactantem Diarrhoea facile corripiet.

§18. Mammas praebeat nutrix, quoties fami vel siti infantis sedandae necessarias intelligit. Sufficiens enim subministrari debet alimentum, non vero copiosum nimis, nec flentem, & saepe etiam renuentem ad ubera cogat. Vomitionem infantum spontaneam summopere laudat vulgus, & tum quidem recte, dum nimio cibo onerantur, quod etiam plerumque fit.

§19. Protinus a cibo sumto mammas haud porrigat. Inter quartam & sextam horam, post duriuscula esculenta ingesta, lac optimum praebetur. Nec post longius jejunium aliud quam noxium serum mammis exprimit infans, ideoque illis non adponendus.

§20. Non saepe nimis nec continue ex eadem mamma lac accipiat, ne in idem semper decumbendo latus, gibber forte evadat.

§21. Fasciis pusillum rite involvat, membris juste dispositis. Caveat vero summo studio, ne arctius adstringantur, inprimis supra thoracem, unde plurima saepe orta mala. Solvat statim fasciam, si illa alligata ejulet infans, & sedulo inquirat, numne fletus aliqua, dum fasciis ligabatur, orta fuerit caussa, quae mox removeatur, e.gr. si plica quaedam alicubi premat, acicula forte pungat, vel brachia aliquo modo distorta fuerint.

§16. DISTURBANCES, finally, that bring about so many changes, both physical and mental, should be carefully observed and to the greatest possible extent avoided.

No just cause for ANGER should be brought about by anyone who keeps company with the wet nurse. But if she ever is excited with anger, *pulvis nitrosus* in water should be offered, but no milk should be pressed from the breasts, which is customary, but be sucked out by someone else, before the child is put to the breasts, which should not even be done until it is clear that the anger has left the mind. That the wet nurse has not been able to restrain her anger is sometimes revealed by a subsequent jaundice or spasm in the child.

Anything that could FRIGHTEN should carefully be avoided. A horror-struck wet nurse should take *liquor cornus cervi succinatus* or a simple mixture with *syrupus floris Papaveris rhoeadis*. Above this the breasts should be sucked as just indicated.

Causes of, and occasions for, SORROW should be eliminated, and the mother should not be to tenacious in correcting the behaviour of the wet nurse, as the latter cannot be expected to adopt customs and behaviour, unfamiliar to her right from the start.

If the wet nurse has a FAMILY, she should be relieved of the care for this, and it should not be permitted to reach her ears, if something has happened in the household, which could disturb her mind.

§ 17. If these things are carefully observed, there is good hope that the health of the wet nurse will remain intact. If, however, be it from neglecting these things or for other reasons, she contracts illness, the child should be left to another lactating woman, who should have more recent milk than the first one, but not be engaged sooner than six weeks after her childbirth, as diarrhoea otherwise easily could afflict the suckling.

§ 18. The wet nurse should offer the breasts as often as she notices that they are necessary for appeasing the child's hunger or thirst, for she has to provide enough nourishment; it should not, however, be too plentiful. Nor should she force a crying, and often even rejectant child to the breast. Spontaneous vomiting of children is much praised among the general public, and quite justly, when they are burdened with to much food, which indeed happens quite often.

§ 19. She should not offer the breast immediately after eating. The best milk is offered from the fourth to the sixth hour after having a rather substantial meal. And after a long fasting, the child does not squeeze anything but harmful whey out of the breasts, and should therefore not be put to them.

§ 20. The child should not to often, or for too long at a stretch, get his milk from the same breast, so that he does not, by always lying on the same side, get a crooked back.

§ 21. She should duly wrap the child in swaddling clothes, with its limbs correctly posed. She should however take care, that it is not too tightly pulled, especially around the chest, from which much evil has often been brought about. She should at once slacken the swaddling clothes if the baby cries as it has been wrapped, and carefully examine, whether any reason for crying has been brought about as the child was wrapped. Such a cause has to be removed immediately, for example, if a crease is applying pressure anywhere, if a pin by chance is pricking, or if the arms have been twisted for some reason.

§22. In fletu dum persistit infans, levi agitatione in brachiis vel cunis, addito jucundo susurro vel cantilena, somnus & quies proliciatur. Si hisce nihil proficimus, alia super alia edantur ludicra spectacula, ut hisce excitatus pusilli animus ad flendi caussas non attendat. Nec vero concedendum est, ut soporandi vim habentibus e.gr. Theriaca Andromachi, Philonio Romano, qualia ad manus habere & furtim ingerere nonnumquam solent nutrices, somnum provocent, hisce enim stuporem, fatuitatem, convulsiones, immo ipsam saepe mortem inferunt.

§23. Mox a sumto lacte brachiis non agitetur infans, nec cunarum unquam sit vehemens & concitatior motus; unde vertigines & vomitus haud aliter ac apud illos, qui navigationi non assueti sunt, oriuntur.

§24. Fascia solvatur & lintea mutentur, quoties naturae obtemperasse cognoscitur infans, quod si negligatur, excoriatio oritur & dolor, ex somnis fit, & in fletum adducitur.

§25. Tegumenta capitis nunquam angusta sint, si igitur arctiora usus reddiderit, nova comparentur, ne tenerum caput prematur, ejusque incremento ponatur obex.

§26. Caput infantis jugi foveatur calore, illa inprimis sincipitis pars, quam Fontanellam dicunt anteriorem, cui propterea singulare linteolum (Fläbb nostri dicunt) adaptare solent. Id vero integumento capitis tantum adhaereat, non vero fasciis circumductis, ut mos est, firmetur.

§27. Caute etiam prospiciat nutrix, ne janua aperiatur, dum fasciis solutus jacet infans, sicque frigidior aura tenello corpori afflet.

§28. Erectus nunquam teneatur infans tenellus adhuc, nec in idem latus diu incumbat, multo minus supinus. E re etiam erit monere, ne somno tradatur capite humili & cum reliquo corpore aequali. Somnos quidem tum capit longiores, sed non adeo dulces & quietos, ac cum capite altiore decumbit.

§29. Candela dum accenditur, non ad latus cunarum ponatur, illuc enim infans oculos inflectit, quod, si diu continuetur, vel saepe repetatur, Strabismum efficit.

§30. E camera omnis spurcitia expurgetur, ne quem redoleat foetorem, munditiisque apparandis magnopere studeat nutrix, & ut aër saepius & circumspecte renovetur operam det. Mundities enim purique aëris copia multa mala avertit.

§ 22. If the child persists in crying, sleep and tranquillity is brought about by gently rocking him, in the arms or in the cradle, combined with a low gentle babbling or a lullaby. If we do not succeed by these, one playful little act after another should be performed, so that the child will be diverted by these pranks, and will not think of the reasons for crying. But it should not be permitted, that sleep is brought about by soporific substances, for example *Theriaca Andromachi* or *Philonium Romanum*, such as wet nurses are quite often wont to have at hand and furtively give, as they thus bring about unconsciousness, confusion, convulsions and often even death.

§ 23. The child should not be rocked in the arms right after having his milk, nor should the movements of the cradle ever be vehement and violent: from this fits of vertigo and vomiting arise, not unlike that among those who are not accustomed to sailing.

§ 24. The swaddle clothes should be unwrapped and the napkins changed as soon as the child is understood to have obeyed nature, as, if this is neglected, abrasion and pain will follow, the child will be woken up and brought to cry.

§ 25. The headgear should never be tight; thus, if the use has made it too narrow, a new one should be provided, so that the child's head will not be compressed, and a hinderance thus set up for its growth.

§ 26. The child's head should be kept warm through continuous warmth, especially the part of the forehead, which is called the anterior fontanel, to which therefore a special cloth (our compatriots call it a "fläbb") usually is applied. This should however merely be attached to the headgear, but not, as is usually done, be fastened by bands wrapped around it.

§ 27. The wet nurse must carefully see to it that the doors are not opened when the child lies without the swaddling clothes, and the cold air as a consequence can blow on the tender little body.

§ 28. The little child should never be held upright as long as he is of tender age, nor be lying for a long time on the same side, let alone on its back. It will also be appropriate to point out, that he should not be put to sleep with the head low, on the same level as the rest of the body. He will certainly sleep longer, but not as well and calmly as when lying with his head higher.

§ 29. When a candle is lit, it should not be placed next to the cradle, as it will attract the child's eyes in that direction, which, if it goes on for a long time, or is frequently repeated, will cause a squint.

§ 30. All dirt should be removed from the room, so that no stench is felt, and the wet nurse should strive to keep it tidy, and see to it that the air is frequently and prudently renewed, as tidiness and plenty of clean air avert much evil.

§31. Hisce observatis, dispiciendum est, quae remedia morbis infantum debeant opponi, si quidem valetudinis quodam genere tentantur. In adversam vero valetudinem illos a RETENTO MECONIO saepe incidere quotidie videmus. Nutritur, sed alvum non deponit, ob respirationis defectum, infans, quamdiu uterum inhabitet. Colligitur igitur in intestinis sordium colluvies, quae, dum aërem haurire incipit, expurgari debet, retenta enim, tormina, agrypniam, convulsiones & ipsam mortem producit. At saepe retinetur primo dum languet vis expellens, secundo dum tenax nimis est haec saburra, & tertio si viarum deest lubricitas. Colostrum matris benigna natura huic fini destinavit, & qui hoc a matre lactante fruuntur beneficio, alio non egent remedio, in primis cum praecedat jejunium, ut novis ingestis interea non obruantur natura. Cum vero hoc saepius destituantur tenelli, alia facienda est medicina. Contra primam caussam pugnare possumus Rhabarbaro vel leni cardiaco. Secunda superatur mellitis vel Manna, tertiae vero opponimus oleosa. Et haec quidem, si omnes tres caussae concurrunt, haud inepte jungimus sequenti Formula: Recipiantur Mannae electae & sacchari albi ana unciae binae solvantur in Aquae Floris Acaciae unciis binis. Per linteum colatis addatur pulveris Radicis Ireos florentinae drachma & olei amygdalarum uncia. Ex mixtis fiat Electuarium, cuius drachma ad unciam semis, sero lactis soluta, propinetur. Si paulo fortior desideratur medicina, in locum radicis Ireos florentinae substitui potest Radix Rhabarbari, & si debilis admodum fuerit infans, addantur guttulae aliquot vini Hispanici vel Hungarici. Magnas etiam utilitates praebent injectae per alvum lotiones. Parari vero illae debent e sero lactis, melle & oleo olivarum vel amygdalarum recenti.

§32. In sano infante residuum assumtorum, & pars adfluentium humorum, inutilis facta, quotidie per alvum aliquoties redditur. Haec si colliguntur, in intestinis & longiori temporis intervallo vel nimis indurata excernuntur ALVUS dicitur OBSTIPATA. Non leve vero hoc est incommodum, unde anxietates, cum doloribus junctae abdominis expansiones, tormina, vomitus & in somno pavores oriuntur. Quae omnia mala vel Clysmate injecto, vel modo dicto Electuario facile levantur, cum vero hujus interdum major requiratur, quam quae commode sumi possit, dosis, facile intra drachmas tres quatuorve subsistere possumus, siquidem Rhabarbari tot addimus grana, quot requirere videantur circumstantiae. Huic etiam malo facilis & celeris medicina est suppositorium, quod e sevo vel passula majori, demtis acinis, tutissime praeparatur.

§ 31. As this has been observed, we shall see, which remedies that are to be put up against the children's diseases, if they are attacked by any kind of illness. We see every day that they often contract illness from RETENTION OF MECONIUM. As long as the child stays in the womb, he is nourished, but does not evacuate his bowels, as there is no respiration. Thus, a mixture of impurities is collected in the intestines, which, as the child begins to breathe the air, should be excreted, but that, when kept, brings about colic, sleeplessness, convulsions and even death. But the retention is often due to 1) power to excrete is lacking; 2) this ballast being to tenacious, and 3) lack of smoothness in the passage. The kind nature has designed the beestings of the mother for this purpose, and those who enjoy this benefit from their lactating mother need no other remedy, especially as fasting has preceded, so that nature is not overwhelmed by new additions. But as little children are often deprived of this, another remedy has to be made up. Against the first cause, we can fight with rhubarb or with some mild cardiac. The second is defeated by preparations with honey or by manna, but against the third one we put up oily preparations. And if all three causes are present, we quite cleverly combine these three remedies in the following recipe: Take of choice manna and of white sugar equally two ounces of each, which is dissolved in *aqua floris Acaciae*, two ounces. This is strained through a linen cloth, and of *pulvis radicis ireos florentinae* is added one drachm, of *oleum amygdalarum* one ounce. From the mixture is made an electuary, of which one drachm to half an ounce, dissolved in whey, is given. If a slightly stronger medicine is desired, rhubarb root could be substituted for the *radix ireos florentinae*, and if the child is somewhat feeble, a couple of drops of Spanish or Hungarian wine is added. Rinsing fluids injected in the bowels are also very useful. These should be prepared from whey, honey and fresh olive oil or almond oil.

§ 32. In the healthy child, the residue of what has been eaten and part of the surplus fluid, made useless, are excreted through the bowels a number of times every day. If this is accumulated in the intestines, and is excreted with longer intervals or too hardened, the BOWELS are said to be CONSTIPATED. This inconvenience indeed is not a slight one, whence unrest, expansion of the stomach accompanied by pains, colic, vomiting, and fits of horror in sleep arise. All this evil is easily mitigated by giving a clyster, or by an electuary as mentioned, but as the dose required is at times larger than could conveniently be taken, we could stop at between three and four drachms, granted that we add as many grains of rhubarb as the circumstances seem to demand. For this evil, a simple and quickly working medicine is also a suppository, which is best prepared with tallow or raisins, with the pips removed.

§33. Contingit etiam frequenter, ut laxa nimis sit infantibus alvis. Bis intra horas 24 beneficio gaudere debent, quod si saepius quam quater fiat, DIARRHŒA laborant. Nuper vero natos excipere fas est, his enim, licet quinquies vel sexies alvum deponant, nihil mali portendit. Cedit facile hoc malum rhabarbaro ex tenui cinamomi aqua a nutrice sumto, cui etiam tum pro cibo sint juscula vel pulmenta ex oryza. Elapsis vero octo circiter horis eidem exhibeatur ex eadem cinamomi aqua Electuarii Diascordii drachma. Si vero his non cedit remediis morbus, regioni umbilici infantis imponi potest linteum quadruplex, calidum, vino rubro, in quo Theriacae Andromachi paullum solutum est, imbutum, vel eidem regioni admoveatur cataplasma Theriacale, quod ex Theriacae Andromachi partibus quatuor, olei macis expressi parte una & guttis aliquot olei stillatitii cumini praeparatur. Scire vero licet, tegi semper debere gossypio umbilicum, dum ejusmodi remedia applicamus.

§34. Haud raro quoque evenit, ut pars intestini recti e sua sede desidat, & foras e corpore prolabatur. Huic vero malo spongiam vino rubro calido (Pontack) imbutam opponimus, quippe quae in praesentissimis remediis habetur. Feliciter etiam adspergitur pulvis e fuligine, vel fumus admittitur accensi Mastichis. Inter haec vero, si sponte sua in locum non restituatur intestinum, arte in pristinam sedem retrudendum est.

§35. Si inquieti sunt infantes, saepius ejulant, idque citato cum fervore, & sine praeviis querelis, corpus contrahunt & varie contorquent, pauco fruuntur & interrupto somno, & dormientibus facies ad risum componitur, lac interdum avide sugunt, mammas mox saepe & fervide arripiunt, mox iterum dimittunt; tum morbo laborant, quem TORMINA VENTRIS, COLICAM SPASMODICAM alii appellant. Quae per alvum ejiciunt, viridia apparent, & lintea eodem colore inficiunt. Acidum spirant, & saepe caseosa sunt. Ipsos etiam ructus gravis & acidus comitatur odor. Malum hoc uti gradu differt, ita raro continue, sed per intervalla affligit. Maxime vero noctu, cito vero curandum est, cum facile post praegressos plerumque in somno, vel quod pejus in vigilantibus, pavores transeat in motus convulsivos & in ipsam denique mortem. Et hoc eo citius contingit, quo debilior sit infans, quo corruptum magis & facilius acescens lac sugat, quo plures in cibo potuque committat errores nutrix, quoque major sit ejus aut cupiditas aliqua, aut pigritia, aut ignavia aut vehementiores concitationes animi.

Sanaturus videat an claussa sit alvus, & tum quidem lotio per alvum quantocius injicienda, & drachmae aliquot olei amygdalarum recentis expressi propinandae, vel si adultior infans Tinctura Rhabarbari exhibenda, simulque ventriculo calens adhuc imponatur, inter lintea, placenta, ex oleo olivarum, farina & ovi vitello in sartagine parata, vel Epithema Aromaticum, aut eidem Balsamum Stomachale, quale est illud SCHERZERI, in cochleari prius super prunas fusum, inungatur. Et hisce quidem per horas aliquot leniuntur tormina, & cessant clamores, ut quiescere possit infans, id quod absorbentibus intus datis raro efficies, ea enim dosi vix exhiberi possunt, quae acido domando sufficiat.

§ 33. It also often happens that the bowels of the children are too loose. Twice every twenty-four hours, they should enjoy the service performed by their bowels, whereas they are suffering from DIARRHOEA if this happens more often than four times. An exception should be made for the newly-born, however, as for them it does not portend anything evil, even when they evacuate their bowels five or six times. This evil will easily yield to rhubarb, taken with weak cinnamon water by the wet nurse, who should also, in this case, have a decoction or porridge of rice for food. After about eight hours, then, she should be offered one drachm of *electuarium Diascordii* in the same cinnamon water. But if the disease does not recede by these remedies, a quadrifold warm linen cloth, soaked in red wine, wherein a little *theriaca Andromachi* has been dissolved, can be applied in the navel region of the child, or else a theriacal poultice, made from four parts *theriaca Andromachi*, one part oil, pressed from mace, and a couple of drops of *oleum stillatitium cumini* is placed in the same area. It should be noticed, however, that the navel should always be covered with a piece of cotton wool when we apply remedies of this kind.

§ 34. It also happens quite often that the rectal part of the intestines leaves its place, and slips out of the body. This evil we treat with a sponge, soaked in warm red wine (Pontack), as this is regarded as one of the most efficient remedies. With good results pulverized soot can also be sprinkled, or the smoke from burning mastic applied. If the intestine does not recede to its proper place by itself from this, however, it has to be pressed back by artificial means.

§ 35. If the children are restless, often cry, and this more and more vehemently, and, without any previous complaining, contract and contort their bodies in various positions, benefit from little and disrupted sleep, and, while asleep, pull their faces to a smile; sometimes greedily suck milk, sometimes vehemently seize the breast, only to immediately let go of it again. In such case, they suffer from a disease, TORMINA VENTRIS, which some call SPASMODIC COLIC. That which is evacuated through the bowels looks green, and colours the napkins the same hue. It smells sour, and is often full of cheese-like lumps. Even their belches are accompanied by a heavy and sour smell. This evil varies in severity, and is seldom continuous, but afflicts at intervals, but especially in the night time; it has to be taken care of quickly, as it easily, after preceding fits of horror, mostly in the sleep, or, which is worse, while being awake, is turned into convulsions, and then into death. And this will come about sooner, the weaker the child is, the more deteriorated and prone to get sour the milk that he sucks, the more the wet nurse errs regarding food and drink, and the greater the passions for something, the greater the indolence, and the inactivity of the wet nurse, or the more vehement her emotions.

Anyone wishing to cure this should see whether the bowels are obstructed, in which case a rinsing fluid should be injected in the bowels as soon as possible, and a couple of drachms of recent *oleum amygdalae* be given, or, if the child is bigger, *tinctura Rhabarbari* could be offered, and at the same time a cake, still hot, made with olive oil, flour, and yolk, in a frying pan, is applied on the stomach, wrapped in a linen cloth, or *epithema aromaticum*, or else could the same region be smeared with *balsamum stomachale*, such as that prescribed by SCHERZERUS, which has first been melted in a spoon over coal. By this the colic is mitigated in a couple of hours, and the crying ceases, so that the child is able to calm down, something that you will seldom achieve by internally administered absorbents, as they could hardly be given in such doses as would be enough to overcome the acid.

Scire vero licet hoc modo inducias tantum factas esse, bellum non compressum, & laetitiam hanc nobis minus fore diuturnam, nisi id agamus, ut lac nutricis corrigatur, & non adeo facile acescat. Nutrici igitur quater aut quinquies quotidie dentur scrupuli aliquot, ex stillatitia Foeniculi aqua, pulveris ex magnesiae albae uncia, conservae Flavedinis corticum auranciorum, seminis Foeniculi dulcis & sacchari albi ana drachmis binis compositi, quo uti illa pergat, usque dum tranquillatae sint penitus res infantis. Diaeta interim nutricis sit acido opposita. Esculenta sint jura & gelatinae carnium juniorum, ipsae etiam carnes, praesertim assae, animalium parum bibentium, aliisque animalibus nutritorum, avium, piscium saxatilium. Ova etiam sorbilia prosunt. Potus sit vel aqua, vel Decoctum album Londinensium. Vitentur interim lacticinia, farinacea, acida, & quaecunque in loco calido sponte sua in acidum vergunt. Hisce vero justa accedat corporis ejus exercitatio. Uti enim motus animalis & vitalis languidus acidi generationi maxime favet, ita etiam exercitia eandem impediunt, acidum subigunt, & efficiunt, ut lac propius, ut ita dicam, accedat ad naturam animalem, ideoque tardius acescat. Tanti vero usus sunt idonea exercitia, ut his per semissem horae ante prandium a nutrice quotidie institutis, sudore provocato, longe certiores viderit fructus Nobilissimus Dominus Doctor & Archiater LINNAEUS, quam ex optimis medicamentis infanti propinatis.

Impetu morbi, ut modo dictum, levato, vix alia opus est medicina praeservatrice, quam laudatis exercitiis. Nec asperum dici potest hoc remedium, cum illo ipso suae valetudini consulat nutrix, quae ceteroquin, ob mutatum vitae genus, inclinatae in deterius principia valetudinis necessario sentiet.

Soli Deo Gratia.

This way is, of course, only a cease-fire achieved, the rebellion having not been quenched, and our joy over this will not last very long if we do not see to it that the milk of the wet nurse is improved, and that it does not so easily become sour. The wet nurse should thus, four or five times a day, be given a couple of scruples of a mixture in *stillatitia foeniculi aqua* of one ounce of *pulvis ex magnesia alba*, two drachms each of *conserva flavedinis corticum aurantiorum*, seeds of *foeniculum dulce*, and white sugar, which she should continue to use until the condition of the child is completely calmed down. Meanwhile, the diet of the wet nurse should be antacid. She should eat broths and aspics of meat from younger animals, even the meat itself, especially roasted, from animals which do not drink much, and from animals, which feed other animals, from birds, and from fish that live among rocks. Raw eggs are also good. For drink, water or *decoctum album Londinense* should be used. Milk dishes should be avoided, on the other hand, as should farinaceous food, acidous food, and anything that turns sour in a warm place by itself. To this should be added appropriate physical exercise, for, as slow motion among living creatures to a large extent promotes the generating of acids, so does physical exercise obstruct it; it overcomes the acids, and makes the milk more resemble animal qualities, so to speak, and thus it will not turn sour so fast. The usefulness of appropriate physical exercise is such, that the most honourable gentleman, doctor and archiater LINNAEUS has seen much more obvious results from this, when performed by the wet nurse for half an hour before breakfast, so that sweating is brought about, than from the best medicines given to the child.

As the fit of disease has been cured, as indicated, no other preservative medicine than these exercises is needed, as mentioned above. Nor could this remedy be called a bitter one, since the wet nurse promotes her own health by it, she, who otherwise, because of the change of life-style, would necessarily notice the first signs of her health verging towards a worse condition.

The Honour to God only

Ad

Pereximium egregiae hujus dissertationis

AUCTOREM

DOMINEM JOHANNEM SCHRÖDER

AMICUM suum suavissimum

Quantos mens valeat Matrum *male sana tenellis*
Foetibus heu! cura neglecta accendere morbos,
Hoc specimen doctum perpulcra comprobat arte.
Gratulor idcirco Tibi *dotes ingeniumque,*
Quo potes a falso verum secernere docte,
Et precor, ut porro benedicat Rector O*lympi*
Dotibus inceptisque Tuis, *mi Candide Frater!*

Pauca haecce manu officiosa
scribere voluit & debuit
M.W.

To
this splendid dissertation's Brilliant
AUTHOR,
Mr JOHANNES SCHRÖDER,
his amiable FRIEND

Alas! what maladies an insane Mother
could give the little child by negligence,
this learned thesis shows with brilliant art.
Therefore, congratulations on Your *talents,*
by which You *sort the false out from the true;*
I pray, may He, *who rules in Heaven, further*
bless all Your *gifts and deeds, my Noble Brother!*

M.W.
wanted to, and was obliged to, write
these few words with wilful hand

Commentary, Schröder

This dissertation, like **Sundius**, above, to a large degree corresponds with parts of Rosén's *Underrättelser* (1753); thus **Schröder 4–30** can be found in Rosén's ch. 1, **Schröder 32** and **34** correspond with Rosén's ch. 2 and 3, respectively, while **Schröder 35** contains much the same information as does Rosén's ch. 7.

ERICO SCHRÖDER] Infantry captain, about whom no further information has been found, however.

ARWIDO KIERULFF] Arvid Kjerrulf (1707–88), magistrate in Gävle, the province of Gästrikland.

MARTINO KIERULFF] Martin/Mårten Kjerrulf (1705–88), had obtained the philosophical degree of *magister* in Lund in 1726 (diss. *De Chao*, praeses Andreas Rydelius); at this time vicar in Tranemo, from 1756 dean.

FREDERICO KIERULFF] Apparently a merchant in S:t Ibb, the island of Ven in the province of Skåne.

LARS SCHRÖDER] Merchant in Gothenburg.

1 *glandulas*] See *Glandula*, Latin word list, p 42.

floridum] *Floridus* in ancient Latin, as e.g. in Apuleius' *Met.* 2.8: *floridae vestis hilaris color*, can have the nuance of 'bright' etc, with respect to colour, which is probably also the sense here; we might note that Eng. "florid" is found in this sense, specifically regarding the blood, e.g. in *Bacon's Life & Death*, p 64: "The lively and floride bloud of the small Arteries" (1650), and in J. Arbuthnot: *An essay concerning the nature of aliments*, p 121: "The Qualities of Blood in a healthy State are to be florid when let out of the Vessel" (1731); cf. OED, s.v. "florid" 5, b.

2 *densiora … infantum funera*] The immediate reason for the publication of Rosén's articles in the calendars (see my commentary to **Sundius 1.1**, *in Calendario Stockholmensi*) was the recent introduction of Swedish population statistics.

In 1686 it had been decreed by law that Swedish parish registers should contain records of all births, christenings, marriages and deaths within the parish, a piece of legislation which had made Sweden the leading European nation as regards demographic matters. In 1736, the bishop of Linköping, Erik Benzelius, had collected information from his parish registers and provided *Kammarkollegium* (the Crown Lands Judiciary Board) with statistics for one decade, which ultimately led to involvement of the Academy of Sciences', and the predecessor of *Statistiska Centralbyrån* (the Central Bureau of Statistics), *Tabellkommissionen* (the Tabular Commission), being instituted in 1749 to publish *Tabellverket* (the Collected Tables); the first official statistics could be published in 1755, much due to the efforts of Pehr Wargentin (1717–83), astronomer – the leading European expert on the moons of Jupiter – and secretary to the Academy of Sciences from 1749 (Lindroth, pp 53sq, 121–124).

Tabellverket also kept a record of death rates among children; according to the figures for 1749, no fewer than 20 % of all children born died before the age of one (Jägervall, p 10) (cf. the figures for 2002, which contain 265 deaths of children under the age of one, while 95 815 births are recorded); since it thus had become obvious that something had to be done about the issue, the Academy asked Rosén to write his articles.

4–8 The guidelines provided in these chapters to a large extent correspond to those found in Soranos' (fl. c. 100 AD) Γυναικεῖα, 2.19–23, which apparently were the standard guidelines in this field for several centuries; cf. e.g. Paolo Bagellardo's *Libellus de egritudinibus infantium*, 1472, 3v–4r, where very much the same advice can be found.

4 *Cum ... interdum ... non possit, quod ... paucis accidit, interdum non debeat, quod de ... pluribus valet, plerumque ... non velit, quod plerisque ... vitio verti potest*] A passage probably influenced by the rhetorical *climax* principle.

adoptitia] This form seems not to be known from ancient Latin; there is, however, an adj. *adopticius*, 'adopted', known from *Diplomata Karoli III* 145 p 232, 29 (876–87) (MLW), and Petri Gothus says, s.v. *Adoptivus*, that it is *Idem quod Adoptitius*.
  Even if the word in Petri Gothus as well as in MLW seems to denote only 'an adopted child', the meaning here is clearly that of 'an adoptive mother'.

si ipsa huic officio vacat] *Vacare* with the dative in the sense of 'take the time to', etc, is known from ancient Latin, e.g. Tacitus *Ann.* 16.22: [*Thraseam*] *triennio non introisse curiam; nuperrimeque ... privatis potius clientium negotiis vacavisse*; cf. OLD s.v. *vaco* 7 b.

hodegi] Hodegos, Gr. ὁδηγός, 'guide', is not known from ancient or mediaeval Latin; cf. footnote (48), p 20, above.

6 *Succulenta magis quam sicca*] According to humoralistic theories (cf. **Sundius 0.1**), the four bodily fluids, viz. blood, phlegm, black bile, and yellow bile, possessed certain combinations of four qualities, namely, hot, cold, humid and dry; the blood was thus considered hot and humid, while the phlegm was cold and humid, the black bile was cold and dry, and the yellow bile was hot and dry; this principle applied not only to the human being in its entirety, but also to the different internal organs, to food and herbs, etc.
  In accordance with these thoughts, thus, the wet nurse should preferrably be a sanguine or phlegmatic person, which, according to my own experience, doesn't seem to be bad advice at all, when it comes to dealing with children.

bene habentium] The absolute *habeo* with an adverb to express conditions of life etc. is used in Classical Latin e.g. by Cicero *Fam.* 16.15.1: *te ... febri carere et belle habere.* K-St, § 26, A.2.a compares this usage to Greek εὖ ἔχειν. Cf. **11** *belle habuisse*]

parvis ...aridisque alimoniis adsueta] *Aridus* in the sense of 'mean', 'frugal', 'parsimonious', etc. is known from ancient Latin, e.g. Plautus, *Per.* 266: *triparcos homines, vetulos, avidos, aridos*; Terence, *Hau.* 526: *habet patrem ... avidum, miserum atque aridum*; Martial, 10.75.11: *sportula nos iunxit ... arida*; Cicero, *Quinct.* 93: *vitam omnino semper horridam atque aridam* and *Sext. Rosc.* 75: *in victu arido*; cf. OLD, s.v. *aridus* 7.

7 *Erigi ... debent*] This is one particular feature of the wet nurse which is not mentioned in Soranus nor in Bagellardo.

8 *Differt ... pro eo ac*] *Pro eo ac* for 'just as', etc, is found in Classical Latin, e.g. in Cicero, *Inv.* 1.54: *pro eo ac si concessum sit concludere oportebit argumentationem*, and *Cat.* 4.3: *debeo sperare deos pro eo mihi ac mereor relaturos esse gratiam*; cf. K-St II, p18sq.

colostri vaccini] The neutre *colostrum* is by OLD regarded as doubtful in ancient Latin, while the normal form seems to be fem. *colostra*, as e.g. in Columella 7.3.17: *exiguum lactis emulgendum est, quod pastores colostram vocant*, and in Pliny *NH* 11.236: *primo semper a partu colostrae fiunt*. For the Neo-Latin period, Petri Gothus has both forms s.v. *colostra*; Noltenius does not mention the word at all, while Zedler has only *colostrum*.

tum enim ... adhaeret] This particular piece of advice is found also in Soranos 2.22, and furthermore in Linnaeus' *Dietetik*, p 13.

9 *sex res non naturales*] Cf. **Martin 19.1**.

10 *Coryza*] Greek word list, p 33.

11 *Potulenta*] See my commentary to **Bergius 5.24**.

Cibum ... dentibus terendo subigat] *Subigo* in the sense of 'knead' etc. is used in different contexts by several ancient Latin authors, e.g. Cato *Agr.* 74: *farinam in mortarium indito, aquae paulatim addito subigitoque pulchre* (on baking); Vitruvius 5.10.3: *earumque camararum superiora coagmenta ex argilla cum capillo subacta liniantur* (on the finishing of walls); Gellius 17.11: *Plutarchus et alii ... scripsere* [- - -] *Erasistratum dicere ... esculenta omnia et posculenta ... ferri in ventriculum ... atque ibi subigi digerique* (on digestion).

The ancient example which most resembles the usage here, however, is Pliny *NH* 11.162: *multis eorum* (sc. *piscium*) *in lingua et toto ore* [*dentes*], *ut turba vulnerum molliant quae adtritu subigere non queunt*.

speciebus] As is pointed out by Hans Helander (*Symbolae Osloenses*, 76, 2001, p 31), genitive and dative/ablative forms in the plural of most nouns of the fifth declension are avoided in classical Latin – *Nolim*, says Cicero in *Topica* 7.30, *ne si Latine quidem dici possit, 'specierum' et 'speciebus' dicere* – but in Neo-Latin, these forms are not only possible to use; Helander's investigations even reveal a certain predilection for the type among scientific authors of the period; there are examples from e.g. Kepler: *in aestimandis figurarum speciebus* (*Harmonice Mundi*, prooem. 5) and Linnaeus: *nondum speciebus ad propria genera redactis* (*De Achrostico*, diss, resp Heiligtag, in *Amoenitates academicae* I, p 145).

cibis flatulentis] *Flatulentus*, 'flatulent', seems to be a Neo-Latin word; Hoven has references to 15-16th century sources; the first occurrences of Eng. "flatulent" in the sense of 'causing flatulence' are found in H. Buttes' *Dyets drie Dinner* (1599): "Cijb, Peaches ... Being soft, moist, and flatulent, they engender humours", and in Th. Blount's *Glossographia* (1674–81): "Pease and Beans are flatulent meat.", according to OED, s.v. "flatulent".

belle habuisse] Cf. **6** *bene habentium*] above.

13 *Rhabarbaro*] See *Pulvis infantum*, Pharmacological word list, p 69.

Diascordii Electuario] See *Electuarium diascordium* Pharmacological word list, p 65.

compesci] *Compesco* is known from ancient Latin in several nuances of 'check', 'restrain', etc; there are also occurrences of a medical sense, as e.g. in Pliny *NH* 24.102: [*Herba sabina*] *collectiones minuit et nomas compescit*, and 34.154: [*squama ferri*] *haemorroidas compescit*.

Purgantia] See "Drug categories", p 58.

Acta Naturae Curiosorum] This is probably the journal of the *Academia Caesarea Leopoldino-Carolina Naturae Curiosorum* of Schweinfurt, Germany, which had been founded in 1652 as *Collegium Naturae Curiosorum*, and which today is known as *Deutsche Akademie der Naturforscher Leopoldina* in Halle.

The full title of the *Acta* would at this time be *Acta Physico-Medica Academiae Caesareae Leopoldino-Carolinae Naturae Curiosorum exhibentia Ephemerides, sive, Observationes Historias et Experimenta Celeberrimis Germaniae et Exterarum Regionum Viris Habita & Communicata, Singulari Studio Collecta.*

radicis hellebori nigri] See *Radix hellebori nigri*, Pharmacological word list, p 70.

carminativis] See *Carminativa*, "Drug categories", p 56.

Semine Anisi] See *Semen anisi*, Pharmacological word list, p 72.

Carvi] See *Semen carvi*, Pharmacological word list, p 72.

perdite amare] Cf. Terence, *Heauton timorumenos*, 97: *filiam ille amare coepit perdite*; Catullus, 45.3: *ni te perdite amo*; 104.3: *nec, si possem, tam perdite amarem*.

jactationes] *Iactatio* in the sense of 'frequent changing of the mind' etc, is found e.g. in Cicero *Tusc.* 2.12: *videre licet alios* [*philosophos*] *tanta levitate et … iactatione*, and in Livy 24.6.9: *hanc levitatem ac iactationem animi neque mirabantur in iuvene furioso*.

14 *plebeculae*] *Plebecula* for 'the common people' is found in Cicero *Att.* 1.16.11: *illa contionalis hirudo aerari, misera ac ieiuna plebecula*; *Att.* 16.8.2: *plebeculam urbanam*; the latter phrase is found also in Horace *Ep.* 2.1.186, and in Persius 4.6, while Suetonius has *praefatus sineret se plebeculam pascere* (*Ves.* 18)

pro re nata] Cf. **Bergius 10.18**.

chylus] See *Chylosus*, Greek word list, p 33.

16 *quoad ejus fieri potest*] Cf. **Bergius 8.23**.

pulvis nitrosus] See *Pulvis nitrosus et camphoratus*, Pharmacological word list, p 70.

icterus] Greek word list, p 35.

liquorem Cornus Cervi succinatum] See *Liquor Cornus Cervi succinatus*, Pharmacological word list, p 66.

Syrupo floris Papaveris Rhoeadis] See *Syrupus floris papaveris rhoeadis*, Pharmacological word list, p 73.

20 *gibber*] Latin word list, p 42.

22 *Theriaca Andromachi*] Pharmacological word list, p 74.

Philonio Romano] See *Philonium Romanum*, Pharmacological word list, p 69.

23 *vertigines*] In the text: *vertigenes*; see *Vertigo* and *Vertiginosus*, Latin word list, p 52

25 *arctiora*] *Arctus* for *artus*, 'tight', 'narrow', etc, is a common Neo-Latin spelling, used e.g. by Petri Gothus, and discussed by Noltenius, col 24, s.v. *artus*, where he basically regards both varieties as equally correct. In Krebs-Schmalz, the word is not mentioned at all.

26 *sincipitis pars*] See *Sinciput*, Latin word list, p 48.

Fontanellam] See *Fontanella*, Latin word list, p 41.

Fläbb] This is, according to SAOL, a headcloth with its corners hanging down; the word is said to belong to dialects of western Sweden, which might have been useful for establishing the authoship of this dissertation, were it not that both Rosén and Schröder were born in this part of the country.

29 *Strabismum*] See *Strabismus*, Greek word list, p 39.

31 *quae remedia morbis ...debeant opponi*] A military metaphor, see p 79sq.

tormina] Latin word list, p 49.

agrypniam] See *Agrypnia*, Greek word list, p 31.

Contra primam ...pugnare possumus ...Secunda superatur ...,tertiae vero opponimus ...] Three more military metaphors, see p 79sq.

Aquae Floris Acaciae] See *Aqua floris acaciae*, Pharmacological word list, p 61

pulveris Radicis Ireos florentinae] See *Pulvis radicis ireos florentinae*, Pharmacological word list, p 70.

olei amygdalarum] See *Oleum amygdalinum* Pharmacological word list, p 68.

Electuarium] See Pharmacological word list, s.v. *Electuarium diascordium*, p 65.

32 *OBSTIPATA*] See *Obstipatio*, Latin word list, p 44.

Clysmate] See *Clysma*, "Drug categories", p 57.

tutissime praeparatur] One example of *tutissime* in a similar, medical context can be found in Pliny NH 25.52: [*Helleborus in Ancyra*] enim tutissime sumitur.

33 *beneficio gaudere debent*] Cf. my commentary to **Bergius 10.29**; cf. also "Language: Variation", p 22.

cataplasma] See "Drug categories", p 56.

macis] Pharmacological word list, p 67.

olei stillatitii cumini] See *Oleum essentialium ex seminibus cymini*, Pharmacological word list, p 69.

34 *Huic...malo...opponimus*] Another military metaphor, see p 79sq.

Mastichis] See *Mastiche*, pharmacological word list, p 67.

35 *COLICAM SPASMODICAM*] Cf. *Tormina [ventris]*, Latin word list, p 49.

Epithema Aromaticum] Pharmacological word list, p 66.

Balsamum Stomachale] Pharmacological word list, p 62.

SCHERZERI] Johann Adam Schertzer (1628–83), Bohemian, who started out as a medical student, during which studies he composed the *balsamum Scherzeri* (see the pharmacological word list, s.v. *Balsamum stomachale*); later, Schertzer changed his subject and held the professorships of Hebrew and subsequently of theology at the university of Leipzig.

hoc modo inducias ... factas ... bellum non compressum] Two more military metaphors, see p 79sq.

magnesiae albae] See *Magnesia alba*, pharmacological word list, p 67.

conserva flavedinis corticum aurantiorum] Pharmacological word list, p 63.

piscium saxatilium] This should be fish which are caught among rocks; according to Magnus Orrelius' *Köpmans- och Material-Lexicon* (1797), p 110sq, a distinction, as regards salt water fish, was made between *pisces pelagii*, which were caught in deep sea, *pisces litorales*, caught from the beach, and *pisces saxatiles*, which Orrelius regards as being the best for food.

Bibliography

The Hippocratic texts are throughout the thesis referred to in accordance with the system used
in Li&Sc, thus:

Acut sp	= περὶ διαίτης ὀξέων		*Loc Hom*	= περὶ τόπων τῶν κατὰ ἄνθρωπον
Aër	= περὶ ἀέρων ὑδάτων τόπων		*Mochl*	= μοχλικόν
Aff	= περὶ παθῶν		*Morb*	= περὶ νούσων
Alim	= περὶ τροφῆς		*Mul*	= γυναικεῖα
Aph	= ἀφορισμοί		*Nat Puer*	= περὶ φύσιος παιδίου
Art	= περὶ ἄρθρων ἐμβολῆς		*Prog*	= προγνωστικόν
Coac	= Κωακαί προγνώσιες		*VC*	= περὶ τῶν ἐν κεφαλῇ τρωμάτων
Cord	= περὶ καρδίης		*Vict*	= περὶ διαίτης
Epid	= ἐπιδημίαι		*VM*	= περὶ ἀρχαίης ἰητρικῆς

1. Latin prints and manuscripts before 1800

Aurivillius, S, praeses/Petri Halenius, J, respondens: *De dentitione difficili*, Upsaliae 1757

Aurivillius, S, praeses/Rydbäck, E.O, respondens: *De doloribus*, Upsaliae 1765

B = Blancardus, S: *Lexicon Medicum ...*, Halae Magdeburgicae 1748

Bagellardo, P: *Libellus de egritudinibus infantium*, Patavii 1472

Benedetti, A: *Anatomice sive de Hystoria corporis humani libri V*, 1528

*Bibliothecae, quam Olim Collegerat ... Nicolaus Rosén ... pars illa, quae libros ad Medicam
Scientiam pertinentes complectebatur*, Upsaliae 1776

Boerhaave, H: *Aphorismi de cognoscendis et curandis morbis ...*, Lugduni Batavorum 1709

Castelli, B: *Lexicon Medicum Graecolatinum*, Venetiis 1607

C = Castelli, B: *Lexicon Medicum Graeco-Latinum*, Lipsiae 1713

Erasmus, D: *Adagiorum opus ... ex postrema autoris recognitione*, Lugduni 1550

Faber Soranus = *Basilii Fabri Sorani Thesaurus eruditionis scholasticae...cura et studio
Christophori Cellarii*, Leipzig 1686

Fahlström, J, respondens: *De variolis*, Parisiis 1685

Floderus, J: *Parentalia Viro, dum in vivis erat, Generoso ac Nobilissimo Domino
Nicolao Rosén à Rosenstein ...*, Upsaliae 1775

Fracastoro, G: *De contagione et contagiosis morbis ...libri III*, Venetiis 1546

Fracastoro, G: *Syphilis, sive morbus Gallicus*, Romae 1531

Franckenius, J, praeses/Lithselius, O, respondens: *De febribus*, Upsaliae 1641

Franckenius, J, praeses/Osander, N.E, respondens: *De corporis humani, in suas partes,
divisione*, Upsaliae 1634

GL (Galenus Latinus) = *Index in tomos omnes operum Galeni*, Basileae 1542

G = Gorraeus, J: *Definitionum Medicarum libri XXIIII literis Graecis distincti*,
Lutetiae Parisiorum 1564

von Haller, A: *Primae lineae physiologiae*, Gottingae 1747

Hoffwenius, P, praeses/Fahlström, J, respondens: *De flatibus*, Upsalae 1681

Hoffwenius, P, praeses/Poppelman, S, respondens: *De concoctione*, Upsaliae 1677

Lindestolpe, J: *Liber de venenis ... corollariis animadversionibus et indice illustratus auctore
Christiano Gottfr. Stentzel*, Francofurti et Lipsiae 1739

Linnaeus, C, praeses/Uddman, I, respondens: *Lepra*, 1763 (In *Amoenitates
academicae*, VII, Holmiae 1769)

Linnaeus, C: *Materia Medica, liber I de plantis*, Holmiae 1749

Magnus, O: *Historia de Gentibus Septentrionalibus*, Romae 1555

Mead, R: *De variolis et morbillis liber*, Londini 1747

Murray, J.A: *Historia insitionis variolarum in Suecia ad novissimum tempus protracta*, Gottingae 1767

Noltenius = Noltenius, J.F: *Lexicon Latinae linguae antibarbarum quadripartitum*, Lipsiae et Helmstadii 1744

Nova Literaria Maris Balthici & Septentrionis, Lubecae 1706

Oosterdijk Schacht, J: *Institutiones medicinae practicae*, Trajecti ad Rhenum 1747

Petri Gothus = Petri Gothus, J: *Dictionarium Latino-Sveco-Germanicum*, Lincopiae 1640

PhHolm = *Pharmacopoeia Holmiensis*, Holmiae 1686

PhLond = *Pharmacopoeia Collegii Regalis Medicorum Londinensis*, Londini 1746

PhSuI = *Pharmacopoea Svecica*, Holmiae 1775

Roberg, L, praeses/Linder, J, respondens: *De foeda lue dicta venerea*, Upsaliae 1705

Roberg, L, praeses/Rosén, N, respondens: *De usu methodi mechanicae in medicina*, Upsaliae 1738

Roberg, L, praeses/Voigtlender, G.F, respondens: *De erroribus in curandis febribus inflammatoriis*, Upsaliae 1738

Rosén, N, praeses/Bergius, P.J, respondens: *De variolis curandis*, Upsaliae 1754

Rosén, N, praeses/Martin, R, respondens: *De variolis praecavendis*, Upsaliae 1751

Rosén, N, praeses/Rosén, E, respondens: *De tussi*, I, Upsaliae 1739

Rosén, N, praeses/Rosén, E, respondens: *De tussi*, II, Upsaliae 1741

Rosén, N, praeses/Schröder, J, respondens: *De morbis infantum pars prima*, Upsaliae 1752

Rosén, N, praeses/Sundius, P, respondens: *De epilepsia infantili*, Upsaliae 1754

Rosén, N, praeses/Wahlbom, J.G, respondens: *Amphimerina catarrhalis*, Holmiae 1750

Rudbeck, O, the Elder, praeses/Figrelius, O, respondens: *De sero eiusque vasis*, Upsaliae 1661

Rudbeck, O, the Younger, praeses/Dalin, J, respondens: *De functionibus corporis humani primariis*, Upsaliae 1695

Rudbeck, O, the Younger, praeses/Detterberg, M, respondens: *De passione hypochondriaca*, (without imprint) 1697

Sydenham, T: *Processus integri in morbis fere omnibus curandis* …, Londini 1695

Wallerius, J.G: *PRAELECTIONES PHARMACEUTICAE, ad normam Pharmacopeae Londinensis, habitae Tempore Autumnali a J.G. Wallerio, Upsaliae A° MDCCLIV* (Ms. UUB D 251)

2 Other references

Annerstedt, C: *Upsala universitets historia*, I–III, Uppsala 1877–1913

Barquet, N and Domingo, P: *Smallpox:* "The Triumph over the Most Terrible of the Ministers of Death" (in *Annals of Internal Medicine*, 127:8, pp 635–642), Philadelphia 1997

Bartal = Bartal, A: *Glossarium mediae et infimae latinitatis regni Hungariae* (1901), Hildesheim – New York 1970

Benner & Tengström = Benner, M. and Tengström, E: *On the Interpretation of Learned Neo-Latin*, Göteborg 1977

Berggren, M: *Andreas Stobaeus Two Panegyrics in Verse*, diss, Uppsala 1994

Dietetik = Linnés föreläsningar i dietetik … samlade och kritiskt ordnade af A.O. Lindfors, Uppsala 1907

Dorland = *Dorland's illustrated Medical Dictionary*, 24th ed, Philadelphia and London, 1965

Du Cange = Du Cange, C. Du Fresne: *Glossarium mediae et infimae latinitatis* (1883–87), Graz 1954

DuCangeGr = Du Cange, C. Du Fresne: *Glossarium ad Scriptores mediae & infimae Graecitatis* ...(1688), Paris 1943

Durling, R.J. and Kudlien, F. (ed.): *Galenus Latinus, II*, Stuttgart 1992

Forcellini = Forcellini, A: *Totius latinitatis lexicon*, Prati 1857–75

Franzén, F.M: "Minne af Archiatern och Medicinae Professoren i Upsala Nils Rosén von Rosenstein "(in *Svenska Akademiens handlingar*), Stockholm 1814

Fredriksson, M: *Esculapius' De stomacho*, diss, Uppsala 2002

Frängsmyr, T: *Svensk idéhistoria. Bildning och vetenskap under tusen år, I*, Stockholm 2000

Fuchs, J.W, Weijers, O, et al. (ed): *Lexicon latinitatis Nederlandicae medii aevi*, Amsterdam/Leiden - Boston - Köln 1970–

GMS = Westerbergh, U and Odelman, E: *Glossarium Mediae latinitatis Sueciae*, Stockholm 1968–2002

Grun, P.A: *Schlüssel zu alten und neuen Abkürzungen*, Limburg/Laun 1966

Haggis, A.W: "Fundamental Errors in the early History of Cinchona" (in *Bulletin of the History of Medicine*, vol X, number 3, p 417–59, 568–92), Baltimore, Md 1941

Helander (95) = Helander, H: *Emanuel Swedenborg, Ludus Heliconius and other Latin poems* ..., Uppsala 1995

Helander, H: "Neo-Latin Studies: Significance and Prospects" (in *Symbolae Osloenses*, vol. 76), Oslo 2001

Henkel, A and Schöne, A (ed): *Emblemata: Handbuch der Sinnbildkunst des XVI. Und XVII. Jahrhunderts* (1967), Stuttgart 1978

Hirsch, A (ed.): *Biographisches Lexikon der hervorragenden Ärzte aller Zeiten und Völker*, 2 auflage, Berlin – Wien 1929–34

Hooke, R: *Micrographia: or some Physiological Descriptions of Minute Bodies made by Magnifying Glasses with Observations and Inquiries thereupon*, London 1665

Hoven, R: *Lexique de la Prose Latine de la Renaissance*, Leiden 1994

Hyrtl, J: *Onomatologia anatomica: Geschichte und Kritik der anatomischen Sprache der Gegenwart*, Wien 1880

IJsewijn, J and Sacré, D: *Companion to Neo-Latin studies*, part II, Leuven 1998

Jarcho, S (ed): *Tractatus Simplex de Cortice Peruviano - A Plain Treatise on the Peruvian Bark*, Boston 1992

Jägervall, M: *Nils Rosén von Rosenstein och hans lärobok i pediatrik*, Lund 1990

Klein, E: *A comprehensive etymological Dictionary of the English Language*, Amsterdam - London - New York, 1966

Knowles Middleton, W.E: *A History of the Thermometer and Its Use in Meteorology*, Baltimore 1966

Krebs-Schmalz = Krebs, J.Ph: *Antibarbarus der lateinischen Sprache, sechste Auflage...von J.H. Schmalz*, I-II, Basel, 1886–88

K-St = Kühner, R. and Stegmann, C: *Ausführliche Grammatik der lateinischen Sprache, Satslehre, dritte Auflage*, Leverkusen, 1955

L&G, Lindgren & Gentz = Lindgren, J. and Gentz, L: *Läkemedelsnamn*, Lund 1918–27

Langslow, D.R: *Medical Latin in the Roman Empire*, Oxford 2000

Lémery, N: *Cours de chymie contenant la manière de faire les opérations qui sont en usage dans la médecine...*, Paris 1675

Lewin, B: *Johan Skytte och de skytteanska professorerna*, Uppsala 1985

Lindeboom, G.A: *Herman Boerhaave The Man and his Work*, Frome and London 1968

Lindfors, A.O: *Minnesord öfver Nils Rosén von Rosenstein ...*, Uppsala 1906

Lindroth, S: *Svensk Lärdomshistoria III, Frihetstiden*, Uppsala 1978

Lindskog, B.I. and Zetterberg, B.L: *Medicinsk terminologi Lexikon*, Stockholm 1981

Li&Sc = Liddell, H.G. and Scott, R: *A Greek-English Lexicon …revised by sir Henry Stuart Jones*, Oxford 1996

L&S = Lewis, Ch.T. and Short, Ch: *A Latin Dictionary* (1879), Oxford 1975

Lundström, S: "Latin" (in Carlsson, L (ed): *Faculty of Arts at Uppsala University – Linguistics and Philology*, pp 47–62, Uppsala 1976)

Maehle, A-H: *Drugs on Trial: Experimental Pharmacology … in the Eighteenth Century* (*Clio Medica* 53), Amsterdam - Atlanta, Ga 1999

Medicinich Chymisch- und Alchemistisches Oraculum, Ulm 1783

MLBr = *Dictionary of medieval Latin from British sources …*, London 1975–

MLW = *Mittellateinisches Wörterbuch*, München 1959–

Müller, I.W: *Iatromechanische Theorie und ärtzliche Praxis*, Stuttgart 1991

Nevéus, T: *En akademisk festsed och dess utveckling*, Uppsala 1986

Nutton, V: "Humoralism" (in Bynum, W.F, and Porter, R (ed): *Companion encyclopedia of the history of medicine, volume 1*, pp 281–91, London and New York 1993)

OED = *Oxford English dictionary* ed. by John Simpson. 3rd. ed. *OED Online.*

OLD = *Oxford Latin dictionary*, ed. by P.G.W. Glare, Oxford 1996

Önnerfors, A: *Pliniana*, diss, Upsaliae 1956

Orrelius, M: *Köpmans- och Material-Lexicon …*, Stockholm 1797

Östlund, K: *Johan Ihre on the Origins and History of the Runes*, diss, Uppsala 2000

Otto, A: *Die Sprichwörter und sprichwörtlichen Redensarten der Römer*, Hildesheim 1962

Ottosson, P-G: *Scholastic medicine and philosophy. A study of Commentaries on Galen's Tegni (ca. 1300–1450)*, Napoli 1984

Pehrsson, A-L: "Nils Rosén von Rosenstein and Iatromechanics" (in Vahlquist, B. and Wallgren, A (ed): *Nils Rosén von Rosenstein and his Textbook on Paediatrics* (*Acta Paediatrica Suppl. 156*), pp 70–102, Uppsala 1964)

Philosophical Transactions [*of the Royal society of London*], London 1665–1886

Renander = Renander, A: *Medicinsk terminologi*, Stockholm 1967

Ridderstad, P.S: *Konsten att sätta punkt*, Lund 1975

Rippinger, L: "Les noms de médicaments en *dia-*" (In *Latomus*, 52:2), Bruxelles 1993

Rosén [von Rosenstein], N: *Compendium anatomicum*, 2nd ed, Stockholm 1738

Rosén [von Rosenstein], N: *Hus- och Rese-Apoteque*, Stockholm 1765

Sacklén, J.F: *Sveriges läkarehistoria*, Nyköping 1822–35

SAOB = *Svenska Akademiens Ordbok* (web edition), 1997–

Sch = Schneider, W: *Lexikon zur Arzneimittelgeschichte* I–VII, Frankfurt a. M. 1968–75

von Schulzenheim, D: *Åminnelse-Tal öfver Kongl. VetenskapsAcademiens framledne ledamot, Välborne Herren, Herr Nils Rosén von Rosenstein*, Stockholm 1773

Sophocles, E.A: *Greek Lexicon of the Roman and Byzantine periods* (1870), Cambridge, Mass 1914

Souter = Souter, A: *A Glossary of later Latin to 600 A.D*, Oxford 1949

Stephanus, H: Θησαυρὸς τῆς ἑλληνικῆς γλόσσης/*Thesaurus Graecae linguae … ediderunt C. B. Hase …G Dindorfius et L. Dindorfius …*, Parisiis 1865

Stotz, P: *Handbuch zur lateinischen Sprache des Mittelalters, zweiter Band*, München 2000

Sz = Leumann - Hofmann - Szantyr: *Lateinische Grammatik II, Lateinische Syntax und Stilistik* (*Handbuch der Altertumswissenschaft 2.2.2*), München 1965

TLL = *Thesaurus linguae Latinae*, Leipzig/Stuttgart/München 1900–

Uggla, A.Hj (ed): *Caroli Linnaei Diaeta naturalis 1733*, Uppsala 1958

UUB D 708b (Case sheets written by, or under the supervision of, Nils Rosén)

Vahlquist, B: "The Diseases of Children and their Remedies" (in *Nils Rosén von Rosenstein and his Textbook on Paediatrics* (*Acta Paediatrica Suppl. 156*), pp 27–69, Uppsala 1964)

Valentinus, B (pseudonym): *Zwölf Schlüssel* (in *Chymische Schriften* ...), Hamburg 1677

Zedler = Zedler, J.H: *Grosses vollständiges Universal-Lexicon aller Wissenschaften und Künste*, Halle und Leipzig 1732–54

Index nominum

Ancient authors

Other persons

Index terminorum technicorum

Index rerum et vocabulorum